MYOCARDIAL VIABILITY

 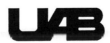

Developments in

Cardiovascular Medicine

VOLUME 226

The titles published in this series are listed at the end of this volume.

Myocardial Viability

2nd Completely Revised Edition

Edited by

AMI E. ISKANDRIAN
Director, Nuclear Cardiology, Division Cardiovascular Disease,
University of Alabama at Birmingham, Birmingham, Alabama, U.S.A.

and

ERNST E. VAN DER WALL
Department of Cardiology, Leiden, University Medical Center,
Leiden, The Netherlands

Kluwer Academic Publishers
Dordrecht / Boston / London

A C.I.P. Catalogue record for this book is available from the Library of Congress

ISBN 0-7923-6161-X

Published by Kluwer Academic Publishers,
P.O. Box 17, 3300 AA Dordrecht, The Netherlands.

Sold and distributed in North, Central and South America
by Kluwer Academic Publishers,
101 Philip Drive, Norwell, MA 02061, U.S.A.

In all other countries, sold and distributed
by Kluwer Academic Publishers,
P.O. Box 322, 3300 AH Dordrecht, The Netherlands.

Printed on acid-free paper

Printed in the Netherlands.

Dedicated

to

Our Wives,

Greta P. Iskandrian and Barbara J. M. van der Wall

and our children

Basil,	Hein,
Susan, and	Sake, and
Kristen	Ernst Lucas

Table of contents

Contributors List

RAGAVENDRA R. BALIGA
University of Texas Southwestern, Medical Center, Dallas, Texas, U.S.A.

J.J. BAX
Department of Cardiology, Leiden University Medical Center, Leiden, The Netherlands

ALBERT V.G. BRUSCHKE
Department of Cardiology, Leiden University Medical Center, Leiden, The Netherlands

FAROOQ A. CHAUDHRY
Echo Lab, Hahnemann University Hospital, Philadelphia, Pennsylvania, U.S.A.

ALBERT DE ROOS
Department of Diagnostic Radiology, Leiden University Medical Center, Leiden, The Netherlands

KATHLEEN GALATRO
MCP Hahnemann School of Medicine, Philadelphia, Pennsylvania, U.S.A.

AMI E. ISKANDRIAN
Director, Nuclear Cardiology, Division Cardiovascular Disease, University of Alabama at Birmingham, Birmingham, Alabama, U.S.A.

JAGAT NARULA
Division of Cardiology, Hahnemann University Hospitals, Philadelphia, Pennsylvania, U.S.A.

JEAN-LOUIS VANOVERSCHELDE
Department of Cardiology, Cliniques Universitaires, St-Luc, Brussels, Belgium

JUTTA SCHAPER
Max Planck Institute, Bad Nauheim, Germany

HEINRICH R. SCHELBERT
Department of Molecular and Medical Pharmacology, UCLA School of Medicine, Los Angeles, California, U.S.A.

ULRICH SCHRICKE
Nuklearmedizinische Klinik und Poliklinik, Klinikum rechts der Isar der TU-München, Münich, Germany

MARKUS SCHWAIGER
Nuklearmedizinische Klinik und Poliklinik, Klinikum rechts der Isar der TU-München, Münich, Germany

ROBERTO SCIAGRÀ
Nuclear Medicine Unit, Department of Clinical Physiopathology, University of Florence, Florence, Italy

ERNST E. VAN DER WALL
Department of Cardiology, Leiden University Medical Center, Leiden, The Netherlands

MARIO S. VERANI
Baylor College of Medicine, The Methodist Hospital, Houston, Texas, U.S.A.

FRANS C. VISSER
Department of Cardiology, Free University Amsterdam, Amsterdam, The Netherlands

HUBERT W. VLIEGEN
Department of Cardiology, Leiden University Medical Center, Leiden, The Netherlands

WILLIAM WIJNS
Department of Cardiology, O.L.Vrouwenziekenhuis, Aalst, Belgium

Introduction

AMI E. ISKANDRIAN & ERNST E. VAN DER WALL

The first edition of this book was published in 1994. Since then important advances have occurred in the field of myocardial viability. This, coupled with increasing interest by the scientific community in the broader issues of its relevance to patient care, suggested to us the need to write the second edition. We are most fortunate to have the help of a distinguished group of experts who have helped shape the field; we appreciate their commitments and contributions.

Almost all chapters have been radically modified. Chapter 1 deals with pathophysiology of myocardial hibernation and stunning; Chapter 2 with apoptosis; Chapter 3 with the role of positron emission tomography; Chapters 4 and 5 with the role of single photon emission computed tomography with thallium-201 and technetium agents, respectively; Chapter 6 with the role of SPECT fatty acid imaging; Chapter 7 with the role of SPECT FDG imaging; Chapter 8 with the role of cardiac catheterization angiography; Chapter 9 with the role of echocardiography; Chapter 10 with the role of magnetic resonance imaging; and Chapter 11 with clinical applications. Finally, Chapter 12 provides a short summary.

This book should prove to be a useful reference for cardiologists, radiologists, nuclear medicine physicians, anesthesiologists, cardiac surgeons, internists and basis scientists, their trainees and medical students who have an interest in this field either from the technical aspects or from the clinical viewpoint. Although the field is changing rapidly, we managed to capture all relevant data since 1994. We are most grateful for the support, understanding and patience of our wives and children. We would like also to thank Amber Tanghe-Neely from Kluwer Academic Publishers for her invaluable help. Renee Brown for secretarial assistance and Jan Schoones from Leiden University library for checking references and providing the index of the book.

1. Hibernating and stunned myocardium: Pathophysiological considerations

MARKUS SCHWAIGER & ULRICH SCHRICKE

Introduction

The mortality from ischemic heart disease has decreased in recent years. The better understanding of risk factors associated with development of coronary artery disease (CAD) has significantly contributed to this decline. Preventive measures such as aggressive therapy of arterial hypertension, diabetes mellitus, lipid disorders and by campaigning against smoking are important components of this medical success. Furthermore, improvements in medical and interventional therapy have reduced the complications associated with acute myocardial infarction as well as revascularization. Patients with advanced CAD appear to benefit most from interventional therapy. Several studies indicate that patients with poor left ventricular function and multivessel disease show improved clinical outcome after surgical revascularization [1-5]. The reversibility of myocardial dysfunction is an important factor contributing to the beneficial effect of revascularization. On the other hand, the risks associated with revascularization are highest in patients with poor left ventricular function [5]. Therefore, noninvasive techniques have been developed to select these patients based on evidence of tissue viability in dysfunctioning myocardium. During the last 30 years, there has been increasing clinical awareness that myocardial dysfunction in patients with CAD does not necessarily reflect scarred tissue [6,7]. In the 1970s, contractile reserve demonstrated in the catheterization laboratory by infusion of catecholamines or postextrasystolic potentiation were parameters, which identified reversibility of left ventricular dysfunction [8,9]. After the introduction of imaging modalities, the noninvasive characterization of regional function, perfusion and metabolism allowed for more sophisticated tissue characterization to identify reversible dysfunction with high diagnostic and prognostic accuracy [10]. At the same time, experimental investigations were initiated to reproduce the clinical observations in the animal laboratory [11]. Although there is no established animal model for chronic CAD associated with left ventricular dysfunction, acute and chronic animal models do successfully reproduce reversible left ventricular dysfunction [12].

A. E. Iskandrian and E. E. van der Wall (eds.), Myocardial Viability, 1-20.

This book chapter summarizes experimental as well as clinical results in order to define the pathophysiology of reversible left ventricular dysfunction. The relationship between observations made clinically using imaging technologies and the hypotheses arising from animal experiments will be discussed in order to provide an improved understanding of the pathophysiological and clinical significance of the imaging results.

Definitions

Various physiological and clinical terms have been used to describe reversible left ventricular dysfunction in patients with CAD. The most commonly used term is 'hibernating myocardium' [6,12]. More recently, the presence of 'stunned myocardium' has been implicated as a consequence of repetitive ischemia in patients with advanced CAD [7]. In addition, pathophysiological concepts such as remodeling, adaptation, dedifferentiation, apoptosis, inflammatory response and pre-conditioning are addressing extent, completeness and time course of functional recovery following revascularization. Aside from the understandable academic desire to develop accurate pathophysiological definitions, one has to accept that acute myocardial ischemia, stunning and hibernation, as well as cell death may dynamically interrelate in the clinical development of left ventricular dysfunction based on the natural history of the disease process.

Acute myocardial ischemia

Occlusion of a coronary artery induced either experimentally or by an acute thrombotic event rapidly leads to left ventricular dysfunction. The degree of wall motion abnormality is related to the severity of ischemia as defined by the reduction of myocardial blood flow [13]. Experimental studies have shown that the reduction of myocardial blood flow, especially in sub-endocardial layers of the left ventricle determines transmural contractile performance [14]. Based on this relationship, a close match between oxygen supply and function has been postulated during myocardial ischemia (Figure 1). Depending on the severity and duration of ischemia, irreversible tissue injury may occur. The irreversible injury begins in the sub-endocardial layer and proceeds transmurally in a wave-front pattern [15]. Myocardial oxygen demand and residual perfusion in the area of risk significantly influences the time course and extent of irreversible tissue injury [16].

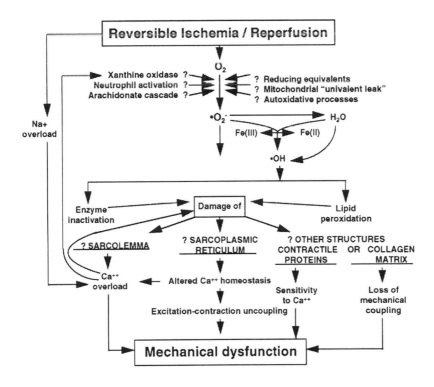

Figure 1. Hypothetical mechanisms in the pathogenesis of postischemic myocardial dysfunction (Kloner *et al.*, reference 11, with permission).

Stunning

If myocardial ischemia is interrupted by reperfusion, myocardial tissue can be salvaged. However, as described first by Heyndrickx *et al.* in 1975, myocardial dysfunction persists after reperfusion despite the return to normal or near normal perfusion [17]. Kloner *et al.* demonstrated in the dog model that 15 minutes of ischemia followed by reperfusion is associated with left ventricular dysfunction over 72 hours [18]. Although the first clinical description included single episode of myocardial ischemia, the term 'stunning' has been extended to left ventricular dysfunction associated with repetitive episodes of regional ischemia [19]. In addition, 'stunning' has been observed after global ischemia during open heart surgery in the arrested heart [20]. Finally, 'stunning' after exercise induced ischemia has been observed experimentally as well as clinically [21]. Thus, several conditions associated with transient ischemia may lead to myocardial 'stunning'. At the present time it is unclear whether all forms of 'stunning' share a common pathogenesis. Multiple factors are thought to contribute to the observed uncoupling of myocardial function in the presence of normal or near normal perfusion and oxygen delivery. The most commonly discussed hypothesis regarding the pathogenesis of 'stunning' is the 'oxygen radical' and the 'calcium hypothesis' [22,23]. Both concepts indicate that left ventricular dysfunction is a consequence of both, ischemic damage during ischemia and reperfusion injury. The oxygen radical hypothesis postulates that 'stunning' is caused by oxygen stress secondary to the generation of oxygen radicals during the reperfusion period. On the other hand, there is considerable evidence that calcium overload during the early phase of reperfusion contributes to the development of left ventricular dysfunction. The molecular mechanism whereby calcium overload causes contractile dysfunction is not well defined (Figure 2).

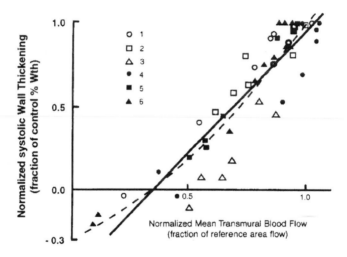

Figure 2. Relationship between systolic wall thickening and transmural blood flow in a conscious, chronic dog model (Gallagher *et al.,* reference 14, with permission).

Hibernation

The term 'hibernating myocardium' has been introduced to describe the clinical observation of reversible left ventricular dysfunction in patients with chronic CAD [6,9]. Several investigations identified subgroups of patients with severe left ventricular dysfunction who demonstrated recovery of regional and global left ventricular function following revascularization. The concept of 'hibernating myocardium', however, does not only include reversibility of dysfunction, but also the hypothesis of reduced resting perfusion in the presence of severe coronary artery stenosis leading to an adaptive downregulation of function [6,12]. This adaptation includes an uncoupling of myocardial contractile function and myocardial blood flow. Uncoupling of contractile work will dramatically decrease the energy demand of myocardial cells, since approximately 60% of oxygen consumption is linked to contractile performance. This energy saving is thought to increase the tolerance of myocardial cells to myocardial ischemia at the expense of regional dysfunction. Furthermore, it is hypothesized that these adaptive processes are associated with dedifferentiation/degeneration of myocardial cells as well as decreased expression of contractile proteins [24,25].

Short term hibernation

There are no established animal models available for myocardial hibernation. On the other hand, there are experimental studies which support the concept of 'adaptation' to myocardial ischemia. Fedele *et al.* have observed that metabolic adaptation occurs following placement of a partial stenosis in the animal model of acute myocardial ischemia with severe dysfunction and production of lactate [26]. The investigators described a significant recovery of metabolic function with reversal of lactate consumption despite unchanged myocardial blood flow in the ischemic myocardium (Figure 3).

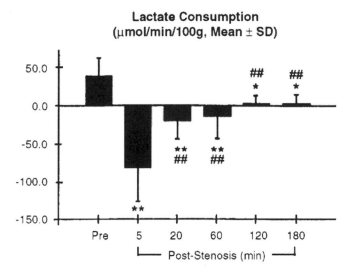

Figure 3. Mean (±SD) myocardial lactate consumption in an anesthetized closed chest pig model, during 3 hours of coronary stenosis. Pre = prestenosis. *p<0.05, **p<0.01 vs prestenosis, ## p<0.01 vs 5 min stenosis (Fedele *et al.*, reference 26, with permission).

Heusch *et al.* extended these experiments demonstrating a contractile reserve during dobutamine-induced pharmacological stress. However, Chen *et al.* showed a deterioration of the metabolic and functional state by the inotropic intervention suggesting recurrence of ischemia [27] (Figure 4). Schulz *et al.* recently indicated that short-term hibernation is characterized by a mismatch of perfusion and function supporting the notion of adaptive processes which uncouple myocardial function resulting in a new balance of oxygen supply and oxygen demand in the presence of reduced myocardial perfusion [28].

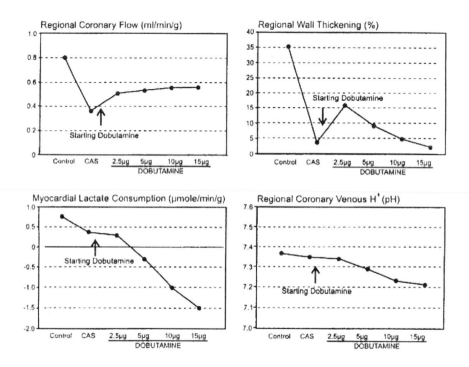

Figure 4. Effect of inotropic intervention with various doses of dobutamine after 24 hours of coronary stenosis (CAS) on regional blood flow, wall thickening, lactate consumption, and coronary venous pH in an anesthetized pig model (Chen *et al.* reference 27, with permission).

Myocardial cell death

As mentioned above, severe ischemia leads to a breakdown of cell membrane function resulting in disruption of ionic hemostasis. Irreversible cell damage is a consequence of oxygen deprivation and build-up of metabolites, which causes irreversible structural changes of the myocytes.

Myocardial necrosis is associated with a release of cytosolic components into the vascular space as well as random fragmentation of the genetic material. Necrosis itself leads to an inflammatory reaction which initiates repair processes within infarcted myocardium. More recently, the concept of 'apoptosis' has been introduced to describe irreversible cell damage in patients with ischemic heart disease. Apoptosis describes 'programmed cell death' which occurs as a consequence of defined signal transduction (Figure 5). Specific signaling pathways have been identified which result in the reorganization of the cyto-skeleton and in cytosolic myolysis as well as the DNA fragmentation [29]. Histological examination of tissue derived from patients with chronic CAD showed evidence of apoptosis which is distinct from acute necrosis. The significance of apoptosis versus acute necrosis in the natural history of ischemic heart disease is not well defined. Experimental data suggest that those processes may occur in parallel; however, the relative contribution of apoptosis is unknown. A number of interventions are being evaluated which interfere with the signaling pathway associated with apoptosis. For example, over-expression of insulin-like growth factor 1 in the mouse protects myocytes after myocardial infarction from death by attenuating ventricular dilatation. Future studies will address the role of apoptosis in chronic left ventricular dysfunction and its inhibition as potential therapeutic strategy [24].

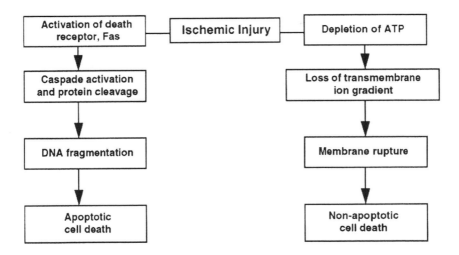

Figure 5. Proposed mechanisms of cell death (Haunstetter *et al.*, reference 29, with permission).

Table 1. Morphological alterations in hibernating myocardium

Cardiomyocyte alteration

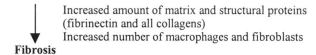

Loss of myofilament (myosin, thin filament complex, titin)
Loss of sarcoplasmic reticulum
Numerous small, doughnutlike mitochondria
Disorganization of cytoskeleton (desmin, tubulin, vinvulin)
Sequestration of cellular particles into extracellular space

Atrophy and apoptosis
Also increased number of glycogen deposits

Interstitial alterations

Increased amount of matrix and structural proteins
(fibrinectin and all collagens)
Increased number of macrophages and fibroblasts

Fibrosis

Remodeling

Following successful myocardial revascularization, left ventricular function will improve depending on the relative distribution of reversible and irreversible myocardial injury. The recovery process involves not only regional function but also global left ventricular geometry. Heart failure associated with chronic ischemic heart disease leads to ventricular dilatation. Increased wall stress is associated with hypertrophy and over-stretching of myocardial cells [30]. It is unknown to which degree remodeling contributes to the clinical presentation of heart failure in patients with chronic CAD. On the other hand, it cannot be expected that regional revascularization leads to immediate changes of left ventricular geometry. Little data are available to describe the relationship of regional function, left ventricular geometry and tissue viability prior to revascularization in order to understand the variables influencing the extent of recovery. On the other hand, several observations indicate that myocardial recovery following revascularization may be prolonged over several months which supports the notion of slow repair processes associated with the beneficial effect of revascularization [31].

The remodeling process is best described after acute anterior infarction. As a consequence of slippage and elongation of non-contractile and necrotic myocyte bundles, wall thinning and dilatation in the infarct region occurs, which leads to infarct expansion, ventricular chamber enlargement and decrease in regional function. The loss of regional function in the infarct region may be compensated partially by hyperkinesis of remote regions. The latter mechanism is less demonstrable in multivessel coronary artery disease. These early changes may be followed by eccentric myocardial hypertrophy, induced by pressure overload and regionally increased wall stress [32]

Pre-conditioning

Pre-conditioning describes the increased tolerance to ischemia following a short interval of ischemia. Murry *et al.* observed that canine myocardium subjected to brief episodes of ischemia and reperfusion tolerates prolonged episodes of ischemia better than myocardium not previously exposed to ischemia [33]. Based on this observation, a large number of studies were initiated to investigate the nature of this protective effect because of its obvious therapeutic implications. The exact mechanism of this process is not yet defined and may differ from species to species [11]. Currently, several studies suggest an important role of protein kinase C, which has first been demonstrated by Downey *et al.* in the rabbit model [34]. The cellular mediators involve activation of nucleotide kinases, which are responsible for dephosphorylation of AMP to adenosine as protective agent [35]. An alternative hypothesis includes an increased calcium influx during the initial ischemia which may be important for cardio-protection during subsequent ischemic episodes. The duration of the beneficial effects of pre-conditioning varies from species to species, but is limited to a few hours after the pre-conditioning event. It is interesting to note, however, that recent investigations also described a late effect of pre-conditioning. The phenomenon of re-appearance of the protective effect has been observed in rabbit, dog and rat. Recent work suggests that the delayed protective effect of pre-conditioning may extend over a period of one to three days [36-38]. The delayed appearance of this increased tolerance suggests the involvement of triggers and signaling pathways responsible for new expression of proteins which may increase the tolerance to myocardial ischemia.

The conditioning process is not only limited to the vascular territory, which has been rendered ischemic, but also involves other territories. Przyklenk *et al.* demonstrated a protective effect in the LAD territory following ischemia in the circumflex territory in the canine heart [39].

Scintigraphic measurements

In the following paragraphs imaging approaches will be discussed in context with the above pathophysiological definitions. Scintigraphic methods provide accurate in-vivo representation of blood flow, membrane function and metabolism, which uniquely allow to investigate the pathophysiology of reversible left ventricular dysfunction in patients.

Assessment of myocardial perfusion

Based on the discussed pathophysiology, stunned and hibernating myocardium can be differentiated by measurements of myocardial perfusion. Animal experiments have demonstrated that myocardial dysfunction (stunning) occurs in the presence of normal myocardial blood flow following transient periods of ischemia [17]. Based on measurements of regional myocardial blood flow in patients with regional dysfunction, a controversy arose whether left ventricular dysfunction represents repetitive stunning or hibernation with chronically reduced resting perfusion. Experimentally, myocardial blood flow can be assessed with high accuracy using the microspheres technique and related to corresponding measurements of function and metabolic performance [14]. This technique cannot be employed clinically. Since the spatial resolution achievable by scintigraphic techniques is limited, transmural flow gradients cannot be adequately resolved. Furthermore, heterogeneity of tissue injury (scar, stunning, hibernation) makes accurate measurements of regional myocardial blood flow with scintigraphic imaging techniques very difficult. In addition, partial volume effects limit the accuracy of flow estimates, especially in areas of myocardial dysfunction (thinning), which result in an underestimation of 'true' myocardial blood flow [40]. Positron emission tomography (PET) provides the most accurate quantitative method for regional flow estimates currently available. However, these measurements require dynamic data acquisition in order to correct for the partial volume effect. New tracer kinetic methods have been introduced to separate perfused from non-perfused myocardium to account for tissue heterogeneity [41,42]. Correction of myocardial blood flow measurements by the perfusible tissue fraction provides highly accurate measurements of perfusion.

Figure 6 summarizes PET blood flow measurements obtained in hibernating myocardium with N-13 ammonia [43]. PET measurements show a decrease in myocardial perfusion in segments which were identified as 'hibernating'. Based on the flow values presented, there is a mismatch between the degree of flow reduction and the severity of wall motion abnormality. Within the limited accuracy of the technology currently available, one can argue that the relative moderate decrease in regional perfusion cannot explain the severity of wall motion abnormality observed in these patients. Therefore, the hypothesis of chronic ischemia does not apply to the clinical presentation of hibernating myocardium. There is no direct evidence that patients with hibernating myocardium display metabolic, electrophysiological or clinical signs of myocardial ischemia. The more likely pathophysiological explanation for reduced myocardial perfusion is the downregulation of myocardial perfusion as a consequence of decreased function and, hence, decreased oxygen demand [44]. Such hypothesis would support the concept of hibernation as an adaptive process to repetitive myocardial ischemia leading to regionally decreased myocardial oxygen demand and, subsequently, myocardial perfusion. Supporting this notion of down-regulation of myocardial perfusion in hibernating myocardium comes from data which demonstrate the presence of coronary reserve in hibernating myocardium [45]. Marzullo *et al.* indicated that dipyridamole causes an increase in regional perfusion in segments which were scintigraphically identified as 'hibernating' [46]. In addition, investigations of contractile reserve demonstrate an improvement in function upon inotropic stimulation [47]. Such stimulation is only possible if blood flow can be increased to meet the increased oxygen demand. The presence of reduced perfusion was also documented by thallium-201 studies with rest/redistribution pattern, which reflect reduced initial uptake of the tracer [48-50].

In summary, current data indicate that left ventricular dysfunction can be associated with either normal or reduced resting perfusion. The degree of flow reduction in hibernating myocardium appears to be small compared to the degree of wall motion abnormality. This mismatch between flow and dysfunction makes the presence of chronic ischemia unlikely, but supports the hypothesis of downregulated perfusion as a consequence of decreased regional oxygen demand.

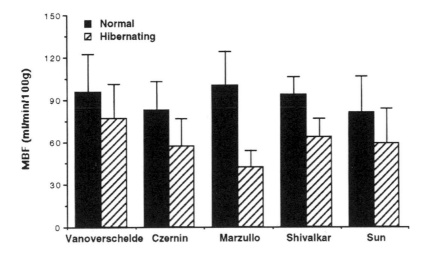

Figure 6. Rest myocardial blood flow (MBF) determined by N-13 ammonia PET studies at various centers comparing areas with hibernating myocardium and areas with normal LV function in the same patients in each study. Vanoverschelde *et al.* (n=17 pts, p<0.001), Czernin *et al.* (n=22 pts, P<0.05), Mazullo (n=14, MBF>2SD below mean in normal subjects), Shivalkar *et al.* (n=18, p<0.005), and Sun *et al.* (n=5, p=0.004).

Assessment of membrane integrity

The potassium analogue thallium-201 is used for the assessment of myocardial perfusion and membrane integrity. After initial myocardial retention, the distribution of the tracer within intra- and extra-cellular space is a function of membrane function. Experimental studies indicate that at least 50% of myocardial thallium-201 uptake occurs by Na/K ATP-ase. Pharmacological interventions, such as ouabain exposure suggest that the thallium-201 gradient between intra- and extra-cellular space is dependent on the integrity of the ionic exchange by ATP-dependent pumps. Therefore, myocardial retention of thallium-201 has been widely accepted as marker of tissue viability.

Thallium-201 redistribution or re-injection studies accurately depict viable myocardium as shown by direct comparison with histology. Zimmerman *et al.* reported that the extent of transmural thallium-201 content closely correlates with the amount of fibrosis [48]. The evaluation of tracer kinetics in isolated hearts and cell cultures as well as the correlation of tracer retention with histological evaluation of tissue samples validate thallium-201 as marker of cell integrity.

Although the uptake of technetium-99m (Tc-99m) sestamibi into the myocardium occurs by passive diffusion, its retention reflects electrochemical gradients maintained by mitochondrial membranes. Pioneering work by Piwnica-Worms, Kronauge and Chiu indicate that tissue retention of Tc-99m sestamibi can be modified by various ionophores and inhibitors, which affect the electrical potential of the plasma and mitochondrial membranes [51-53]. There are several indications that Tc-99 sestamibi tissue retention depends on ionic hemostasis. Incubation of cells with a high external concentration of potassium which depolarizes plasma membranes, lowers cellular uptake of Tc-99 sestamibi to about 17% of control levels. In addition, valinomycin which annihilates the mitochondrial potential, decreases cellular uptake of Tc-99 sestamibi to a background level [54]. Current knowledge about the tracer kinetics in myocardial cells suggests that Tc-99 sestamibi concentrates in the cell as a function of trans-membrane electrical potentials. Due to the negatively charged membranes at the mitochondrial level, the tracer concentrates preferentially in the mitochondria.

Correlation of Tc-99 sestamibi tissue retention with histological examination of tissue revealed similar relationships between tracer retention and fibrosis as has been observed with thallium-201 [55,56]. These data indicate that tissue retention under resting conditions can be used as marker of tissue viability. The use of nitroglycerine has been shown to increase the predictive value for the identification of tissue viability. Nitrates can improve regional myocardial blood flow in ischemic areas through a combination of vasodilation of epicardial coronary arteries and recruitment of collateral flow into the ischemic zone. Galli *et al.* reported that the size and severity of the resting perfusion defect following nitrate application decreased in 56% of the patients studied [57]. The exact mechanism of observations made by Galli and other investigators is not known. Increased blood flow, unloading of the left ventricle and improved wall motion may lead to an improved appreciation of sestamibi retention. Further studies are needed to confirm these initial observations and to elucidate the underlying mechanisms.

Assessment of myocardial metabolism

Myocardial metabolism is markedly altered during acute myocardial ischemia. Oxidative metabolism, especially the oxydation of fatty acids, is reduced during ischemia while myocardial glucose utilization may be increased as a consequence of anaerobic glycolysis [58,59]. Lactate production has been used as a sensitive metabolic marker for the presence of myocardial ischemia [26]. There are few data concerning metabolic alterations in stunned myocardium. Upon reperfusion, fatty acid metabolism recovers rapidly and oxidative metabolism resumes [60,61]. Myocardial oxygen consumption of stunned myocardium is normal or slightly reduced while data regarding glucose utilization are inconsistent [62]. Based on the existing literature, there is no evidence for metabolic abnormalities in stunned myocardium. This is supported by ultra-structural analysis which shows only mild changes in the mitochondria.

In contrast, hibernating myocardium displays specific metabolic abnormalities which are characterized by increased glucose extraction and increased glucose utilization. Scintigraphic evidence of maintained or even increased FDG uptake in comparison to myocardial blood flow is being clinically used to identify reversible left ventricular dysfunction [63, 64]. The mechanism of this regional alteration of glucose metabolism is not yet defined, because appropriate animal models reproducing hibernating myocardium are not available. However, repetitive ischemia leading to chronic left ventricular dysfunction in the animal model is associated with increased glycolytic flux [60]. Furthermore, animal data indicate that the transport of glucose is enhanced by increased expression of glucose transport proteins, especially GLUT 1 [65,66]. GLUT 1 is the insulin-independent glucose transporter which may explain the presence of FDG uptake in hibernating myocardium in fasted state as well as in patients with diabetes mellitus (Figure 7). In addition, myocardial ischemia induces translocation of glucose transporters [66,67]. This translocation of GLUT proteins during and after ischemia occurs via a different signaling pathway than that of insulin. Inhibition of the PI3-kinase (which is involved in the insulin-dependent cell signaling) by Wortmannin, does not block GLUT translocation during ischemia [67]. Histological examinations support the notion of dysregulated glucose metabolism by the demonstration of increased glycogen storage in hibernating cells. Further studies are required to investigate the molecular mechanism regulating glycogen stores in hibernating myocardium [68].

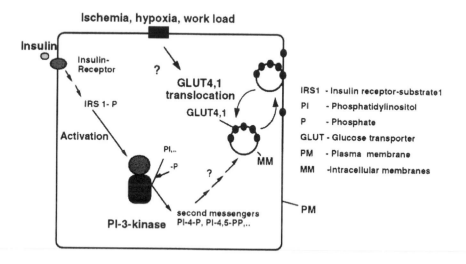

Figure 7. Schematic diagram illustrating the effects of insulin, ischemia, and workload on the translocation of glucose transporter proteins.

As in stunned myocardium, the oxidative metabolism does not seem to be impaired in hibernating myocardium. Studies using carbon-11 (C-11) acetate have shown tracer kinetics similar to that of normal myocardium [69]. Based on these results, C-11 acetate kinetics have been proposed as a predictor for the reversibility of left ventricular dysfunction in patients with advanced CAD. Myocardial uptake and kinetics of C-11 acetate are independent of substrate interaction because it enters the mitochondria directly in the form of C-11 acetyl CoA. Limited information can be derived from C-11 acetate regarding beta oxydation, but the clearance of C-11 activity in form of C-11 CO_2 reflects the flux of acetyl CoA through the tricarboxylic acid (TCA) cycle [28]. There are few studies available evaluating the long-chain fatty acid metabolism in hibernating myocardium. However, iodinated fatty acid analogs have been used to describe the metabolic integrity of hibernating myocardium. Since these radiopharmaceuticals are avidly extracted by the myocardium, scintigraphic information primarily reflects myocardial blood flow and, thus, can be seen indirectly as marker of cardiac metabolism. The only exception is the radioiodinated long-chain fatty acid beta-methylpentadecanoic acid (BMIPP), which identifies distinct metabolic patterns in patients with hibernating myocardium. This tracer has been shown to display reduced retention in reversibly dysfunctioning myocardium. Studies comparing thallium-201 and BMIPP in the same patients following acute myocardial infarction, as well as in animal experiments, suggest that BMIPP tissue retention is reduced in ischemically injured myocardium. Mismatch of thallium-201 and BMIPP uptake has been proposed as a marker of reversible tissue injury. The underlying mechanism for this scintigraphic pattern is not defined. The most likely explanation is rapid back diffusion after initial uptake as observed with C-11 palmitate in acutely ischemic myocardium [70]. See chapter by Verani on fatty acid imaging.

Assessment of myocardial hypoxia

The use of hypoxia seeking agents for the identification of ischemic tissue injury has been propagated [71-73]. Misonidazol and its analogs are retained in tissue with low oxygen retention while they rapidly clear from normoxic tissue. Animal data in acutely ischemic and reperfused myocardium have shown increased retention of radiolabeled misonidazol. Currently, there are no clinical data available to document feasibility of such radiopharmaceuticals to identify reversible left ventricular dysfunction. The question arises if hibernating myocardium displays chronically reduced tissue oxygen retention. Studies with such tracers may be useful in challenging the hypothesis of chronic ischemia or hypoxia in hibernating myocardium.

Myocardial necrosis

Following myocardial infarction and interventional therapy (lysis, coronary angioplasty), left ventricular dysfunction usually reflects an admixture of myocardial necrosis, stunned and hibernating myocardium. The use of metabolic tracers such as F-18 deoxyglucose may be limited because of inflammatory reactions in acutely injured myocardium [74]. Several studies have shown that the predictive accuracy of F-18 deoxyglucose for identification of reversible tissue injury is limited during the sub-acute phase of an acute myocardial infarction [69,74]. Therefore, the combination of flow tracers and marker of acute myocardial necrosis may identify the extent of reversible tissue injury. Johnson *et al.* applied dual isotope techniques using indium-111 labeled antimyosin and thallium-201 in patients with acute myocardial infarction [75]. Segments which displayed reduced thallium-201 uptake but no retention of indium-111 antimyosin displayed reversible tissue injury. Few data exist defining the incidence of acute myocardial necrosis in patients with chronic left ventricular dysfunction. With the increasing consideration of apoptosis being important in the development of heart failure in patients with ischemic or non-ischemic heart disease, the use of radiopharmaceuticals identifying myocardial cell death appears to be attractive [76]. With the better understanding of the signal pathways leading to apoptosis, new radiopharmaceuticals may be developed to study the process in in-vivo conditions.

Conclusion

Chronic and advanced coronary artery disease is frequently associated with impaired left ventricular function. The reversibility of dysfunction represents an important clinical target for therapeutic interventions. Several techniques have shown to accurately predict functional recovery following revascularization. The underlying pathophysiology of dysfunction remains the focus of intense research which is expected to lead to the development of new therapeutic strategies in heart failure patients.

References

1.   Kaul TK, Angihotri AK, Fields BL, Riggins LS Wyatt DA, Jones CR. Coronary artery bypass grafting in patients with an ejection fraction of twenty percent or less. J Thorac Cardiovasc Surg 1996;111:1001-12.
2.   Miller DC, Stinson EB, Alderman EL. Surgical treatment of ischemic cardiomyopathy: is it ever too late? Am J Surg 1981;141:688-93.
3.   Luciani GB, Faggian G, Razzolini R, Livi U, Bortolotti U, Mazzucco A. Severe ischemic left ventricular failure: coronary operation or heart transplantation. Ann Thorac Surg 1993;55:719-23.
4.   Mickleborough LL, Maruyma H, Takagi Y, Mohamed S, Sun Z, Ebisuzaki L. Results of revascularization in patients with severe left ventricular dysfunction. Circulation 1995;92(9 Suppl):II73-9.
5.   Passamani E, Davis KB, Gillespie MJ, Killip T. A randomized trial of coronary artery bypass surgery. Survival of patients with a low ejection fraction. N Engl J Med 1996;312:1665-71.
6.   Rahimtoola SH. The hibernating myocardium. Am Heart J 1989;117:211-21.
7.   Wijns W, Vatner SF, Camici PG. Hibernating myocardium [Review]. N Engl J Med 1998;339:173-81.
8.   Dyke SH, Cohn PF, Gorlin R, Sonnenblick EH. Detection of residual myocardial function in coronary artery disease using post-extra systolic potentiation. Circulation 1974;50:694 - 9.
9.   Diamond GA, Forrester JS, deLuz PL, Wyatt HL, Swan HJ. Post extrasystolic potentiation of ischemic myocardium by atrial stimulation. Am Heart J 1978;95:204-9.
10. Bax JJ, Wijns W, Cornel JH, Boersma E, Fioretti PM. Accuracy of currently available techniques for prediction of functional recovery after revascularization in patients with

left ventricular dysfunction due to chronic coronary artery disease: comparison of pooled data. J Am Coll Cardiol 1997;30:1451-60.

11. Kloner RA, Bolli R, Marban E, Eeinlib L, Braunwald E. Medical and cellular implications of stunning, hibernation, and preconditioning: an NHLBI Workshop. Circulation 1998;97:1848-67.

12. Heusch G. Hibernating myocardium. Physiol Rev 1998;78:1055-85.

13. Theroux P, Franklin D, Ross J Jr, Kamper WS. Regional myocardial function during acute coronary artery occlusion and its modification by pharmacological agents in the dog. Circ Res 1974;35:896-908.

14. Gallagher KP, Matsuzaki M, Koziol JA, Kamper WS, Ross J Jr. Regional myocardial perfusion and wall thickening during ischemia in conscious dogs. Am J Physiol 1984;247:H727-38.

15. Reimer KA, Jennings RB. The "wavefront phenomenon" of myocardial ischemic cell death. II. Transmural progression of necrosis within the framework of ischemic bed size (myocardium at risk) and collateral flow. Lab Invest 1979;40:633-44.

16. Schaper W, Frenzel H, Hort W, Winkler B. Experimental coronary artery occlusion. II. Spatial and temporal evolution of infarcts in the dog heart. Basic Res Cardiol 1979;74:233-9.

17. Heyndrickx GR, Millard RW, McRitchie RJ, Maroko PR, Vatner SF. Regional myocardial function and electrophysiological alterations after brief coronary artery occlusion in conscious dogs. J Clin Invest 1975;56:978-85.

18. Kloner RA, De Boer LW, Darsee JR et al. Prolonged abnormalities of myocardium salvaged by reperfusion. Am J Physiol 1981;1981:H591-9.

19. Kloner RA, Allen J, Cox TA, Zheng Y, Ruiz CE. Stunned left ventricular myocardium after exercise treadmill testing in coronary artery disease. Am J Cardiol 1991;68:329-34.

20. Stewart JR, Blackwell WH, Crute SL, Loughlin V, Greenfield LJ, Hess ML. Inhibition of surgically induced ischemia/reperfusion injury by oxygen free radical scavengers. J Thorac Cardiovasc Surg 1983;86:262-72.

21. Homans DC, Sublett E, Dai XZ, Bache RJ. Persistence of regional left ventricular dysfunction after exercise-induced myocardial ischemia. J Clin Invest 1986;77:66-73.

22. Bolli R. Role of oxygen radicals in myocardial stunning. In: Kloner RA, Przyklenk, editors. Stunned myocardium. New York: Marcel Dekker; 1993. p. 155-95.

23. Kusuoka H, Marban E. Cellular mechanisms of myocardial stunning. Annu Rev Physiol 1992;54:243-56.

24. Elsässer A, Schlepper M, Klovekorn WP et al. Hibernating myocardium: an incomplete adaptation to ischemia. Circulation 1997;96:2920-31.

25. Schwarz ER, Schoendube FA, Kostin S et al. Prolonged myocardial hibernation exacerbates cardiomyocyte degeneration and impairs recovery of function after revascularization. J Am Coll Cardiol 1998;31:1018-26.

26. Fedele FA, Gewirtz H, Capone RJ, Sharaf B, Most AS. Metabolic response to prolonged reduction of myocardial blood flow distal to a severe coronary artery stenosis. Circulation 1988;78:729-35.

27. Chen C, Li L, Chen LL et al. Incremental doses of dobutamine induce a biphasic response in dysfunctional left ventricular regions subtending coronary stenoses. Circulation 1995;92:756-66.

28. Schulz R, Kappeler C, Coenen H, Bockisch A, Heusch G. Positron emission tomography analysis of $[1-^{11}C]$ acetate kinetics in short-term hibernating myocardium. Circulation 1998;97:1009-16.

29. Haunstetter A, Izumo S. Apoptosis: basic mechanisms and implications for cardiovascular disease. Circ Res 1998;82:1111-29.

30. Gerdes AM, Kellerman SE, Moore JA et al. Structural remodeling of cardiac myocytes in patients with ischemic cardiomyopathy. Circulation 1992;86:426-30.

31. Niehaber CA, Brunken RC, Sherman CT *et al.* Metabolic and functional recovery of ischemic human myocardium after coronary angioplasty. J Am Coll Cardiol 1991;18:966-78.
32. Weber KT, Brilla CG, Janicki JS. Myocardial remodeling and pathologic hypertrophy. Hosp Pract (Off Ed) 1991;26:73-80.
33. Murry CE, Jennings RB, Reimer KA. Preconditioning with ischemia: a delay of lethal cell injury in ischemic myocardium. Circulation 1986;75:1124-36.
34. Armstrong S, Downey JM, Ganote CE. Preconditioning of isolated rabbit cardiomyocytes: induction by metabolic stress and blockade by the adenosine antagonist SPT and calphostin C, a protein kinase C inhibitor. Cardiovasc Res 1994;28;72-7.
35. Ytrehus K, Liu Y, Downey JM. Preconditioning protects ischemic rabbit hearts by protein kinase C activation. Am J Physiol 1994;226:H1145-52.
36. Kuzuya T, Hoshida S, Yamashita N *et al.* Delayed effects of sublethal ischemia on the acquisition of tolerance to ischemia. Circ Res 1993;72:1293-9.
37. Marber MS, Latchman DS, Walker JM, Yellon DM. Cardiac stress protein elevation 24 hours after brief ischemia or heat stress is associated with resistance to myocardial infarction. Circulation 1993;88:1264-72.
38. Yamashita N, Hoshida S, Taniguchi N, Kuzuya T, Hori M. A 'second window of protection' occurs 24 hours after ischemic preconditioning in rat heart. J Mol Cell Cardiol 1997;30:1181-9.
39. Przyklenk K, Bauer B, Orize M, Kloner RA, Whittaker P. Regional ischemic 'preconditioning' protects remote virgin myocardium from subsequent sustained coronary occlusion. Circulation 1993;87:893-9.
40. Parodi O, Schelbert HR, Schwaiger M, Hansen H, Selin C, Hoffmann EJ. Cardiac emission computed tomography: underestimation of regional tracer concentrations due to wall motion abnormalities. J Comput Assist Tomogr 1984;8:1083-92.
41. Iida H, Rhodes CG, de Silva R *et al.* Myocardial tissue fraction--correction for partial volume effects and measure of tissue viability. J Nucl Med 1991;32:2169-75.
42. Hutchins GD, Schwaiger M, Rosenspire KC, Krivokapick J, Schelbert H, Kuhl DE. Noninvasive quantification of regional blood flow in the human heart using N-13 ammonia and dynamic positron emission tomographic imaging. J Am Coll Cardiol 1990;15:1032-42.
43. Rahimtoola SH. Hibernating myocardium has reduced blood flow at rest that increases with low-dose dobutamine. Circulation 1996;94:3055-61.
44. Schulz R, Rose J, Vahlhaus C, Post H, baukenkohler U, Heusch G. No maintenance of perfusion-contraction matching during 24 hours sustained moderate myocardial ischemia in pigs [abstract]. FASEB J 1997;11(3 Suppl):A432.
45. Lee HH, Davida-Roman VG, Ludbrook PA *et al.* Dependency of contractile reserve on myocardial blood flow. Circulation 1997;96:2884-91.
46. Marzullo P, Parodi O, Sambuceti G *et al.* Residual coronary reserve identifies segmental viability in patients with wall motion abnormalities. J Am Coll Cardiol 1995;26:342-50.
47. Sun KT, Czernin J, Krivokapick J *et al.* Effects of dobutamine stimulation on myocardial blood flow, glucose metabolism, and wall motion in normal and dysfunctional myocardium. Circulation 1996;94:3146-54.
48. Zimmermann R, Mall G, Rauch B *et al.* Residual 201Tl activity in irreversible defects as a marker of myocardial viability. Clinicopathological study. Circulation 1995;91:1016-21.
49. Ragosta M, Beller GA, Watson DD, Kaul S, Gimple LW. Quantitative planar rest-redistribution 201TI imaging in detection of myocardial viability and prediction of improvement in left ventricular function after coronary bypass surgery in patients with severely depressed left ventricular function. Circulation 1993;87:1630-41.

50. Udelson JE, Coleman PS, Metherall J *et al*. Predicting recovery of severe regional ventricular dysfunction. Comparison of resting scintigraphy with 201Tl and 99mTc-sestamibi. Circulation 1994;89:2552-61.
51. Piwnica-Worms D, Kronauge JF, Holman BL, Davison A, Jones AG. Comparative myocardial uptake characteristics of hexakis (alkylisonitrile) technetium(I) complexes. Effect of lipophilicity. Invest Radiol 1989;24:25-9.
52. Piwnica-Worms D, Kronauge JF, Delmon L, Holman BL, Marsh JD, Jones AG. Effect of metabolic inhibition on technetium-99m-MIBI kinetics in cultured chick myocardial cells. J Nucl Med 1990;31:464-72.
53. Piwnica-Worms D, Kronauge JF, Chiu ML. Enhancement by tetraphenylborate of technetium-99m-MIBI uptake kinetics and accumulation in cultured chick myocardial cells. J Nucl Med 1991;32:1992-9.
54. Piwnica-Worms D, Kronauge JF, Chiu ML. Uptake and retention of hexakis (2-methoxysobutyl isonitrile) technetium(I) in cultured chick myocardial cells. Mitochondrial and plasma membrane potential dependence. Circulation 1990;82:1826-38.
55. Medrano R, Lowny RW, Young JB *et al*. Assessment of myocardial viability with 99mTc sestamibi in patients undergoing cardiac transplantation. A scintigraphic/ pathological study. Circulation 1996; 94:1010-7.
56. Maes AF, Borgers M, Flameng W *et al*. Assessment of myocardial viability in chronic coronary artery disease using technetium-99m sestamibi SPECT. Correlation with histologic and positron emission tomographic studies and functional follow-up. J Am Coll Cardiol 1997;29:62-8.
57. Galli M, Marcassa C, Imparato A, Campini R, Orrego PS, Gianuzzi P. Effects of nitroglycerin by technetium-99m sestamibi tomoscintigraphy on resting regional myocardial hypoperfusion in stable patients with healed myocardial infarction. Am J Cardiol 1994;74:843-8.
58. Kalff V, Schwaiger M, Nguyen N, McLanakan TB, Gallagher KP. The relationship between myocardial blood flow and glucose uptake in ischemic canine myocardium determined with fluorine-18 deoxyglucose. J Nucl Med 1992;33:1346-53.
59. Neely JR. Metabolic disturbances after coronary occlusion. Hosp Pract (Off Ed) 1989;24:81-5,90-6.
60. Liedtke AJ. Alterations of carbohydrate and lipid metabolism in the acutely ischemic heart. Prog Cardiovasc Dis 1981;23:321-36.
61. Lopaschuk GD. Advantages and limitations of experimental techniques used to measure cardiac energy metabolism. J Nucl Cardiol 1997;4:316-28.
62. Hacker TA, Renstrom B, Nellis SH, Liedtke AJ. Effect of repetitive stunning on myocardial metabolism in pig hearts. Am J Physiol 1997;273:H1395-402.
63. vom Dahl J, Eitzman DT, al Aouar ZR *et al*. Relation of regional function, perfusion, and metabolism in patients with advanced coronary artery disease undergoing surgical revascularization. Circulation 1994;90:2356-66.
64. Tillisch J, Brunken R, Marshall R *et al*. Reversibility of cardiac wall motion abnormalities predicted by positron tomography. N Engl J Med 1986;314:884-8.
65. Brosius FC 3rd, Liu Y, Nguyen N, Sun D, Bartlett J, Schwaiger M. Persistent myocardial ischemia increases GLUT 1 transporter expression in both ischemic and non-ischemic heart regions. J Mol Cell Cardiol 1997;29:1675-85.
66. Sun D, Nguyen N, DeGrado TR, Schwiager M, Brosius RC 3rd. Ischemia induces translocation of the insulin-responsive glucose transporter GLUT4 to the plasma membrane of cardiac myocytes. Circulation 1994;89:793-8.
67. Egert S, Nguyen N, Brosius FC 3rd, Schwaiger M. Effects of wortmannin on insulin- and ischemia- induced stimulation of GLUT4 translocation and FDG uptake in perfused rat hearts. Cardiovasc Res 1997;35:283-93.

68. Borgers M, Thone F, Wouters L, Ausma J, Shivalkar B, Flameng W. Structural correlates of regional myocardial dysfunction in patients with critical coronary artery stenosis: chronic hibernation? Cardiovasc Pathol 1993;2:237-45.
69. Gropler RJ, Geltman EM, Sampathkumaran K *et al*. Functional recovery after coronary revascularization for chronic coronary artery disease is dependent on maintenance of oxidative metabolism. J Am Coll Cardiol 1992;20:569-77.
70. Taki J, Khikawa A, Nakajima K, Kawasuji M, Tonami M. Comparison of flow capacities of arterial and venous grafts for coronary artery bypass grafting: evaluation with exercise thallium-201 single-photon emission tomography. Eur J Nucl Med 1997;24:1487-93.
71. Martin GV, Caldwell JH, Rasey JS, Grunbaum Z, Cerqueira M, Krohn KA. Enhanced binding of the hypoxic cell marker [3H]fluoromisonidazole in ischemic myocardium. J Nucl Med 1989;30:194-201.
72. Okada RD, Nguyen KN, Strauss HW, Johnson G 3rd. Effects of low flow and hypoxia on myocardial retention of technetium-99m BMS181321. Eur J Nucl Med 1996;23:443-7.
73. Okada RD, Johnson G 3rd, Nguyen KN, Edwards B, Archer CM, Kelly JD. 99mTc HL91. Effects of low flow and hypoxia on a new ischemia-avid myocardial imaging agent. Circulation 1997;95:1892-9.
74. Schwaiger M, Brunken R, Grover-McKay M *et al*. Regional myocardial metabolism in patients with acute myocardial infarction assessed by positron emission tomography. J Am Coll Cardiol 1986;8:800-8.
75. Johnson LL, Seldin DW, Backer LC *et al*. Antimyosin imaging in acute transmural myocardial infarctions: results of a multicenter clinical trial. J Am Coll Cardiol 1989;13: 27-35.
76. Vriens PW, Blankenberg FG, Stoot JH *et al*. The use of technetium Tc 99m annexin V for in vivo imaging of apoptosis during cardiac allograft rejection. J Thorac Cardiovasc Surg 1998;116:844-53.

2. Role of apoptosis in myocardial hibernation and myocardial stunning

RAGAVENDRA R BALIGA, JUTTA SCHAPER & JAGAT
NARULA

Introduction

Clinicians have long recognized that left ventricular dysfunction in patients
with coronary disease is a reversible condition [1,2]. In 1975 Vatner and
associates first described post-ischemic myocardial dysfunction in
conscious dogs produced by brief coronary occlusions followed by
reperfusion [3]. In 1982, Braunwald and Kloner [4] coined the term
'myocardial stunning' to describe prolonged but reversible myocardial
dysfunction following restoration of myocardial blood flow. In 1985,
Rahimtoola observed progressive recovery of chronic left ventricular
dysfunction following coronary artery bypass grafting in the absence of
transmural necrosis [5]. He described these findings as 'hibernating
myocardium' reflecting a state of persistently impaired myocardial function
at rest due to reduced coronary blood flow that can be partially or
completely restored to normal if the net balance between myocardial
oxygen supply and demand is favorably altered [6]. The major difference
between stunned and hibernating myocardium is the level of myocardial
perfusion which is chronically reduced in hibernating myocardium but
normal in stunned myocardium. Until recently, the observation of
functional recovery was thought to imply that the structural morphology of
stunned and hibernating myocardium must be essentially normal. However,
increasing evidence from analysis of myocardial biopsy specimens
obtained during coronary artery bypass surgery have revealed that stunned
and hibernating myocardium are accompanied by several structural changes
including apoptotic cell death.

Apoptosis or programmed cell death

Historically pathologists have viewed cell death using light and electron
microscopy, and have described morphologic characteristics of necrosis.
In 1910 von Recklinghausen proposed the term oncosis (Gk. *óncosis*, =
swelling) precisely to mean cell death with swelling. As early as 1885
another morphological form of cell death was recognized by Walter

Flemming who called it chromatolysis. He noticed that the epithelial lining of regressing ovarian follicles were littered with cells, the nuclei of which were breaking up. A few months later the same observations were made by Franz Nissen who observed chromatolysis in lactating mammary glands. By 1914 enough data were available for a German anatomist, Ludwig Graper to publish a paper entitled (in translation) " A new point of view regarding the elimination of cells". In 1967, Frans Wackers used the term 'bionecrosis' to describe changes in human mammary gland [7]. He noticed that dead and dying cells existed among living cells *without provoking cellular reaction*. He also commented that although the cells were dead it was still *possible to recognize them as cells*. These milestone papers made no significant impact until 'chromatolysis' and 'bionecrosis' resurfaced in 1971 when Kerr described what he called at first 'shrinkage necrosis' and a year later apoptosis (Greek *apo-ptosis*= "falling off", as in petals of a flower or leaves of a tree). Apoptosis leads to necrosis with karyorhexis and cell shrinkage and stands in contrast to oncosis, which leads to necrosis with karyolysis and cell swelling. Wyllie *et al.* in 1984 demonstrated discrete inter-nucleosomal DNA fragmentation in apoptosis and thereby added a specific biochemical marker to the distinctive morphological changes of apoptosis.

DNA fragmentation is the hallmark of apoptosis and its demonstration remains the most widely used test for the detection of apoptosis. The specific DNA cleavage results in nucleosomal or polynucleosomal fragments (180 bp or multiples) and these low molecular weight fragments provide rungs-of-ladder pattern upon electrophoretic resolution of tissue homogenates. The fragmentation of DNA has been demonstrated in the individual cell nuclei by the TUNEL (terminal deoxynucleotidyl transferase-mediated deoxyuridine triphosphate nick end-labeling) technique. During this process, nicked ends of DNA fragments are tacked by nucleotides in the presence of terminal deoxynucleotidyl transferase (tdT). The incorporation of tdT in the nucleus is then identified by histochemical techniques. In addition to TUNEL staining other nuclear stains particularly in flow cytometric analysis have been described. Included in the list of nuclear stains are propidium iodide, Hoechst and acridine orange. More recently, plasma membrane changes have been noted to occur in apoptosis. In early apoptosis, there is a conformational change in the plasma membrane of the cell resulting in predominance of the phosphatidylserine (PS) groups on outer face of the plasma membrane secondary to loss of membrane enzymes that flip PS to the inner side of the membrane [8]. Strauss and co-workers showed that the PS neoexpression can be identified using a radiolabeled ligand annexin-V [9]. Finally, occurrence of apoptosis is supported by the identifcation of its biochemical mediators such as Fas, caspases or BCl2 family apoptotic proteins.

Cellular and molecular basis of apoptosis

Apoptosis is a genetically programmed and tightly controlled process. Execution of apoptosis requires specific involvement of interaction of cell surface receptors or intracellular signaling pathways with extra- or intracellular inducers of apoptosis followed by serial activation of proteolytic caspases. The caspase activation leads to fragmentation of various cytoplasmic proteins, and RNAs, as well as DNA and DNA repair enzymes. Fragmentation of intracellular and nuclear constituents facilitates condensation of the cell. The process of apoptosis can proceed through two major pathways to activate terminal caspases 3, 6 and 7 (See schematic diagram). These pathways are not essentially exclusive. In the first pathway, cytokines or related inducers of apoptosis such as TNF and Fas-ligand through binding to death receptors [10], whereas granzyme B in association with sublytic action of perforins directly interact with caspases 8 and 10.

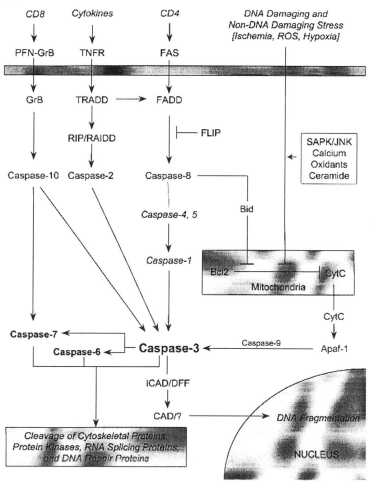

Death receptors activate caspase cascade via death domain proteins. The activation of caspases 8 and 10 eventually converge into terminal caspase activation. The second pathway is initiated by DNA damaging and non-DNA damaging stress that leads to release of cytochrome C from mitochondrial compartment [11] by activation of stress signaling pathways, ceramide, calcium excess or reactive oxygen species. The release of cytochrome c is modulated by BCl2 family proteins (which may both be pro and anti-apoptotic), p53, ADP-ATP carrier proteins etc. The presence of cytochrome C in the cytoplasm interacts with ced-4 homologue and caspase 9 induces a caspase-3 activation and intensification loop [12]. The two pathways can interact at the level of caspase 8 which leads to translocation of Bid to mitochondria which in turn releases the cytochrome c from mitochondria [13].

Apoptosis in cardiac disease

Apoptosis is most often associated with cells progressing through the cell cycle and, for this reason, it has generally been believed that apoptosis does not occur in terminally differentiated adult cells such as the cardiac myocyte. Narula *et al.* provided the evidence that apoptosis occurs in the myocardium in patients with end-stage heart failure [14]. In the adult heart apoptosis has also been observed in normal cardiac aging, acute myocardial infarction, chronic heart failure, tachycardia-induced cardiomyopathy and in right ventricular dysplasia. In the first few hours after the onset of ischemia, apoptosis predominates followed by necrosis. A second wave of apoptosis follows about a week later and has been reported to contribute to post-infarction remodeling [15]. However, these clinical reports of apoptosis have been supported by several animal models suggesting that apoptosis can be induced in the myocardium by a variety of insults including ischemia-reperfusion [16], myocardial infarction [17], rapid ventricular pacing [18], mechanical stretch [19], and pressure overload due to aortic constriction [20], as well as spontaneously hypertensive rats (SHR) [21].

Apoptosis in acute myocardial infarction and reperfusion

Although necrosis is the predominant mode of death of cardiac myocytes after acute myocardial infarction, there is growing evidence that apoptotic cell death precedes necrosis in acute myocardial infarction. In animal models of myocardial infarction apoptosis contributes substantially to cell death as 5% to 33% of the cardiac myocytes demonstrate positive staining for DNA fragmentation [22-25]. Post-mortem studies of myocardial infarction in the human hearts have shown that apoptosis is predominantly localized in the hypoperfused border zone between the central infarct area and non-compromised myocardial tissue [15,26]. It has been suggested that milder degrees of ischemia not sufficient to result in necrosis leads to apoptosis. Although the precise mechanism of induction of apoptosis is not clear, ischemia does lead to activation of stress-activated protein kinases [14] and release of cytochrome c from mitochondria [27]. The two processes of SAPK activation and cytochrome release may be interrelated. Cytochrome c once released facilitates activation of caspase cascade leading to apoptotic cell death [11]. In addition, ischemia may lead to upregulation of cytokines such as TNFα and NO as also Fas receptors on cardiomyocytes which in turn may contribute to apoptosis.

In addition to the fact that prolonged periods of myocardial ischemia lead to tissue injury and cell death, early reperfusion although vital for myocardial tissue salvage, can also lead to increased loss of myocytes in response to activation of inflammatory mediators and the formation of reactive oxygen species [28-30]. The role of apoptosis has been recently reported in animal models, where reperfusion was shown to accelerate the occurrence of apoptotic cell death in cardiac myocytes [16,23]. The augmentation of apoptotic processes following reperfusion may result from release of superoxide or intracellular calcium excess. Both events may lead to mitochondrial release of cytochrome c and caspase activation.

Ischemic preconditioning, in addition, in order to reduce infarct size and ventricular arrhythmias has been shown to ameliorate myocardial stunning and post-ischemic contractile dysfunction [31,32]. A more recent study has shown that ischemic preconditioning decreases apoptosis in rat hearts in vivo [33]. The possible mechanisms of prevention of apoptosis may include reperfusion mediated induction of survival factors [34] such as stress-activated protein kinase translocation to the nucleus.

Apoptosis in hibernating myocardium

Although growing role of apoptosis has been reported by numerous experimental and clinical studies of acute myocardial infarction, DNA fragmentation occurs in the myocytes that had already shown irreversibly oncotic, but not apoptotic ultrastructures with ischemia and/or reperfusion. DNA fragmentation itself does not always mean apoptosis and so called apoptotic myocytes may belong to a category of cell death other than apoptosis. It has been traditionally believed that the cardiac myocytes in the hibernating myocardium are essentially healthy cells [35-37]. However, transmural biopsies obtained during surgery have revealed that hibernating myocardium is characterized by dedifferentiation, degeneration and replacement fibrosis. Potentially reversible 'dedifferentiating changes' include loss of contractile sarcomeres, expression of smooth muscle actin, cardiotin, titin, intracellular glycogen plaques, increase in small mitochondria, heterogeneous distribution of chromatin in the nucleus and disorganization and loss of sarcoplasmic reticulum [38-40]. It is assumed, but not proven, that some cellular dedifferentiation alterations will be corrected when function is recovered.

Borgers *et al.* using electron microscopic analysis of left ventricular biopsies demonstrated structural alterations [36,38,41,42]. The hibernating myocardium was associated with an alteration of all structural proteins resulting in disorganization of cytoskeleton, loss of myofilaments and the occurrence of large areas filled with glycogen. The disorganization of the cytoskeleton results from desmin accumulation and the lack of titin and α-actinin whereas the loss of myofilaments caused an impairment in the contractile capacity of the cardiac myocytes. The decrease in titin filaments caused a change in cardiac compliance as titin is one of the elastic filaments of the sarcomere. These structural changes in cardiac myocytes are associated with fibrosis. The pathogenesis of fibrosis is unclear but has been postulated to be due to replacement or reparative process by some investigators whereas others have suggested that it is a 'reactive' phenomenon [43].

Schwarz *et al.* obtained transmural biopsy specimens from the hibernating regions of myocardium of 24 patients during coronary artery bypass surgery [39]. Hibernating regions of myocardium were determined by preoperative technetium-99m sestamibi uptake and 18-F fluorodeoxyglucose uptake on positron emission tomography and intraoperatively by hypocontractile regions of myocardium. Viable myocytes were found in all biopsy samples from the hypocontractile regions. There was no evidence for previous transmural infarction. Using electron microscopy they found that cardiac myocytes showed signs of severe degeneration with loss of myofilaments, occurrence of cellular degeneration with loss of myofilaments, decreased sizes of mitochondria and cellular debris. An increased degree of extracellular fibrosis was present. The myocyte nuclei were abnormally shaped and sized and displayed cytoplasmic inclusions or the occurrence of fine filaments. The mitochondria had a different appearance; many were small and some showed a reduced number of cristae. Other abnormalities such as presence of glycogen deposits, fat droplets, lipofucsin and degenerative vacuoles were common. Immunohistochemical analysis was used to study titin and α-actinin. In this study there was loss of these structures. Staining for collagen VI was used as an indicator of fibrosis and varying degrees of fibrosis was noted. The loss of contractile material and severity of fibrosis assessed by immunohistochemical staining paralleled the degree of degenerative changes detected by electron microscopy in each patient. The most important finding was that all biopsy specimens showed signs of long-term degeneration, most probably due to ischemia without evidence of transmural infarction. Interestingly, the severity of morphologic changes did not correlate with regional wall abnormalities, with FDG uptake, nor with functional or clinical outcome. These authors recognized that the severe cellular degeneration may have resulted in cell death in their biopsy specimens. They proposed that hibernating myocardium may represent an adaptive process insufficient to maintain cell integrity for the entire hypoperfused myocardium. They concluded that not all myocardial cells can survive, and functional recovery is partially incomplete or delayed, or both [39]. In a more recent study the same group of investigators have shown that prolonged myocardial hibernation exacerbates cardiomyocyte degeneration and impairs recovery of function after revascularization [44]. Subsequent investigators demonstrated that apoptosis occurs in hibernation [43,45]. Chen *et al.* created a stenosis in the left anterior descending coronary artery in 13 pigs to reduce coronary blood flow by about a third for a period of 24 hours to 4 weeks which resulted in severe systolic dysfunction by echocardiography [45]. In 5 pigs there was no myocardial infarction whereas in the remaining pigs there was minimal patchy infarction (<60%). In all experimental pigs, apoptosis was detected in the hibernating region supplied by the stenotic left anterior descending coronary artery (LAD) with the in situ end-labeling method and 'DNA laddering'. Apoptosis was patchy and seen predominantly in the subendocardial region. Apoptosis was rare in the subepicardial region of the hibernating region. If the apoptotic cells in the subendocardial and subepicardial myocardium were averaged for each of the pigs there were 4.8±2.3% apoptotic myocytes. Apoptosis was observed both in the regions adjacent to the patchy fibrosis or in the regions from fibrosis. There was no difference in the number of apoptotic cells in the hibernating region with different duration of hibernation at 24 hours, 7 days, and 4 weeks. However, a large number of animals are needed to determine whether apoptosis increases with time, stabilizes or eventually decreases with the duration of hibernation. No apoptosis was found in the normal control regions. The percentage of cells with apoptosis correlated significantly with the severity of myocardial hypoperfusion. Apoptosis was more severe in animals with patchy infarction than in those without patchy infarction. No apoptosis was found in sham-operated animals. Chen *et al.* suggest that the ongoing myocardial cell death in their study may in part be responsible for myocyte loss and increased fibrosis in long-term hibernating left ventricular regions [45]. Their conclusions have been partly supported by a more recent study where hibernating myocardium exhibited time-dependent deterioration due to progressive structural degeneration with enhanced fibrosis [44].

Elässer *et al.* studied 38 patients with hibernating myocardium, which was identified by a combination of angiography, multigated radionuclide ventriculography, thallium-201 scintigraphy and low-dose dobutamine echocardiography [43]. They obtained transmural biopsies from these patients during cardiac surgery. Using electron microscopy, immunohistochemistry and in situ hybridization they observed disorganization of the contractile and cytoskeletal proteins myosin, actin, desmin, titin, α-actinin, and vinculin (Figures 1-3). In addition, there was upregulation of extracellular matrix proteins resulting in significant fibrosis (Figure 1). The mRNAs corresponding to cellular proteins were reduced and those of the extracellular space increased, indicating changes at the transcriptional level because expression of the respective genes seemed to be predominantly regulated at the transcriptional level (Figure 2). The most obvious changes in myocytes were the loss of myofilaments, disorganization of the cytoskeleton, and the occurrence of large areas filled with glycogen (Figure 1). The lack of titin and α-actinin, components of the sarcomeric skeleton added to the structural disorganization (Figure 2). As a consequence, the loss of myofilaments causes a reduction of the contractile capacity of the myocytes, the disarrangement of the cytoskeleton results in loss of cellular stability, and the defects of the sarcomeric skeleton leads to sarcomeric instability. In addition, the reduction in titin filaments produces a change of compliance since titin is the 'third' elastic filament of the sarcomere.

The pathophysiologic abnormality of the cardiomyocytes becomes more aggravated by the development of fibrosis. Elässer et al. reported that all constituents of the basement membrane, i.e., laminin, collagen IV and VI, and fibronectin, were present in large amounts, which will encapsulate the myocytes [43]. Furthermore, the matrix protein fibronectin and the fibrillar collagens I and III fill the enlarged interstitial space, and macrophages and fibroblasts are present in large numbers. Macrophages proceed to phagocytose the cellular debris, and the fibroblasts produce the different extracellular matrix proteins. Elässer et al. [43] believed that the combination of cellular degeneration with the development of fibrosis in hibernating myocardium significantly determined the degree and speed of recovery after coronary artery bypass operation, which is a view slightly different from that postulated by Borgers and co-workers [38].

Earlier workers have noted the lack of necrosis in hibernating myocardium [46,47]. Elässer and co-workers reported typical ultrastructural lesions of apoptosis and the TUNEL reaction confirmed the presence of DNA fragments in myocyte nuclei (Figure 3). They found that apoptosis not only occurred in myocytes but also in interstitial cells. Although they were, unable to quantify the apoptosis since the biopsy specimens were small, they observed that apoptosis occurred mainly in the cells with severe cellular degenerative alterations. They found that inflammation with cellular infiltration of mononuclear cells was absent and excluded this as a stimulus for cell death in the hibernating myocardium. In their patients there was recovery of regional function 3 months after CABG surgery confirming that their patients indeed had hibernating myocardium.

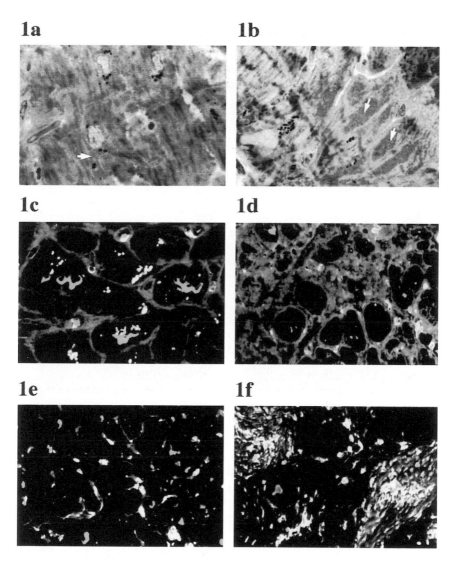

Figure 1. Mycocytic and interstitial changes in hibernating myocardium. Very small quantities of glycogen are usually seen perinuclearly in normal myocytes (A, arrow), whereas large amount of glycogen is observed in the hibernating myocardium (B, arrows). There was no correlation between severity of degeneration and glycogen accumulation. (PAS stain for glycogen, pink). While the normal myocytes are separated by very small quantities of collagen (C), progressively large amount of collagen accumulates as the severity of degeneration increases in hibernating myocardium (D). (Immunohistochemical staining with collagen type I antibody, green; Bioscience Laboratory). In hibernating myocardium (F) interstitial fibroblasts increase proportionally to the severity of degeneration; compare with the minimal fibrocytic activity in the normal myocardium (E). (Immunostaining for vimentin, yellowish-green; Dianova Laboratory). (Figure by permission from Dr. Jutta Schaper and American Heart Association; Elässer *et al.* 1997).

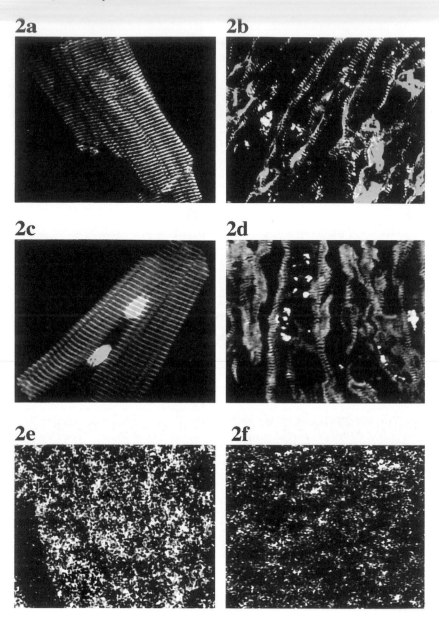

Figure 2. Changes in the contractile proteins in hibernating myocardium. Severe loss of contractile proteins occurs in the hibernating myocardium. A normal isolated myocyte shows regular cross-striations of alpha-actinin (A), whereas severe lack of actinin is observed in hibernating myocardium with severe degeneration (B). (Immunostaining with anti-α-actinin antibody, yellowish green; Sigma Laboratory). Red color in figure B denotes double staining for collagen VI and represents widening extracellular spaces. Similar to loss of α-actinin, titin is also lost in hibernating myocardium (D) as compared to the normal isolated myocytes (C). (Immunohistochemical staining with titin T12 antibody, greenish-yellow; Boehringer-Mannheim). Myosin mRNA is similarly reduced in hibernating myocardium (F) as compared to normal myocytes (E). (In situ hybridization with cRNA probe). (Figure by permission from Dr. Jutta Schaper and American Heart Association; Elässer *et al.* 1997)

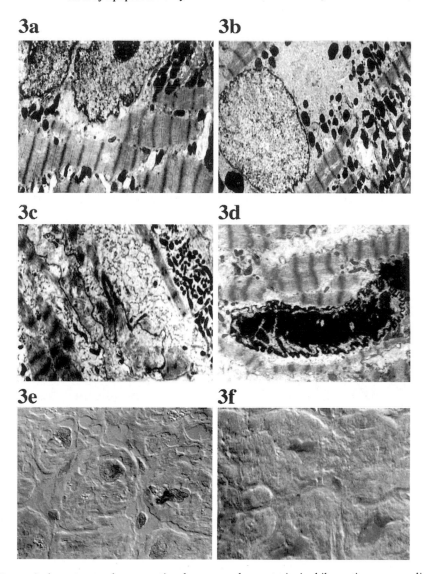

Figure 3. lntrastructural mycocytic changes and apoptosis in hibernating myocardium. Normal myocardium shows regularly distributed sarcomeres, a normal nucleus and mitochondria (A). Moderate degeneration in hibernating myocardium demonstrates loss of myofilaments in perinuclear area, prominent sarcoplasmic reticulum and abbreviated mitochondrial shadows (B). The ultrastructural changes are either exaggerated (C) or demonstrate apoptotic changes (nuclear chromatin clumping in presence of preserved organelles, D) in hibernating myocardium associated with severe degeneration. Association of apoptosis in hibernating myocardium is demonstrated by *TUNEL* staining and interference contrast microscopy (E). Nuclei with fragmented DNA are demonstrated by brown color staining compared to normal nuclei in blue color (F). (Immunostaining for vimentin, yellowish-green; Dianova Laboratory). (Figure by permission from Dr. Jutta Schaper and American Heart Association; Reference Elässer *et al.*)

Inducers of apoptosis in hibernation

The possible inducers of apoptosis in hibernating myocardium include oxidative stress induced by ischemia, heat shock proteins induced by ischemia, withdrawal of growth factors, and cytokines produced by macrophages and fibroblasts. It must be remembered that in hibernating myocardium inflammatory mononuclear cell infiltration is characteristically absent and hence cannot be implicated in apoptosis of the hibernating myocardium.

The identification of reactive oxygen species as a mediator of myocardial ischemia including hibernating myocardium is well known. Apoptosis may occur as a consequence of generation of oxygen containing free radicals, which induce DNA damage and apoptosis. However, the role of oxygen-free radicals in hibernation remains to be established. Oxygen-free radicals can induce the expression of immediate early genes associated with apoptosis [48]. In addition to oxygen-free radicals, several growth factors have been shown to play a role in apoptosis. Apoptosis has been described in cardiac myocytes with angiotensin II stimulation, which is reversed using an angiotensin type I receptor antagonist [49,50]. Dzau and co-workers have shown that angiotensin type 2 receptors mediate apoptosis [51,52]. The group of Lakatta demonstrated in *in vivo* studies that there is a 4.5 fold increase in apoptosis in failing SHR hearts over control animals and the administration of captopril reduced the amount of apoptosis [53]. Similar results have been obtained by Sabbah and coworkers in dogs where angiotensin converting enzyme (ACE) inhibition attenuated cardiomyocyte apoptosis [54]. Overexpression of IGF-1 has been shown in *in vivo* infarct models to promote myocardial salvage and apoptosis occurs less commonly in animals that overexpress IGF-1. Chien and associates have shown that cardiotrophin-1 (CT-1) a novel growth factor, which reduces apoptosis in neonatal rat ventricular myocytes [55]. The anti-apoptotic action of CT-1 has been shown to require the activation of Ras/Raf/MEK/mitogen-activated protein kinase pathway, since inhibition of extracellular signal regulated kinase 1 and 2 activation with the MEK inhibitor PD98059 prevented CT-1s anti-apoptotic activity [55]. Another mechanism by which cardiotrophin-1 treated cardiac myocytes are protected from ischemic apoptosis is by upregulation of heat shock proteins [56]. More recently, the late Thomas W. Smith and colleagues reported that neuregulins (a family of locally acting peptide autocoids known to be important in the development of the central and peripheral nervous system) promoted survival and inhibited apoptosis in neonatal and adult rat ventricular myocytes [57,58]. Interestingly, neuregulins also activated mitogen-activated protein kinase pathways in myocytes [59]. However, the activation of this mitogen-activated protein kinase pathway alone was sufficient for the anti-apoptotic effects of these ligands since several other growth factors including angiotensin II [60], interleukin-1ß and interferon-gamma, activated this signal transduction cascade, all of which have been shown to promote apoptosis in both adult and neonatal rat ventricular myocytes [17]. Further studies are required to determine how these peptide growth factors influence cellular degeneration and the accompanying apoptosis in hibernating myocardium.

Inflammatory cytokines such as tumor necrosis factor (TNF-α) can induce apoptosis. Serum TNF-α is produced within the heart by cardiac myocytes and is elevated in acute myocardial infarction. It has been shown that serum TNF-α can induce apoptosis in rat cardiac myocytes. Two major receptor subtypes of TNF-α are TNFR-1 and TNFR-2 are expressed by cardiac myocytes and it has been shown that apoptosis is specifically induced by TNFR-1 agonists [61]. The Fas receptor is markedly upregulated in cardiomyocytes during ischemia and hypoxia, and cardiomyocytes may thus become susceptible to apoptosis by interactions with Fas ligand. Under control conditions only less than 1% of the cardiac myocytes express Fas antigen, but within a few hours of ischemia and ischemia/reperfusion Fas becomes detectable in more than 50% of the cardiac myocytes [22,62]. A second mechanism by which inflammatory cytokines might act is through the induction of increased nitric oxide production in the myocardium.

Williams and associates and other investigators have described the induction of heat shock proteins Hsp70 by ischemia, the potential role of Hsp70 in ischemic preconditioning and inverse correlation between expression of Hsp70 induced by ischemic preconditioning and infarct size in animal models [63-66]. The overexpression of Hsp70 in transgenic mice improves myocardial function, and preserves metabolic function and reduced infarct size after ischemia/reperfusion [67,68]. Ferrari and co-workers [69] demonstrated that hibernation was accompanied by the myocardial expression of heat shock protein 72 (*hsp*72). Maneuvers that increase Hsp70 expression inhibit apoptosis in a variety of cell types [70-72]. Tissue-specific expression of Hsp70-2 prevents apoptosis in various cell types through a mechanism involving cell cycle control [73]. Hsp70 chaperone function in regulating apoptosis may be at the level of signal transduction, as it has been implicated in the stress-activated pathway [74]. Given their strategic locations in all major cellular organelles, it has been proposed that Hsp may combat oxidative stress/damage by refolding damaged repressors of the cell death pathway or preventing their degradation [66]. Alternatively, repressing the release of suicide activators, such as cytochrome *c*, could occur through interactions with mitochondrial chaperones and chaperonins. Results of several recent studies have implicated the small molecular weight Hsp25/27 in cell survival pathways involving cell differentiation and oxidative stress/damage. Antisense reduction of Hsp25/27 accelerates apoptosis suggesting that during proliferation and differentiation of myocardial cells, the Hsp25/27 chaperone, and others can reduce oxidative stress/damage and prevent apoptosis through a redox-dependent mechanism [75,76]. Identification of small molecules, potentially suitable for use as drugs that trigger expression of heat shock proteins is being sought [65].

Nitric oxide (NO) plays a central role in normal myocardial biology. It has the ability to exert both beneficial and deleterious effects on the cardiac myocytes. At higher concentrations it induces apoptosis. One mechanism by which NO causes apoptosis is by the formation of reactive oxygen and nitrogen species. It reacts with superoxide anion to generate peroxynitrate, a free radical that may be more toxic and long-live than NO or O_2^- [77]. Eroxynitrate can react with tyrosine residues of susceptible proteins, in some cases causing irreversible inactivation [78]. At lower concentrations NO may protect myocyte apoptosis from deleterious stimuli such as norepinephrine and mechanical stress. Cheng *et al.* [19] reported that mechanical strain induced apoptosis in myocytes was completely inhibited by the addition of an NO donor. The protective effect of NO correlated with its ability to decrease the level of superoxide in the myocardium, suggesting that it might exert its beneficial action by scavenging superoxide generated by mechanical stretch. However, further studies are required to elucidate the mechanism by which NO protects myocytes from apoptosis. In other cell types, NO can prevent apoptosis by inhibiting specific enzymes in the apoptotic pathway [79]. The direct role of NO induced apoptosis in the pathogenesis of hibernating myocardium is not known.

Intracellular acidification is a feature of ischemic myocytes and develops as a result of anaerobic metabolism, net hydrolysis of ATP and CO_2 retention [80]. There is now growing evidence that acidification is a common feature of apoptotic cells [81]. Cardiomyocytes possess various mechanism for regulating intracellular pH. Well recognized mechanisms include the sodium-hydrogen exchange, sodium-bicarbonate cotransporter [82] and one sodium independent chloride-bicarbonate exchanger [83]. Although sodium-hydrogen exchange is considered to play the most important role in the recovery of intracellular pH from acute acid load such as that induced by ischemia, in fact, its beneficial role for the ischemic/reperfused myocardium is limited. Paradoxically, the inhibition rather than the activation of the sodium-hydrogen exchange is beneficial for the ischemic/reperfused myocardium. Inhibition of the exchanger or low pH reduces the activity of the sodium-hydrogen exchanger and the detrimental calcium overload via consequent sodium-calcium exchange protects myocardium. A third proton-extruding process ATP-dependent, vacuolar proton pump (VPATPase) may operate in cardiomyocytes [84]. VPATPases have been described in a variety of cell types, being responsible for the acidification of intracellular compartment, such as synaptic vesicles, lysosomes and endosomes. More recently, it has been postulated that the VPATPase may play a role in hypoxia-induced myocyte apoptosis suggesting that alterations in intracellular pH is critical for the triggering the death signal to cardiac myocytes in vivo. Impairment of the VPATPase affects extrusion of protons from the cytoplasm to intracellular acidic complexes, decreasing intracellular pH and abolishes the protective influence of attenuation of the sodium-hydrogen exchanger on calcium overload. In contrast, VPATPase-mediated proton efflux may spare sodium overload via the sodium-exchange and thereby attenuate calcium influx via the sodium-calcium exchange [85]. VPATPase plays an important accessory role in cardiomyocyte protection by reducing acidosis and sodium-hydrogen exchange-induced calcium overload.

Another metabolic abnormality well recognized in the hibernating myocardium is insulin resistance [86-88]. Hearts from hyperinsulinemic, insulin-resistant rats do not properly regulate intracellular calcium concentration and these hearts show increased sensitivity to ischemic myocardial injury [89]. It is well known that development of hibernation is related to the severity of ischemia [90] suggesting that hibernation and the accompanying apoptosis is more likely to develop in the insulin resistance state especially in non-insulin dependent diabetes mellitus. Using positron emission tomography and FDG uptake it has been shown that patients without left ventricular dysfunction were less likely to have myocardial insulin resistance [91] when compared to a group of patients which included those left ventricular dysfunction [92]. Camici *et al.* have suggested that hibernating myocardium is associated with increased myocardial insulin resistance [88]. It remains to be explored whether diabetics treated with traglitazone which ameliorates insulin resistance, will develop less severe apoptosis and consequently less hibernation following ischemic-reperfusion injury.

Apoptosis in stunned myocardium

Although there is scant evidence in literature about apoptosis in the stunned myocardium it may very well play a role in its pathogenesis because currently two viable hypothesis regarding the pathogenesis of myocardial stunning, including oxyradical generation and the calcium excess, also constitute the substrates for induction of apoptosis.

Myocardial stunning is characterized by decreased myofilament calcium responsiveness. Marban and associates have proposed that stunned myocardium undergoes limited proteolysis by calcium-activated protease, namely calpain I during early reperfusion [93]. They also showed that the observed decrease of calcium responsiveness is stunned myocardium is due to changes in myofilaments themselves. The phenotype of stunning could be mimicked by direct exposure of skinned cardiac muscles to calpain I. In separate studies they found that troponin I is partially and selectively degraded in stunned myocardium; the changes were reproduced by calpain I and was prevented by calpastatin, an endogenous calpain I inhibitor. The investigators concluded that myocardial stunning is caused by partial degradation of troponin I as a result of the activation of calcium-dependent protease during reperfusion [93].

Also Sonnenblick and co-workers have suggested that profound structural alterations of the extracellular collagen matrix occur in stunned myocardium [94]. The dilatation and expansion of stunned myocardium would suggest acute ischemic alterations in the collagen matrix of the heart. In a subsequent study this group found that a nonuniform transmural loss of collagen occurred in the stunned tissue associated with 73.6% increase in collagenase activity [95]. In addition, this group found that the aminophenylmercuric acetate-activated procollagenase and the lysosomal enzymes elastase and cathepsin G were not different in the stunned and normal zone tissue, and thus the exogenous sources of protease appear to be unlikely at the time of measurement (90-minute final reperfusion period) in their model of ischemia. They also found that dansyl chloride labeling of exposed N-terminal amino acid residues was 9% greater in stunned than normal zone isolated collagen fibers indicating that there was greater in vivo cleavage of the stunned collagen matrix. Myocardial dysfunction was produced by multiple coronary occlusion protocol, a procedure that has been demonstrated to produce myocardial dysfunction without any irreversible cellular damage. Thus, it appears that myocardial ischemia affects the extracellular compartment of the heart before irreversible structural changes in the cellular compartment. Damage to matrix integrity during ischemia and post-ischemic reperfusion can be due to several mechanisms: mechanical, degradative processes, and detachment of collagen from its anchoring sites on the sarcolemma. The extracellular collagen network is extensive and is felt to have an important influence on the passive properties of the heart. The adult cardiac matrix is highly insoluble and cross-linked. The extent of the linkage in the collagen network is clearly indicated by the ability to remove the collagen mesh as a unit. At the cellular level, myocytes are connected to myocytes and to the vasculature by collagen struts. These struts are observed to inert onto the sarcolemma just lateral to the Z-disk [96]. The collagen attaches at these specific membrane sites onto adhesion molecules, termed integrins. The integrin receptors are a family of heterodimeric transmembrane glycoproteins involved in a wide range of cell-cell and cell-matrix interactions [97]. Terracio et al. have demonstrated localization of the collagen integrins to the sarcolemma of adult rat myocytes, in a discrete pattern presumably at the Z disk [98]. The expression of the integrin protein is increased in cardiac hypertrophy [98-100]. The intracellular domain of the integrins is thought to the linked to the contractile apparatus via several cytoskeletal proteins (talin, vinculin, alpha-actinin). Thus, integrins are likely to play an important role in the transduction of extracellular stress (signals) into the cell, to the contractile apparatus, and possibly to the nucleus via the cytoskeleton. Ischemic reperfusion injury could affect this attachment in several ways, resulting in loss of collagen binding to its receptor and/or impairment of the force transduction pathway. The multiple occlusion/reperfusion model of stunning is characterized by both intracellular and extracellular edema [95,101]. The significant changes in ionic environment could affect the receptor-ligand interaction. Scanning electron microscopy reveals extensive loss of collagen struts. Whether this loss is due to a degradative process or to a dissociation of the integrin from the collagen is not clear. Sonnenblick *et al.* group [94] found regions of densely clumped stained matrix in fields devoid of matrix staining. This pattern contrasts with a fine uniform staining pattern of the collagen weave in the normal myocardium [102]. The regions of clumped matrix may represent receptor dissociated matrix still tethered to the main collagenous network. The sarcomeres in a normal myocardium are aligned in an well ordered array. It is felt that the cytoskeleton protein and desmin tether the Z disks to maintain sarcomere registration. The stunned myocardium demonstrates significant mis-registration of the sarcomeres [103]. An immunofluorescent study was performed on stunned myocardium to assess for cytoskeletal abnormalities [104]. Conjugated monoclonal antibodies to desmin and vimentin revealed a regular striated pattern in normal tissue, compatible with their localization at or near the Z disks. In contrast, anti-vinculin antibodies stained the sarcolemma and cell junctions with no striation pattern. In the stunned myocardium, there was marked attenuation or loss of normal patterns. The alterations in vinculin staining suggests a potential abnormality in the intracellular integrin transduction system. A further observation in these studies was the finding of strong anti-vimentin staining in the perinuclear region of normal tissue, with a halo-like appearance. This was not observed in the stunned tissue. It is conceivable that this protein represents the final pathway of external force transmission to the nucleus. Sonnenblick and associates have described several changes in cardiac myocytes and interstitium but have not described apoptosis in the stunned myocardium [94]. It is conceivable that apoptosis occurs both in myocytes and non-myocytes such as cardiac fibroblasts and microvascular endothelial cells. However, further studies are required to determine the role of apoptosis in stunned myocardium.

Numerous studies have shown that brief periods of acute myocardial ischemia protect the heart from detrimental consequences of ischemia-reperfusion injuries in different animal species including humans. In addition to reducing ventricular arrhythmias and reduction in infarct size, ischemic preconditioning reduces postischemic contractile dysfunction [31,32]. Ischemic preconditioning reduces irreversible ischemic injury in part by decreasing apoptosis after prolonged ischemia and reperfusion

[33,84] as evidenced by internucleosomal DNA fragmentation. The basic mechanism by which ischemic preconditioning could prevent apoptosis remains unknown. Recent experiments have demonstrated that apoptosis could be delayed in neutrophils [81], and in hematopoietic stem cells [105] by preservation of intracellular pH homeostasis. On the basis of these findings, Gottlieb *et al.* [84] suggested that activation of vacuolar proton ATPase by PKC during preconditioning may attenuate intracellular acidification during metabolic inhibition and thereby protect mycoytes from apoptosis in vitro. Consistent with this hypothesis are studies that have demonstrated that ischemic preconditioning was accompanied by a reduction in intracellular acidosis in rat hearts [106-109]. In addition to increased proton export through vacuolar proton ATPase by PKC activation, reduced proton production from anaerobic glycolysis may also contribute to prevent myocyte apoptosis in rat hearts in vivo.

Myocardial stunning has been described with elevated catecholamines in pheochromocytoma [110,111]. Colucci *et al.* have demonstrated that catecholamines can induce apoptosis in cardiac myocytes [112]. The role of catecholamine induced apoptosis in myocardial stunning needs to be explored.

Prevention of apoptosis for therapeutic intervention

It has been shown that trimetazidine [50] reduces ischemic apoptosis by exerting a protecting effect against acidosis, the preservation of intracellular pH may have interfered with the induction of myocyte apoptosis [113].

Kharbanda and co-workers [27] have shown that family of cysteine, asparatyl-specific proteases known as caspases are required for the execution of apoptosis in the heart. Caspase activation itself is clearly one of the final steps required for the execution phase of apoptosis. Presumably, degradation of intracellular proteins that are caspase targets, either specifically or in total, results in a cell demise. Further work in this area is required to determine whether cleavage of many proteins together or only a select few is critical for apoptosis of myocytes remains to be defined. Caspases are attractive potential targets for the treatment of ischemia-reperfusion injury and the appealing prospect of small-molecule inhibitor therapy. Peptidyl caspase inhibitors have been found to be effective in animal models of myocardial ischemia-reperfusion injury. What are the best caspase targets for inhibition of apoptosis? To answer this requires a better understanding of the role of individual caspases in cardiac myocytes. Tissue-specific delivery of the selective caspase inhibitor is required. On a more practical level, can caspase inhibitor be identified that is suitable for use in vivo? Although ACE inhibitors work by inhibiting proteases, there are few other examples. This reflects, in part, formidable difficulties in generating small molecule, non-peptide inhibitors of proteolytic enzymes that are selectively, stable and penetrate membranes effectively. This notwithstanding, elegant work on cysteine protease inhibition has provided a starting point, leading to the identification of several classes of potent reversible and irreversible caspase inhibitors [114]. Studies with these compounds will no doubt provide answers to may questions regarding the therapeutic potential of caspase inhibition. Although the relative importance of apoptotic and non-apoptotic cell death in myocardial ischemia is not unknown, use of caspase inhibitor zVAD.fmk leads to reduction in acute functional parameters after myocardial infarct. However, these changes were recorded within 24 hours of infarction, and it is unclear whether the effects of zVAD.fmk persists for longer periods of time [25]. The role of caspase inhibitors in preventing or ameliorating myocardial hibernation needs to be investigated.

The work ahead necessary to develop and refine clinically useful anti-apoptotic therapy is daunting. There are many unanswered questions. What will be the most practical method to deliver this therapy to the cardiac myocyte? Will anti-apoptotic agents act selectively on affected myocytes to provide clinical efficacy? Will anti-apoptotic agents be effective or will they be limited by dose heterogeneity? If anti-apoptotic is proven to have long lasting efficacy should it be used for all patients with myocardial infarction or confined only to patients with left ventricular dysfunction. Will anti-apoptotic therapy be so effective that it replaces ACE inhibitors or will it always be used as an adjunct to a ACE inhibitors? These questions will lay the foundation for the next decade of investigation.

Conclusions

Although there is a growing evidence for the role of apoptosis in pathogenesis of myocardial damage in various cardiovascular disorders, its importance in altered myocardial states is not well established. The hibernating myocardium is characterized by a reduction in contractile apparatus and cytoskeleton, and by an increase in glycogen content and degeneration of mitochondria associated with structural abnormalities reminiscent of cell dedifferentiation and cellular degeneration. Unlike an increase in intracellular calcium content in myocardial stunning [115], hibernating myocardium is a low demand-low supply situation with a low intracellular calcium level. It can be imagined that in an initial stages of hibernation, the contractility of the myocytes is suppressed because of stunning, and subsequently, the repeated insults may reduce the calcium sensitivity of the myofibrils and/or reduce the storage capacity for calcium of the sarcoplasmic reticulum. This leads to an atrophy-of-inactivity of the sarcomeres and the consequent loss of contractile material [43]. This reduction in myocyte constituents and size reduces the demand for oxygen of the individual cells and is initially a protective mechanism aimed primarily at survival of the cell but not at the maintenance of its function. Subsequent progressive ischemia should further disturb the new delicate balance between supply and demand causing further cellular degeneration until apoptosis occurs [116]. The apoptosis is almost always associated with severe myocyte degenerative alterations which adversely affects the potential reversibility of systolic function after restoration of blood supply [117]. The importance of apoptosis in myocardial hibernation can only be established if intervention with inhibitors of apoptosis should be able to avoid irreversible structural changes in ischemic myocardium after mechanical or surgical revascularization.

References

1. Rees G, Bristow JD, Kremkau EL *et al.* Influence of aortocoronary bypass on left ventricular performance. N Engl J Med 1971;284:1116-20.
2. Chatterjee K, Swan HJC, Parmley WW, Sustaita H, Marcus HS, Matloff J. Influence of direct direct myocardial revascularization on left ventricular asynergy and function in patients with coronary artery disease: with and without previous myocardial infarction. Circulation 1973;47:276-86.
3. Heyndrickx GR, Millard RW, McRitchie RJ *et al.* Regional myocardial function and electrophysiological alterations after brief coronary artery occlusion in conscious dogs. J Clin Invest 1975;56:978-85.
4. Braunwald E, Kloner RA. The stunned myocardium: prolonged, postischemic ventricular dysfunction. Circulation 1982;66:1146-9.
5. Rahimtoola SH. A perspective on the three large multicenter randomized clinical trials of coronary bypass surgery for chronic stable angina. Circulation 1985;72:123-35.
6. Rahimtoola SH. The hibernating myocardium. Am Heart J 1989;117:211-52.
7. Wackers FJ, Vogt-Hoerner G. Presence of focal bionecrosis in the epithelium of the acini in the human mammary gland. Ann Anat Pathol 1967;12:21-34.
8. Maulik N, Kagan VE, Tyurin VA, Das DK. Redistribution of phosphatidylethanolamine and phosphatidylserine precedes reperfusion-induced apoptosis. Am J Physiol 1998;274:H242-8.
9. Blankenberg FG, Katsikis PD, Tait JF *et al.* In vivo detection and imaging of phosphatidylserine expression during programmed cell death. Proc Natl Acad Sci USA 1998;95:6349-54.
10. Nagata S. Apoptosis by death factor. Cell 1997; 88:355-65.
11. Liu X, Kim CN, Yang J, Jemmerson R, Wang X. Induction of apoptotic program in cell-free extracts requirements for dATP and Cytochrom C. Cell 1996;86:147-57.
12. Li P, Nijhawan D, Budihardjo I *et al.* Cytochrome C and dATP dependent formation of Apaf-1/Caspase 9 complex initiates an apoptotic protease cascade. Cell 1997;91:479-89.
13. Luo X, Budihardjol I, Zon H, Slaughter C, Wang X. Bid, a Bcl-2 interacting protein, mediates Cytochrome c release from mitochondria in response to activation of cell surface death receptors. Cell 1998;94:481-90.
14. Narula J , Haider N, Virmani *et al.* Apoptosis in myocytes in end-stage heart failure. N Engl J Med 1996;335:1182-9.

15. Olivetti G, Abbi R, Quaini F *et al.* Apoptosis in the failing human heart. N Engl J Med 1997;336:1131-41.
16. Gottlieb RA, Buresldon KO, Kloner RA, Babior BM, Engler RL. Reperfusion injury induces apoptosis in rabbit cardiac myocytes. J Clin Invest 1994;74:86-107.
17. Kajustura J, Cigola E, Malhotra A *et al.* Angiotensin II induces apoptosis of adult ventricular myocytes in vitro. J Mol Cell Cardiol 1997;29:859-70.
18. Liu Y, Cigola E, Cheng W *et al.* Myocyte nuclear mitotic division and programmed myocyte cell death characterize the cardiac myopathy induced rapid ventricular pacing in dogs. Lab Invest 1995;73:771-87.
19. Cheng W, Li B, Kajstura J *et al.* Stretch-induced programmed myocyte cell death. J Clin Invest 1995;96:2247-59.
20. Teiger E, Than VD, Richard L, *et al.* Apoptosis in pressure overload induced heart hypertrophy in the rat. J Clin Invest 1996;97:2891-7.
21. Hamet R, Richard L, Dam TV *et al.* Apoptosis in target organs of hypertension. Hypertension 1995;26:642-8.
22. Kajustura J, Cheng W, Reiss K *et al.* Apoptotic and necrotic myocyte cell deaths are independent contributing variables of infarct size in rats. Lab Invest 1996;74:86-107.
23. Fliss H, Gattinger D. Apoptosis in ischemic and reperfused rat myocardium. Circ Res 1996;79:949-56.
24. Bialik S, Geenen DL, Sasson IE *et al.* Myocardial apoptosis during acute myocardial infarction in the mouse localizes to hypoxic regions but occurs independently of p53. J Clin Invest 1997;100:1363-72.
25. Yaoita H, Ogawa K, Maehara K, Maruyama Y. Attenuation of ischemia/perfusion injury in rats by a caspase inhibitor. Circulation 1998;97:276-81.
26. Saraste A, Pulkki K, Kallajoki M, Henriksen K, Parvinen M, Voipio-Pukki LM. Apoptosis in human myocardial infarction. Circulation 1997;95:320-3.
27. Kharbanda S, Arbustini E, Kolodgie FD *et al.* Release of cytochrome c from mitochondria, activation of caspases and apoptosis in explanted cardiomyopathic hearts from cardiac allograft recipients [abstract]. Circulation 1997;96(8 Suppl):I-115.-6
28. Kloner RA, Pryzklenk K, Whittacker P. Deleterious effects of oxygen radicals in oxygen/reperfusion: resolved and unresolved issues. Circulation 1989;80:1115-27.
29. Entman ML, Smith CW. Post-reperfusion inflammation: a model for reaction to injury in cardiovascular disease. Cardiovasc Res 1994;28:1301-11.
30. Jeroudi MO, Hartely CJ, Bolli R. Myocardial perfusion injury: role of oxygen radicals and potential therapy with antioxidants. Am J Cardiol 1994;73:2B-7B.
31. Urabe K, Miura TM, Iwamoto TI *et al.* Pre-conditioning enhances myocardial resistance to post-ischemic myocardial stunning via adenosine receptor activation. Cardiovasc Res 1993;27:657-62.
32. Cohen MV, Liu GS, Downey JM. Preconditioning causes improved wall motion as well as smaller infarcts after transient coronary occlusion in rabbits. Circulation 1991;84:341-9.
33. Piot CA, Padmanabhan D, Ursell PC, Sievers RE, Wolfe CL. Ischemic preconditioning decreases apotosis in rat hearts in vivo. Circulation 1997;96:1598-604.
34. Mizukami Y, Yoshioka K, Morimoto S, Yoshida K. A novel mechanism of JNK activation: nuclear translocation and activation of JNK1 during ischemia and reperfusion. J Biol Chem 1997;272:16657-62.
35. Nayler WG. Calcium, calcium antagonists, stunning and hibernation: on overview. In: Opie LH, editor. Stunning, hibernation and calcium in myocardial ischemia and reperfusion. Boston: Kluwer Academic Publishers, 1992. p. 226-34.
36. Ausma J, Cleutjens J, Thone F, Falmeng W, Raemaekers W, Borgers M. Chronic hibernating myocardium: interstitial changes. Mol Cell Biochem 1995;147:35-42.
37. Vanoverschelde JL, Depre C, Wijns M, Bol A, Dion R, Gerber B, Borgers M, Melin J. Physiopathologie de l'hibernation chronique: apports de la tomographie par emissions positrons. Med Sci 1995;11:1315-22.

38. Borgers M, Thone F, Wouters L, Ausma J, Shivalkar B, Flameng W. Structural correlates of regional myocardial dysfunction in patients with critical coronary artery stenosis: chronic hibernation? Cardiovasc Pathol 1993;2:237-45.
39. Schwarz ER, Schaper J, vom Dahl J, et al. Myocyte degeneration and cell death in hibernating human myocardium. J Am Coll Cardiol 1996;26:1577-85.
40. Shivalkar B, Maes A, Borgers M et al. Only hibernating myocardium invariably shows early recovery after coronary revascularization. Circulation 1996;94:308-15.
41. Vanoverschelde JL, Wijns W, Depre C et al. Mechanism of chronic regional postischemic dysfunction in humans: new insights from the study of noninfarcted collateral-depednent myocardium. Circulation 1993;87:1513-23.
42. Ausma J, Schaart G, Thone F et al. Chronic ischemic viable myocardium in man: aspects of dedifferentiation. Cardiovasc Pathol 1995;4:29-37.
43. Elässer A, Schlepper M, Klovekorn WP et al. C, Munkel B, Schaper W, Schaper J. Hibernating myocardium: an incomplete adaptation to ischemia.   Circulation 1997;96:2920-31.
44. Schwarz ER, Schoendube FA, Kostin S, et al. Prolonged myocardial hibernation exacerbates cardiomyocyte degeneration and impairs recovery of function after revascularization. J Am Coll Cardiol 1998;31:1018-26.
45. Chen C, Lijie MA, Linfert DR et al. Myocardial cell death and apoptosis in hibernating myocardium. J Am Coll Cardiol 1997;30:1407-12.
46. Jennings RB, Somers HM, Herson PB, Kaltenbach JP. Ischemic injury of myocardium. Ann N Y Acad Sci 1969;156:61-78.
47. Schaper J, Mulch J, Winkler B, Schaper W. Ultrastructural, functional, and biochemical criteria for estimation of reversiblity of ischemic injury: a study on the effects of global ischemia on the isolated dog heart. J Mol Cell Cardiol 1979;11:521-41.
48. Webster KA, Discher DJ, Bishoporic NH. Regulation of fos and jun immediate-early genes by redox or metabolic stress in cardiac myocytes. Circ Res 1994;74:679-86.
49. Pierzchalski P, Reiss K, Cheng W et al. p53 induces myocyte apoptosis via the activation of the renin-angiotensin system. Exp Cell Res 1997;234:57-65.
50. Kajustura J, Liu Y, Baldini A et al. Coronary artery constriction in rats: necrotic and apoptotic myocyte death. Am J Cardiol 1998;82:30K-41K.
51. Yamada T, Horiuchi M, Dzau VJ. Angiotension II type 2 receptor mediates programmed cell death. Proc Natl Acad Sci USA 1996;93:156-60.
52. Horiuchi M, Yamada T, Hayashida W, Dzau VJ. Interferon regulatory factor-1 up-regulates angiotensin II type 2 receptor and induces apoptosis. J Biol Chem 1997;272:11952-8.
53. Li Z, Bing OH, Long X, Robinson KG, Lakatta EG. Increased cardiomyocyte apoptosis during transition to heart failure in the spontaneously hypertensive rat. Am J Physiol 1997;272:H2313-9.
54. Goussev A, Sharov VG, Shimoyama H et al. Effects of ACE inhibition on cardiomyocyte apoptosis in dogs with heart failure. Am J Physiol 1998;275:H626-31.
55. Sheng Z, Knowlton K, Chen J, Hoshijima M, Brown JH, Chien KR. Cardiotrophin 1 (CT-1) inhibition of cardiac myocyte apoptosis via a mitogen-activated protein kinase-dependent pathway. Divergence from downstream CT-1 signals for myocardial cell hypertrophy. J Biol Chem 1997;272:5783-91.
56. Stephenou A, Brar B, Heads R et al. Cardiotrophin-1 induces heat shock protein accumulation in cultured cardiac cells and protects from stressful stimuli. J Mol Cell Cardiol 1998;30:849-55.
57. Sawyer DB, Baliga RR, Schneider J, Marchionni, MA, Kelly RA, Smith TW. Neuregulin stimulates ErB4 receptor phosphorylation in neonatal rat ventricular myocytes [abstract]. Circulation 1996;94(8 Suppl):I-644.

58. Zhao YY, Sawyer DR, Baliga RR *et al.* Neuregulins promote survival and growth of cardiac myocytes: persistence of ErbB2/ErbB4 expression in neonatal and adult ventricular myocytes. J Biol Chem 1998;273:10261-69.

59 Baliga RR, Simmons WW, Sawyer DB *et al.* The Role of MEK-MAPK-RSK pathway, PI3 kinase pathway, and p70S^{6}K in neuregulin induced growth of cardiac myocytes [abstract]. Circulation 1997;96(8 Suppl):I-362.

60. Sadoshima J, Qiu Z, Morgan JP, Izumo S. Angiotensin II and other hypertrophic stimuli mediated by G protein-coupled receptors activate tyrosine kinase, mitogen-activated protein kinase, and 90-kD S6 kinase in cyardiac myocyte. The critical role of CA(2+)-dependent signaling. Circ Res 1995;76:1-5.

61. Krown KA, Page MT, Nguyen C *et al.* Tumour necrosis factor α-induced apoptosis in cardiac myocytes. Involvement of the sphingolipid signaling cascade in cardiac cell death. J Clin Invest 1996;98:2854-65.

62. Yue TL, Ma XL, Wang X *et al.* Possible involvement of stress activated protein kinase signaling patwhay and Fas receptor expression in prevention of ischemia/reperfusion induced cardiomyocyte apoptosis by carvedilol. Circ Res 1998;82:166-74.

63. Radford NB, Fina M, Benjamin IJ *et al.* Cardioprotective effects of 70-kDa heat shock protein in transgenic mice. Proc Natl Acad Sci USA 1996;93:2339-42.

64. Hutter JJ, Mestril R, Tam EK, Sievers RE, Dillmann WH, Wolfe CL. Overexpression of heat shock protein 72 in transgenic mice decreases infarct size in vivo. Circulation 1996;94:1408-11.

65. Williams RS. Heat shock proteins and ischemic injury to the myocardium. Circulation 1997;96:4138-40.

66. Benjamin IJ, McMillan DR. Stress (heat shock) proteins: molecular chaperones in cardiovascular biology and disease. Circ Res 1998;83:117-32.

67. Plumier JC, Rossie BM, Currie TW, Angelidis CE, Kazlaris H, Kollias G, Pagoulatos GN. Transgenic mice expressing the human heat shock protein 70 have improved post-ischemic myocardial recovery. J Clin Invest 1995;95:1854-60.

68. Marber MS, Mestril R, Chi SH, Sayen MR, Yellon DM, Dillmann WH. Overexpression of the rat inducible 70-kD heat stress protein in a transgenic mouse increases the resistance of the heart to ischemic injury. J Clin Invest 1995;95:1446-56.

69. Ferrari R, Bongrazio M, Cargnoni A *et al.* Heat shock protein changes in hibernation: a similarity with heart failure. J Mol Cell Cardiol 1996;28:2383-95.

70. Demeester S, Buchman T, Qiu Y *et al.* Heat shock induces Iκß and prevents stress-induced endothelial cell apoptosis. Arch Surg 1997;132:1283-7.

71. Garcia-Bermejo L. Vilaboa N, Perez C, Galan A, De Blas E, Aller P. Modulation of heat-shock protein 70 (HSP 70) gene expression by sodium butyrate in U-937 promonocytic cells: relationships with differentiation and apoptosis. Exp Cell Res 1997;236:268-74.

72. Mosser D, Caron A, Bourget L, Denis-Larose C, Massie B. Role of the human heat shock protein hsp70 in protection against stress-induced apoptosis. Mol Cell Biol 1997;17:5317-27.

73. Dix DJ, Allen JW, Collins BW *et al.* Targeted gene disruption of Hsp70-2 results in failed meiosis, germ cell apoptosis and male fertility. Proc Natl Acad Sci USA 1996;93:3264-8.

74. Gabai V, Merin A, Mosser D *et al.* Hsp 70 prevents activation of stress kinases. J Biol Chem 1997;272:18033-7.

75. Mehlen P, Schulze-Osthoff K, Arrigo AP. Small stress proteins as novel regulators of apoptosis: heat shock protein 27 blocks Fas/APO-1 and staurosporine-induced cell death. J Biol Chem 1996;271:16510-4.

76. Mehlen P, Mehlen A, Godet J, Arrigo AP. Hsp27 as a switch between differentiation and apoptosis in murine embryonic cells. J Biol Chem 1997;272:31657-65.

77. Radi R, Beckman JS, Bush KM, Freeman BA. Peroxynitrate oxidation of sulfhydryls. The cytotoxic potential of superoxide and nitrixc oxide. J Biol Chem 1991;266:4244-50.
78. Ischiropoulos H, Zhu L, Chen J *et al.* Peroxynitrate-mediated tyrosine nitration catalyzed by superoxide dismutase. Arch Biochem Biophys 1992;298:431-7.
79. Mannick JB, Miao XQ, Stamler JS. Nitric oxide inhibits Fas-induced apoptosis. J Biol Chem 1997;272:24125-8.
80. Dennis SC, Gevers W, Opie LH. Protons in ischemia: where do they come from; where do they go? J Mol Cell Cardiol 1991;23:1077-86.
81. Gottlieb RA, Giesing HA, Zhu JY, Engler RL, Babior BM. Cell acidification in apoptosis: granulocyte colony-stimulating factor delays programmed cell death in neutrophils by up-regulating the vaculor hydrogen-ATPase. Proc Natl Acad Sci USA 1995;92:5965-8.
82. Lagadic-Gossmann D, Buckler KJ, Vaughan-Jones RD. Role of bicarbonate in pH recovery from intracellular acidosis in guinea-pig ventricular myocyte. J Physiol (Lond) 1992;458:361-84.
83. Vaughan-Jones RD. An investigation of chloride-bicarbonate exchanger in the sheep cardiac Purkinje fibres. J Physiol (Lond) 1986;379:377.
84. Gottlieb RA, Gruol DL, Zhu JY, Engler RL. Preconditioning in rabbit cardiomyocytes: role of pH, vacuolar proton ATPase and apoptosis. J Clin Invest 1996;97:2391-8.
85. Karwatowksa-Prokopczuk E, Nordberg JA, Li H-L, Engler RL, Gottlieb RA. Effect of vaculolar proton ATPase on pH$_i$, calcium and apotosis in neonatal cardiomyocytes during metabolic inhibition/recovery. Circ Res 1998;82:1139-44.
86. Gerber B, Melin JA, Bol A, Vanoverschelde JL. Attenuated response of myocardial glucose utilization to insulin stimulation in hibernating myocardium [abstract]. Circulation 1995;92(8 suppl):I-313.
87. Maki M, Luotoolahti M, Nuutila P *et al.* Glucose uptake in the chronically dysfunctional but viable myocardium. Circulation 1996;93:1658-1666.
88. Marinho NVS, Keogh BE, Costa DC *et al.* Pathophysiology of chronic left ventricular dysfunction: new insights from the measurement of absolute myocardial blood flow and glucose utilization. Circulation 1996;93:737-44.
89. Maddaford TG, Russell JC, Pierce GN. Postischemic cardiac performance in the insulin resistant JCRLLA-cp rat. Am J Physiol 1997;273:H1187-92.
90. Schultz R, Rose J, Martin C Brodde OE, Heusch G. Development of short-term myocardial hibernation: its limitation by the severity of ischemia and inotropic stimulation. Circulation 1993;88:684-95.
91. Baliga R, Lammertsma A, Rhodes CJ, Aitman TJ, Scott J, Kooner JS. Positron emission tomography localises insulin resistance to skeletal muscle in premature coronary heart disease [abstract]. Circulation 1995;92(8 Suppl);I16-7.
92. Paternostoro G, Camici PG, Lammertsmaa A *et al.* Cardiac and skeletal muscle insulin resistance in patients with coronary artery disease. A study with positron emission tomography. J Clin Invest 1996;98:2094-9.
93. Gao WD, Atar D, Liu Y, Perez NG, Murphy AM, Marban E. Role of troponin I in the pathogenesis of stunned myocardium. Circ Res 1997;80:393-9.
94. Zhao M, Zhang H, Robinson TF, Factor SM, Sonnenblick EH, Eng C. Profound structural alterations of the extracellular collagen matrix in postischemic dysfunctional ('stunned') but viable myocardium. J Am Coll Cardiol 1987;10:1322-34.
95. Charney RH, Takahashi S, Zhao M, Sonnenblick EH, Eng C. Collagen loss in the stunned myocardium. Circulation 1992;85:1483-90.
96. Borg T, Johnson LD, Lill PH. Specific attachment of collagen to cardiac myocytes: in-vivo and in-vitro. Dev Biol 1983;97:417-23.
97. Hynes RO. Integrins: a family of cell surface receptors. Cell 1987;48:549-54.
98. Terracio L, Rubin K, Gullberg D *et al.* Expression of collagen binding integrins during cardiac development and hypertrophy. Circ Res 1991;68:734-44.

99. Ross RS, Pham C, Shai S-Y *et al.* ß1 integrins participate in the hypertrophic response of rat ventricular myocytes. Circ Res 1998;82:1160-72.

100. Baliga RR, Brooks WW, Bing OH, Singh K, Colucci WS. Beta-1 integrins in cardiac hypertrophy and failure. Accepted for the 72nd annual scientific sessions of the American Heart Association, Dallas, Nov, 1999. Circulation. In press 1999.

101. Zhao M, Sonneblick EH, Zhang H, Eng C. Increase in myofilament separation in the 'stunned' myocardium. J Mol Cell Cardiol 1992;24:269-76.

102. Robinson BL, Morito T, Toft DO, Morris JJ. Accelerated recovery of postischemic stunned myocardium after induced expression of myocardial heat-shock protein (Hsp 70). J Thorac Cardiovasc Surg 1995;109:753-64.

103. Zhao M, Forman R, Sonnenblick EH *et al.* Sarcomere mis-registration in the stunned myocardium: evidence for intracellular slippage [abstract]. Circulation 1989;80(4 Suppl):II513.

104. Zhao M, Sonnenblick EH, Zhang H, Factor SM, Eng C. Cytoskeletal alterations in the stunned myocardium [abstract]. FASEB J 1992;6:A1245.

105. Caceres-Cortes J, Rajotte D, Dumouchel J, Haddad P, Hoang T. Product of the Steel locus suppresses apoptosis in hemopoietic cells: comparison with pathways activated by granulocyte macrophage colony-stimulating factor. J Biol Chem 1994;269:12084-91.

106. Kida M, Fujiwara H, Ishida M *et al.* Ischemic preconditioning preserves creatine phosphate and intracellular pH. Circulation 1991;84:2495-503.

107. Wolfe CL, Sievers RE, Visseren FL, Donnelly TJ. Loss of myocardial protection after preconditioning correlates with the time course of glycogen recovery within the preconditioned segment. Circulation 1993;87:881-92.

108. de Albuquerque CP, Gerstenblith G, Weiss RG. Importance of metabolic inhibition and cellular pH in mediating preconditioning contractile and metabolic effects in rat hearts. Circ Res 1994;74:139-50.

109. Schaefer S, Carr LJ, Prussel E, Ramasamy R. Effects of glycogen depletion on ischemic injury in isolated rat hearts: insights into preconditioning. Am J Physiol 1995;268:H935-44.

110. Yamanaka O, Yasumasa F, Nakamura T *et al.* Myocardial stunning like phenomenon during a crisis of phechromocytoma. Jpn Circ J 1994;58:737-42.

111. Quigg RJ, Om A. Reversal of severe cardiac systolic dyfunction caused by pheochromocytoma in a heart transplant candidate. J Heart Lung Transplant 1994;13:525-32.

112. Communal C, Singh K, Pimentel DR, Colucci WS. Norepinephrine stimulates apoptosis in adult rat ventriclar myocytes by activation of the ß-adrenergic pathway. Circulation 1998;98:1329-34.

113. Lagadic-Gossmann D, Le Prigent K, Feuvray D. Effects of trimetazidine on intracellular pH regulation in the rat isolated ventricular myocyte. Br J Pharmacol 1996;117:831-8.

114. Thornberry NA. Caspases: Key mediators of apoptosis. Chem Biol 1998;5:R97-103.

115. Bolli R. Mechanism of myocardial stunning. Circulation 1990;82:723-38.

116. Olivetti G, Quaini F, Sala R *et al.* Acute myocardial infarction in humans is associated with activation of programmed myocyte cell death in the surviving portion of the heart. J Mol Cell Cardiol 1996;28:2005-16.

117. Kerr JFR, Wyllie AH, Currie AR. Apoptosis: a basic biologic phenomenon with wide-ranging implications in tissue kinetics. Br J Cancer 1972;26:239-57.

3. Assessment of myocardial viability with positron emission tomography

HEINRICH R. SCHELBERT

Introduction

The assessment of myocardial viability in patients with chronic coronary artery disease but well preserved left ventricular performance is of interest but often remains without significant impact on therapy. More often than not do investigations on myocardial viability in such patients appear to explore a paradigm and to test and validate a particular diagnostic approach. The lack of clinical outcome data on viability assessment in patients with normal or near normal left ventricular function and the absence of compelling arguments for why viability should be determined in such patients appear in support of this contention. However, the search for myocardial viability appears critical and often pivotal in the management of patients with end-stage coronary artery disease and severe depression of cardiac function. In fact, several investigations confirm the often considerable impact myocardial viability studies have on the management of such patients [1-5]. Viability assessments aid in predicting cardiac morbidity and mortality as well as in identifying those patients who are likely to benefit most from surgical revascularization. Demonstration of viable myocardium in ischemic cardiomyopathy can therefore substantially contribute to the pre-surgical assessment of the risk to benefit ratio. Viability studies have therefore become in many institutions an integral part of the diagnostic work-up of heart failure patients with ischemic cardiomyopathy [6,7].

This chapter reviews the rationale for using positron emission tomography (PET) in the search for myocardial viability, discusses approaches that have been extensively validated and are currently in use, and reviews clinical observations and their implications for the use of PET in the management of patients with ischemic cardiomyopathy.

Identification of viable myocardium by PET

Rather than being an exotic imaging modality PET has become an integral component of the nuclear medicine armamentarium. While more versatile

A. E. Iskandrian and E. E. van der Wall (eds.), Myocardial Viability, 47-72.
© 2000 *Kluwer Academic Publishers. Printed in the Netherlands.*

but also more complex, it takes advantage of the unique decay characteristics of positron-emitting radionuclides. This permits reconstruction of transaxial images of regional tissue radioactivity concentrations in organs in a fashion similar to that employed in x-ray computed tomography. The images are quantitative representations of true tissue radioactivity concentrations and depict anatomical detail with higher spatial, contrast and temporal resolution than available through standard single photon emission computed tomography (SPECT). Besides radiotracers for qualitative and quantitative evaluations of regional myocardial blood flow and its distribution throughout the myocardium, PET employs radiotracers for probing the myocardium's substrate metabolism, neuronal control and membrane properties or myocardial tissue state.

The search for myocardial viability with PET follows the two major pathophysiologic concepts of "myocardial viability" or, using a clinically more meaningful term, "potentially reversible contractile dysfunction." By exploring first the regional distribution of blood flow in dysfunctional myocardium, initial information is gained on whether "hibernation" or "repetitive stunning" might account for the regional wall motion abnormality. Thought of as a downregulation of contractile function in response to diminished substrate supply and blood flow, "hibernation" characteristically reveals a reduction in myocardial blood flow [8,9]. In contrast, "repetitive stunning" as a consequence of a marked reduction in myocardial flow reserve characteristically demonstrates normal levels of blood flow at rest [10,11]. However, patterns of blood flow alone identify reversible contractile dysfunction only incompletely. Except for both ends of the spectrum of flow reductions in dysfunctional myocardium where normal levels are consistent with stunning and very low levels with irreversible injury, intermediate degrees of flow reductions can be associated with either reversibility or irreversibility of contractile function [12]. Therefore, moderately diminished flow may represent in addition to hibernation also myocardial necrosis or tissue fibrosis. If contractile dysfunction is to be reversible, then cellular homeostasis and membrane integrity must be preserved. Both can be demonstrated with [201]Thallium$^+$ (^{201}Tl) as a cationic potassium analog. Both processes require energy and thus depend on metabolic activity as the source of energy. It is this particular aspect of viability that can be elucidated with PET. Radiotracers like fluor-18(^{18}F)-deoxyglucose identify the persistence of exogenous glucose utilization or, like carbon-11(^{11}C)-palmitate or ^{11}C-acetate the persistence of substrate oxidation and, to some extent, the initial energy dependent sequestration step of free fatty acid from plasma into the myocyte. Augmented use of exogenous glucose or persistent substrate oxidation in hypoperfused dysfunctional myocardium indicate "viability" or "reversibility " whereas a reduction in substrate metabolism in parallel to a reduction in blood flow reflects loss of viable myocardium and thus, scar tissue and/or necrosis.

Oxidative metabolism and viability

It is the amount of residual metabolic activity in hypoperfused myocardium that distinguishes between reversibility and irreversibility of contractile dysfunction. PET explores either residual oxidative or enhanced anaerobic glucose utilization. To study oxidative metabolism ^{11}C acetate is administered intravenously and its uptake in and clearance from myocardium measured from serially acquired PET images. The radiotracer ^{11}C acetate becomes rapidly incorporated into the tricarboxylic acid (TCA) cycle. After two turns through the cycle, the radiolabel is liberated from the cycle in the form of [11]CO_2; its rate of release from the myocardium then parallels the rate of TCA cycle activity [13]. Clearance rates of ^{11}C acetate from myocardium yield estimates of the TCA cycle activity and, by inference, of the rate of oxidative phosphorylation [14-18]. Regional rates of oxidative metabolism within two standard deviations of those in remote myocardium have been found to predict accurately post-revascularization improvements in regional wall motion [19,20]. Compared to regional blood flow, oxidative rates offered greater predictive accuracy, probably because oxygen consumption as the product of blood flow and the extraction fraction of oxygen more realistically reflects the regional oxygen availability.

Thought initially to parallel myocardial blood flow, more recent studies demonstrated disparities between oxygen consumption and blood flow. In fact, a non-linear or bi-phasic correlation appears to describe best the relationship between both [21-23]. It is therefore that measurements of oxygen consumption more accurately than estimates of flow alone identify the presence or absence of viable myocardium. However, recent observations challenge these initial observations on the predictive accuracy of ^{11}C-acetate studies [23,24]. Relative flow reductions rather than ^{11}C acetate clearance rates predicted more accurately the long-term outcome in regional contractile function. Only the "oxidative reserve" assessed by ^{11}C-acetate during low-dose dobutamine infusion stimulation completely separated reversible from irreversible contractile dysfunction [24]. Thus, the ultimate value of ^{11}C-acetate for assessing myocardial viability remains unresolved. Perhaps, as suggested previously [25], it will be important to combine the assessment of oxidative metabolism with that of blood flow to achieve optimum predictive accuracies.

Glucose utilization and viability

Most of the search for myocardial viability with PET has relied on ^{18}F-deoxyglucose. The agent traces the initial transmembranous exchange of glucose from blood into the myocardium and the initial hexokinase mediated phosphorylation step to glucose-6-phosphate. Once administered intravenously, imaging is delayed for 30 minutes to allow for metabolic trapping of the ^{18}F-deoxyglucose in the myocardium. At that time, the myocardial ^{18}F activity concentrations represent mostly phosphorylated glucose tracer and thus regional rates of exogenous glucose utilization [26-28].

Again, the initial step of the viability examination with ^{18}F deoxyglucose entails the evaluation of regional myocardial blood flow using nitrogen-13 (^{13}N) ammonia, [82]Rubidium[+], or in other instances, oxygen-15 (^{15}O)-water. The evaluation of regional myocardial glucose utilization with ^{18}F deoxyglucose follows. Three different patterns of blood flow and metabolism in dysfunctional myocardium may be present. First, normal blood flow associated with normal or enhanced glucose uptake; second, reduced blood flow but normal or augmented glucose utilization and, third, reduced blood flow and proportionately reduced glucose utilization [29-31]. Under ideal conditions, the normal flow and normal glucose uptake pattern seems consistent with "repetitive stunning" [32], the reduced flow but preserved glucose uptake ("mismatch") with "hibernation" [33] and the concordant reduction of flow and metabolism ("match") with scar tissue and/or necrosis. It is these flow metabolism patterns that have been employed first for identifying viable myocardium and that have established PET's role as a clinical tool in cardiology.

Patterns of blood flow and glucose metabolism

Under ideal conditions, each of the two patterns of reversibly dysfunctional myocardium might correlate to each of the two pathophysiologic mechanisms of reversible contractile dysfunction. Normal levels of blood flow and of glucose utilization then represent "repetitive stunning" and reduced flow associated with normal or enhanced rates of glucose utilization "hibernation" (Figure 1). Both conditions represent the two ends of a continuum of abnormalities associated with reversible contractile dysfunction. In human coronary artery disease however, stunning and hibernation probably coexist almost invariably in addition to scar tissue and/or necrosis and normal myocardium. For example, fibrosis alone causes a regional reduction in transmural blood flow even when flow per unit viable myocardium is normal. Such normal flows per unit myocardium would be encountered in normal or in "repetitively stunned myocardium"

Normal	Mismatch	Match

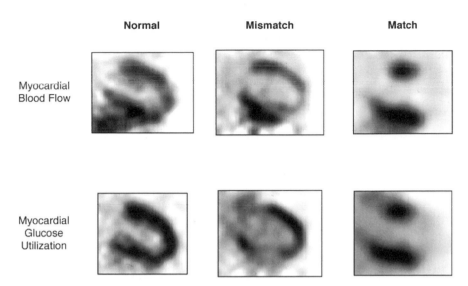

Myocardial Blood Flow

Myocardial Glucose Utilization

Figure 1. Patterns of blood flow and metabolism on positron emission tomography. Horizontal long axis cuts through the left ventricular myocardium are shown. The upper row depicts images of myocardial blood flow obtained with ^{13}N-ammonia, the lower row of glucose metabolism with ^{18}F deoxyglucose. The images on the left show normal, homogeneous blood flow and glucose metabolism. This pattern is seen in normal individuals but also in dysfunctional myocardium due to stunning. As shown in the center panel, blood flow is decreased in the dysfunctional anterior wall while, as shown at the bottom, glucose metabolism is preserved. This pattern is referred to as a blood flow metabolism mismatch and predicts functional improvement following revascularization. Lastly, the images on the right depict a reduction in blood flow in the dysfunctional anterior wall associated with a proportionate decrease in regional glucose metabolism. This pattern is referred to as a blood flow metabolism match.

[34,35]. Diminished flow per volume unit myocardium would be consistent with "hibernation" but is likely to be associated with augmented rates of glucose utilization. Further, transient increases in demand met by inadequate increases in substrate supply cause acute ischemic episodes that could superimpose "stunning" on hibernation [36].

The terms "viable" and "nonviable" can be misleading within the context of blood flow metabolism patterns. With the exception of a complete loss of flow and metabolism as a consequence of transmural necrosis and replacement by scar tissue that renders a segment truly "nonviable," most dysfunctional segments contain mixtures of fibrosis and/or necrosis and normal or ischemically injured myocardium (Figure 2). In a strict sense, there is then "viable myocardium" even though contractile function may be irreversibly impaired. The amount of regional tissue fibrosis, either diffuse or discrete, is another determinant of "contractile dysfunction." Even when substantial amounts of normal and/or of reversibly dysfunctional myocardium exist, fibrosis presumably precludes a complete recovery of segmental wall motion. If fibrosis dominates and occupies more than 30 to 35% of a myocardial segment, then segmental wall motion is likely to be irreversibly impaired [37-40].

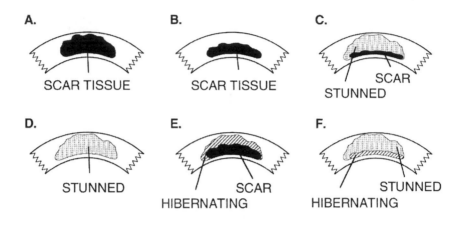

Figure 2. Different patterns that might account for potentially reversible and irreversible contractile dysfunction associated with either normal or reduced myocardial blood flow (see text).

The amount of fibrosis can be estimated with PET. The vascular space is measured with $^{15}0$ labeled red blood cells and the myocardial space with $^{15}0$ labeled water and the so called "water perfusable tissue index" is derived [41]. Assuming only viable but not fibrotic/necrotic myocardium exchanges water, then the fraction unable to exchange water represents the fraction of irreversibly injured tissue. Thus, the perfusable tissue index as the ratio of the fraction of the myocardial volume that exchanges water to the total volume of the myocardium approaches unity in normal myocardium. Conversely, it will be less than unity in segments with substantial amounts of fibrosis. Consistent with morphometric findings in dysfunctional myocardium, a water perfusable tissue index of less than 0.7 designates a segmental wall motion abnormality as irreversible [35,42,43]. Clinical observations confirm the value of the water perfusable tissue index as an alternative means for assessing myocardial viability. Furthermore, the index provides a measure of viable myocardium to which flow and substrate metabolism can be related. This is different from the more commonly used approach for deriving average transmural rates of blood flow and metabolism [35].

The accuracy of blood flow and glucose metabolism patterns for identifying reversible or irreversible contractile dysfunction has been measured against post-revascularization outcomes in regional wall motion as the "gold standard." In 295 patients in 13 investigations, the pattern of normal flow and metabolism and the pattern of reduced flow but enhanced glucose utilization demonstrate positive predictive accuracies ranging from 67 to 100% [20,31,32,44-53]. Conversely, a concordant reduction in both, blood flow and glucose metabolism was 75 to 100% accurate in predicting that wall motion would not improve following revascularization.

Several factors probably account for the considerable interstudy differences in predictive accuracy. They include patient selection, criteria for image analysis, standardization of study conditions, especially of the dietary state, and the time from revascularization to re-evaluation of regional myocardial wall motion.

Image analysis

In addition to visual inspection, many laboratories apply quantitative criteria to the image analysis. Using circumferential activity profiles of short-axis images and polar maps, flow defects are defined as regional reductions in tracer uptake by for example more than two standard deviations below the normal mean. The second step, the analysis of the ^{18}F-deoxyglucose images alone and in relation to the flow images remains less well standardized. In one approach, myocardium with apparently normal blood flow at rest is defined as "reference myocardium." The ^{18}F activity concentration in these regions is normalized to the flow tracer concentrations in the same myocardial region. Disparities between glucose metabolism and flow are defined by either the difference or the ratio of ^{18}F to, for example, ^{13}N (for ^{13}N ammonia) concentrations. Ratios or differences that exceed the normal differences or ratios as established from databases of normal by more than two standard deviations are then considered abnormal and categorized as "mismatches." Variations to this particular analysis program include modifications for normalizing the blood flow to the metabolic images or different threshold values for discriminating between abnormal and normal patterns [23,49]. Other approaches again rely only on the relative myocardial ^{18}F activity concentrations. For example, reductions in metabolic activity of less than 40 to 50% below normal are considered to reflect myocardial viability [54]. Absolute rates of exogenous glucose utilization in µmoles glucose.min^{-1}.g^{-1} have also been used. The average glucose metabolic activity in these studies was correlated with the post-revascularization increase in left ventricular function [55]. Yet, it seems that in the clinical routine, the direct correlation between glucose metabolism rates with regional myocardial perfusion markedly facilitates and strengthens the diagnostic interpretative process.

Standardization of study and dietary conditions

Glucose utilization and consequently, ^{18}F-deoxyglucose uptake in normal myocardium depends largely on hormonal factors and plasma substrate concentrations [56]. Low plasma free fatty acid together with high insulin concentrations promote myocardial uptake of ^{18}F-deoxyglucose while high plasma free fatty acid and low insulin levels shift myocardial substrate usage from glucose to free fatty acid and result in low ^{18}F-deoxyglucose uptake. Ischemically compromised myocardium does not fully participate in this regulatory mechanism [57,58]. While uptake of ^{18}F deoxyglucose in normal myocardium may be low or even undetectable in the fasting state, it is selectively enhanced in ischemically compromised myocardium. If a patient is therefore studied under fasting conditions, reversibly compromised myocardium is seen on the ^{18}F-deoxyglucose image as a region of strikingly increased activity [44]. While conceptually ideal because it selectively targets ischemically compromised myocardium, the approach identifies also small fractions or islands of viable myocardium that are without little if any consequence on regional wall motion. A decline in specificity for predicting improvements in segmental wall motion results. Poor image quality is another confounding factor [59]. The slow clearance of ^{18}F-deoxyglucose from the blood pool produces low myocardium to background uptake ratios and thus low signal to noise ratios that often preclude adequate image interpretation. Most laboratories therefore administer oral glucose to stimulate insulin secretion [30] or inject supplemental doses of regular, short-acting insulin [60] or, alternatively, employ the hyperinsulinemic-euglycemic glucose clamp to accelerate clearance of ^{18}F-deoxyglucose from blood and to drive the tracer into the myocardium [61-63]. Images of high diagnostic quality with good visualization of remote and presumably normal myocardium result. The relative ^{18}F-deoxyglucose concentration in viable dysfunctional myocardium may then be increased, be normal or be reduced but, importantly, always less than regional myocardial blood flow. The glucose loading or clamp approach may not uncover small amounts of viable myocardium that are of little if any consequence on regional wall motion. The approach is therefore more specific for identifying those myocardial segments that are likely to improve wall motion after restoration of blood flow.

Rate of recovery of contractile function

The rate of recovery of contractile function can vary considerably between myocardial regions and between patients. Blood flow and contractile function also may recover at markedly different rates. Following coronary angioplasty for example, regional blood flows had significantly improved within three days while contractile function remained unchanged [64]. On re-examination nine weeks later, no further improvements in blood flow were observed but now regional wall motion had improved or fully recovered. Also, variable rates of recovery of contractile dysfunction have been observed following surgical revascularization. For example, 76% of myocardial regions with initially only mild flow reductions (designated by the authors as "stunned") improved or fully recovered function within ten days after revascularization as compared to only 50% of segments with more severely reduced flows (designated by the authors as "hibernating") [65]. Only after an additional four to twelve months had the "hibernating" segments reached similar percentages of functional improvement (73 and 83%). The differences in the magnitude flow reductions suggest differences in the severity of the "functional compromise" and, perhaps, "ischemic" injury.

The varying degrees of structural abnormalities uncovered in dysfunctional myocardium might possibly explain the marked differences in the rates of recovery of contractile function [39,40,66] as well as the at times markedly delayed improvement of congestive heart failure symptoms and cardiac performance [67]. Repair or rebuilding of contractile protein requires time. A slow but progressive recovery of contractile function in a region of reversible contractile dysfunction possibly accompanied by reversal of left ventricular remodeling might explain the at times slow functional and symptomatic improvement [66].

Morphologic and metabolic correlates of "hibernation"

Long before the emergence of the concept of "myocardial hibernation" had specific structural alterations of myocytes in dysfunctional human myocardium been observed [68]. Characteristically, such myocytes reveal peri-nuclear loss of contractile protein and replacement by glycogen deposits. The structure of the cell nucleus is usually preserved; there are numerous small mitochondria of normal morphologic appearance. Other features include re-expression of proteins known to be present in the fetal state [69]. This then raised the possibility of "dedifferentiation" of terminally dedifferentiated myocytes rather than "degeneration" accounting for the morphologic changes. Correlating the degree of structural changes with patterns of blood flow and metabolism demonstrated a disproportionately greater fraction of abnormal myocytes in myocardium with flow metabolism mismatches, or myocardium expected to recover contractile function [32,37,39,53]. Such abnormal myocytes were therefore referred to as "hibernating" [69]. By contrast, segments with normal flow and metabolism contained mostly normal myocytes with some abnormal cells and fibrosis while myocardial segments with concordant reductions in flow and metabolism, considered therefore as irreversibly dysfunctional, contained large amounts of fibrosis and scar tissue.

Similar structural abnormalities occur also in myocytes obtained from myocardium designated as "repetitively stunned" because of normal or near normal blood flows at baseline but a severely reduced flow reserve [32]. These "abnormal myocytes" therefore do not appear to be unique to hibernation nor to stunning. The structural abnormalities therefore have been suspected to result from (a) loss of contractile function or "inactivity", (b) mechanical stretch and stress; and (c) altered substrate metabolism [69]. Of interest, mechanical immobilization of atrial myocardium due to experimentally induced atrial fibrillation produced comparable structural changes [70,71], supporting the notion that they result from "immobility" rather than from an adaptation to a state of limited substrate supply.

The relative uptake of the flow marker ^{13}N-ammonia correlates inversely with the percent fibrosis [32,37,53]. Also, some studies demonstrate a direct and statistically significant correlation between the fraction of abnormal myocytes and the relative ^{18}F-deoxyglucose uptake [37], implicating such cells as the structural correlate of enhanced glucose uptake. However, the lack of such correlation between the severity of structural changes and ^{18}F-deoxyglucose in another study [72] points to other or additional mechanisms of the enhanced glucose utilization.

One possible mechanism involves membrane glucose transporters (GLUT). Increased expression of the insulin-independent GLUT1 and of the insulin-dependent GLUT4 has been found in dysfunctional human myocardium [73]. Other, acute experimental studies in animals have reported translocation of GLUT1 and GLUT4 from the cytoplasma to the cell membrane in response to acute myocardial ischemia [74]. Besides an augmented inward transfer of glucose, an uncoupling of anaerobic from aerobic or oxidative metabolism of glucose has been suggested as an additional explanation [75]. Pyruvate as the end product of glycolysis then cannot proceed into mitochondria and is released from myocardium in the form of lactate. In this scenario, an enhanced transmembranous transport capacity for glucose might act as flux-generating step with glucose being diverted into the glycogen pool or channeled into the glycolytic pathway.

Consistent with clinical observations [1-3], assays of human myocardium suggest that "hibernation" does not represent a steady state but rather an "incomplete adaptation to ischemia" [40]. Complicating this condition further is superimposition of transient episodes of acute myocardial ischemia on hibernation [36]. Reduced transcriptional activities for contractile and cytoskeletal proteins have been found in dysfunctional human myocardium while transcriptional activities for connective tissue were augmented [40]. This then argues in favor of a progressive deterioration of the myocytal structure together with connective tissue formation. An additional confounding factor includes a possible continued loss of myocytes through apoptosis or oncosis or both [40,76,77]. If true, then "hibernation" does not represent a steady state condition that can be sustained indefinitely but a progression to irreversible injury.

Clinical use of blood flow metabolism imaging

The management of end-stage coronary artery disease patients with severe depression of left ventricular function often represents a formidable challenge. Despite impressive improvements in pharmacologic options, the long-term survival of such patients on conservative medical regimen while improving remains relatively low [78]. Cardiac transplantation on the other hand can markedly enhance the quality of life and long-term survival. Yet, the availability of donor hearts continues to be limited so that this treatment modality has not become widely accessible. This leaves coronary revascularization often as the only alternative.

However, the decision for surgical revascularization often presents both, patient and physician with a considerable dilemma. The high risk of surgical mortality especially when co-morbidities are present must be weighed against uncertain or unpredictable benefits. Surgical revascularization can significantly enhance long-term survival and reduce angina symptoms [79,80]. Less predictable are potential improvements in left ventricular function and in congestive heart failure related symptoms and thus in the quality of life. In fact, the Coronary Artery Surgery Study (CASS registry) demonstrated statistically significant five-year survival benefits and amelioration of anginal symptoms in low left ventricular function patients but no definite improvement in congestive heart failure symptoms [79,80]. Evidence forthcoming from clinical investigations suggest that PET based assessment of myocardial blood flow and metabolism can contribute substantially to predicting short- and long-term post-surgical outcomes and thus profoundly influence the risk benefit ratio. Specifically, patterns of blood flow and metabolism can identify those patients at the highest risk for cardiac events, and conversely, those patients likely to benefit most from surgical revascularization in terms of improvements in global left ventricular function, symptoms related to congestive heart failure and long-term survival.

Global left ventricular function

Several clinical investigations in coronary artery disease patients with left ventricular ejection fractions of less than 35% reported substantial improvements in left ventricular ejection fractions when flow metabolism studies on PET had demonstrated substantial amounts of potentially reversible contractile dysfunction. Average increases in ejection fraction units ranged in the studies from 8 to 51% [431,37,46-48,53,55,60,72,81-85]. A meta-analysis of these studies in a total of 292 patients reveals an average 30±15% increase in average ejection fractions. The left ventricular ejection fractions averaged 36±10% prior to and 46±10% at 3-12 months after surgery. No such improvement occurred in patients without or with only small blood flow metabolism mismatches (LVEF 40±10% to 39±12%).

The degree of left ventricular functional compromise varied considerably and ranged from normal to severely reduced. If, as shown in figure 3, the data were analyzed according to the left ventricular functional depression prior to surgery, then the studies show a more dramatic benefit in left ventricular function in patients with ischemic cardiomyopathy (an increase in LVEF by 42% as compared to only 19% in patients with LVEF greater than 35%).

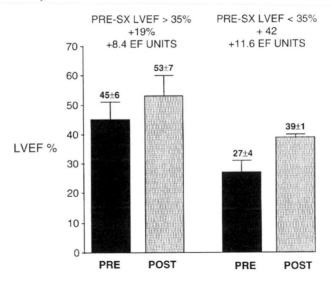

Figure 3. Responses of global left ventricular ejection fractions (LVEF) following surgical revascularization (SX). The figure summarizes the observations in 14 clinical studies. Studies are grouped according to the level of left ventricular function prior to surgery. The panel on the left summarizes studies in patients with average ejection fractions of greater than 35%, the panel on the right studies with average ejection fractions less than 35%. Note that the percent increase in left ventricular function is greater in patients with more severely depressed left ventricular function as compared to those with only moderate reductions.

Further, the functional improvement ranges from about 5% to more than 50% in one study [86]. A prime reason for this variability is the extent of the pre-surgical mismatch. It now appears that the magnitude of the functional improvement depends among other factors on the amount of reversibly dysfunctional myocardium (Figure 4) [60,86]. Further, the increase in left ventricular ejection fraction has been found to correlate inversely and non-linearly with the size of the perfusion defect (Figure 5) [87].

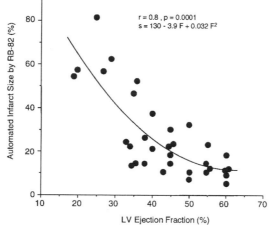

Figure 4. Correlation between the extent of myocardial perfusion defects and the global left ventricular ejection fraction. Note the non-linear correlation with the steepest decline in ejection fraction for large flow defects. Reproduced with permission from Yoshida *et al.* [87], with permission. LV = left ventricle; Rb-82 = rubidium-82.

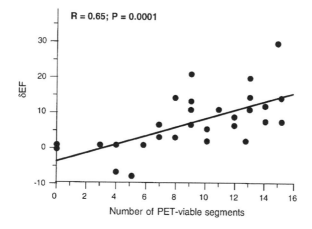

Figure 5. Correlation between the extent of blood flow metabolism mismatches and the improvement in left ventricular function. The number of segments demonstrating blood flow metabolism mismatches correlate linearly with the delta percent increase in the ejection fraction (δ EF). Reproduced from Pagano *et al.* [86] with permission.

If this non-linear correlation can be confirmed by other studies, then a small revascularization dependent reduction in the extent of a perfusion defect in a patient with a very low ejection fraction would result in a disproportionately greater rise in the ejection fractions and in patients with only mildly decreased ejection fractions. Conversely, the same studies noted that left ventricular ejection fractions remained unchanged or declined even further in the absence in reversibly dysfunctional myocardium with only flow metabolism matches. It is of interest that, though still reported in preliminary form [66], revascularization of reversibly dysfunctional myocardial regions may also lead to significant decreases in left ventricular and enddiastolic and endsystolic volumes. This then raises the question of whether restoration of contractile function in a discrete myocardial region also causes changes in the left ventricular geometry perhaps through a reversal of left ventricular remodeling.

Congestive heart failure symptoms

Though mostly retrospective, several studies report significant post-revascularization changes in heart failure symptoms in patients with reversible dysfunctional myocardium [1,3,4]. In one study, the percentage of patients in NYHA Congestive Heart Failure Classes III and IV declined from 81% prior to surgery to 23% after surgery (Figure 6) [1].

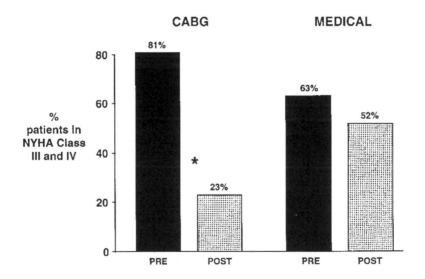

Figure 6. Changes in congestive heart failure class in patients with blood flow metabolism mismatches as a function of treatment. Adopted from Di Carli *et al.* [1] with permission of the American Heart Association.

All patients had reversibly dysfunctional myocardium on PET. Conversely, the percentage of patients with severe heart failure symptoms remained relatively unaffected by surgical revascularization in the absence of blood flow metabolism mismatches (66% versus 62%). Similarly, it may be possible to predict the improvement in physical activity in response to surgical revascularization in a more quantitative fashion. For example, measuring physical activity in unites of metabolic activity with a specific activity scale [88], the post revascularization gain in physical activity was found to be correlated directly with the extent of the blood flow metabolism mismatch on PET (Figure 7) [89]. Large flow metabolism mismatches were associated with substantial gains in physical activity while only small gains were achieved when no or only small amounts of flow metabolism mismatches were present.

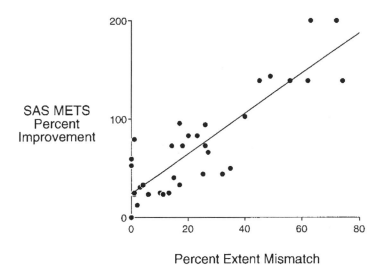

Figure 7. Post-surgical improvement in physical activity as a function of the pre-surgical extent of the blood flow metabolism mismatch. Physical activity is expressed in metabolic units using a specific activity scale (SAS METS). Reproduced with permission from Di Carli *et al.* [89] with permission.

Long-term survival

Patterns of blood flow and glucose metabolism on PET contain predictive information on long-term survival after surgery [1,3]. Coronary artery bypass grafting appears to have little effect on the long-term survival of ischemic cardiomyopathy patients without PET evidence of reversible contractile dysfunction. Survival rates in such patients seem relatively high; the 82% two to three year survival as reported in one study is similar to that in patients without mismatches on PET but treated only conservatively (94%) [1]. While other reports confirm the high survival rates others conversely indicate a poorer long-term outcome. This especially applies to patients with extensive matching blood flow metabolism defects involving 40% to 50% of the left ventricle. The latter observation is more in line with findings on ^{201}Tl SPECT studies [90]. Importantly however, an otherwise poor long–term prognosis of patients with extensive blood flow metabolism mismatches can be reversed through revascularization with a substantial reduction in future cardiac events including death.

Peri-operative course and operative mortality

Besides their predictive value for the long-term post surgical outcome, PET blood flow metabolism patterns also seem of more immediate value for gauging the operative mortality and the peri-operative course. Ischemic cardiomyopathy patients with left ventricular ejection fractions of less than 35% submitted to revascularization based on only standard clinical criteria had an 11.4% peri-operative (30-day) mortality; two-thirds of the patients experienced peri-operative complications ranging from low cardiac output, need for inotropic support and cardiac arrest [4]. If revascularization was performed only after the patients were found to have substantial amounts of reversibly dysfunctional myocardium and met all other standard clinical criteria, then the peri-operative mortality declined to zero. Also, PET selected patients experienced fewer peri-operative complications. They occurred only one-third of patients; the remaining two-thirds of patients could be transferred out of the postsurgical intensive care unit within less than two days.

Risk assessment and prediction of cardiac events

Consistent with the notion of an "inadequate adaptation to ischemia," the blood flow metabolism mismatch may not necessarily represent a steady state where the diminished demand matches the diminished supply. Rather, it appears to be often an unstable state with a propensity for fatal and non-fatal cardiac events. Monitored over time periods of two to three years, patients with mismatches were more likely to sustain non-fatal myocardial infarctions, to develop unstable angina or to require interventional revascularization than patients without mismatches [1,3,4,85,86,91,92]. The blood flow metabolism mismatch emerged as the most powerful predictor of future non-fatal and fatal cardiac events. A meta-analysis of these studies suggests cardiac events in 33% of the 144 patients with mismatches as compared to only 13% of 171 patients without mismatches. Left ventricular ejection fractions in these patients ranged from normal to severely depressed; in one study, a low left ventricular ejection fraction continued to be highly predictive of subsequent mortality [92]. In patient populations with uniformly depressed left ventricular ejection fractions, the flow metabolism mismatch emerged as a powerful predictor of cardiac death. In two studies for example, a flow metabolism mismatch was associated with a 41% and 50% mortality over a 12 month period; the corresponding mortalities were 13% and 9% for patients without mismatches but with similarly depressed left ventricular function [1,3]. Death was sudden in most patients while congestive heart failure ranked second.

The key points of these clinical observations with blood flow imaging in ischemic cardiomyopathy can be summarized as follows: first, a blood flow metabolism mismatch identifies a high risk for future cardiac events including death. Second, patterns of blood flow metabolism are predictive of peri-operative cardiovascular complications including death; and, thirdly, PET based evidence of potential reversible contractile dysfunction has predictive value for post surgical improvement in global left ventricular function, congestive heart failure related symptoms and importantly, long-term survival.

The surgical PET studies can therefore considerably influence the risk-benefit ratio of surgical revascularization. Conversely, the absence of reversibly dysfunctional myocardium on PET can lend additional support for deciding against coronary revascularization in favor of conservative treatment or cardiac transportation as alternative therapeutic strategies. This is also why PET based myocardial perfusion in metabolism imaging in some institutions has become already or is being advocated as integral part of the diagnostic work-up in ischemic cardiomyopathy. Specific criteria for proceeding with coronary revascularization have been established [6]. They include the following:

- left ventricular end diastolic dimension of less than 70 mm/m^2,
- a left ventricular ejection fraction of greater than 20%;
- a mismatch least 20% of reversibly dysfunctional myocardium; and
- suitable coronary vessels.

Other institutions employ slightly modified criteria. For example, blood flow metabolism matches in excess of 40-50% of the left ventricle are considered as contraindications for surgical revascularization [4]. Once these criteria have been fulfilled, it appears important to proceed with revascularization promptly. This is because of a continued loss of reversibility (as discussed above) which adversely affects the expected post-surgical benefits. In one study, a delay of revascularization by several months was in addition to pre-surgical death associated with a loss in an improvement in left ventricular function. The continued loss of reversibility is further confirmed by the reported time dependent decline in the prevalence of viable myocardium following an acute myocardial infarction.

The routine use of PET based evaluations of blood flow and glucose metabolism can significantly impact therapy planning. For example, PET findings altered treatment decisions in 57% of all 87 patients evaluated at the Cardiac PET Centre of the University of Ottawa Heart Institute between February and December 1995 [5]. About half of the patients had an ejection fraction less than 30%. After the PET study, 63% of the 11 patients considered initially for transplantation were submitted to CABG. While 42% of patients assigned initially to surgical revascularization received medical treatment; about half of the eighteen patients considered initially for conservative therapy were now referred to CABG. Of note, PET findings had an even greater impact on patients with severely depressed left ventricular function (LVEF < 30%); it altered the treatment plan in 71% of the patients.

The UCLA Heart Failure and Cardiac Transplantation Program reports a similar experience. In 112 patients with ejection fractions of less than 35% referred to UCLA between April 1987 and July 1994 for cardiac transplant evaluation [93], the PET blood flow metabolism examination identified reversibly dysfunctional myocardium of more than 20% of the left ventricle in 38 patients. Of these, 30 patients underwent surgical revasculariaztion rather than cardiac transplantation; eight patients were treated conservatively because of poor target vessels or refusal to leave the transplant list. Of the remaining patients without or with only small amounts PET based reversibility, thirty received cardiac allografts and 41 were treated conservatively. Peri-operative mortality was similar for coronary artery bypass grafting (10%) and transplantation (6.1%). Of note, actuarial survival rates of patients after revascularization were similar to those of patients after transplantation (71.4 % and 80.1%); both patient groups had higher survival rates than patients treated conservatively (42.4%).

In reviewing 288 patients with congestive heart failure (LVEF 26+9%) studied at UCLA, PET demonstrated blood flow glucose metabolism mismatches in 54% [94]. Half of the mismatches involved more than 25% of the left ventricle; these mismatches were therefore considered "functionally significant" as they are likely to result in post-revascularization gains in left ventricular function. The remaining mismatches were smaller in size. As they could predict a greater risk for future cardiac events, they were referred to as "prognostically significant." Whether they warrant revascularization requires further study. Also, not all of patients with functionally significant mismatches proceeded to have coronary revascularization. Reasons for not performing surgery included significant co-morbidities, failure to meet other criteria required for revascularization or the desire to remain on the transplant waiting list.

Current and future developments

Technical innovations promise to expand the availability of PET based assessments of reversible contractile dysfunction. Arguments against PET have included its complexity and its expense. Yet, most laboratories providing clinical PET services do so at cost that is competitive with conventional ^{201}Tl redistribution/reinjection or ^{99m}Tc Sestamibi SPECT imaging. Gated PET imaging acquisition is also feasible so that functional in addition to metabolic and flow parameters can be obtained [95,96]. Even though somewhat more expensive, PET offers superior diagnostic accuracy because of better spatial and contrast resolution; visualization of greater anatomical detail at higher myocardium to background activity ratios identifies reversibly dysfunctional myocardium more accurately and more precisely delineates its extent. This may be the reason why nearly 50% of patients with very low ejection fractions and extensive regions of surgically confirmed reversible contractile dysfunction demonstrated equivocal results on ^{201}Tl SPECT imaging which subsequently were correctly identified on PET imaging [2]. It also might account for the over- estimation of irreversible contractile dysfunction by ^{201}Tl SPECT redistribution imaging as reported previously [97]. Therefore, the somewhat higher cost of PET is offset by often substantial gains in diagnostic quality and information.

Furthermore, imaging of positron labeled radiopharmaceuticals is now expanding beyond dedicated PET systems to hybrid and to modified SPECT systems. Even during the early stages of cardiac PET did some institutions employ hybrid imaging approaches [47]. Myocardial perfusion was assessed with ^{201}Tl or ^{99m}Tc-sestamibi or tetrofosmin SPECT and myocardial ^{18}F-deoxyglucose uptake with PET. Recent studies report the feasibility of myocardial ^{18}F-deoxyglucose imaging with modified or specifically designed SPECT systems [98-100]. Indeed, SPECT-like devices appear to yield diagnostic findings with an accuracy approaching that of PET [101]. Initial studies have demonstrated the feasibility of identifying blood flow metabolism patterns with SPECT-like devices alone, with predictive accuracies approaching those as reported previously by dedicated PET systems. For example, one study in 17 patients with ^{201}Tl and ^{18}F-deoxyglucose SPECT imaging using high energy photon collimators reports predictive accuracies similar to those for PET and exceeding those for low dose dobutamine echocardiography [101]. The SPECT ^{18}F-deoxyglucose approach also appears to outperform the conventional SPECT ^{201}Tl approach. Image artifacts with for example apparent reductions in flow tracer uptake especially in the inferior wall of the left ventricle complicate the correlative interpretation of SPECT perfusion and ^{18}F-deoxyglucose images [102]. However, correction for photon attenuation on SPECT imaging is now possible and is likely to overcome this limitation [103]. With the anticipated more widespread availability of ^{18}F-deoxyglucose through regional distribution centers blood flow metabolism imaging for the identification of viable myocardium is likely to become clinically more widely accessible and at a lower cost.

Conclusion

The assessment of myocardial blood flow and glucose metabolism with PET has proved to be clinically useful especially in patients with ischemic cardiomyopathy. Patterns of blood flow and metabolism identify those patients with the highest risk for future cardiac events ranging from unstable angina, surgical revascularization, non-fatal myocardial infarction and death. Conversely, the same blood flow metabolism patterns identify patients who are likely to gain most from surgical revascularization in terms of improved long term survival, increases in left ventricular function and amelioration of congestive heart failure related symptoms.   PET findings also have an impact on the immediate perioperative course; PET demonstrated viability results in a lower perioperative mortality and fewer postoperative complications. Clinical investigations have demonstrated PET's impact on therapy planning, on stratifying patients to medical therapy or cardiac transplantation or, especially, to surgical revascularization.   Current developments with lower cost imaging instrumentation and more widespread availability of positron labeled metabolic tracers are likely to expand the clinical use of this powerful diagnostic imaging modality.

Acknowledgments

The author wishes to thank David Twomey for the illustrations and Eileen Rosenfeld and Julie Kuhns for their skillful secretarial assistance.

References

1.   Di Carli MF, Davidson M, Little R *et al*. Value of metabolic imaging with positron emission tomography for evaluating prognosis in patients with coronary artery disease and left ventricular dysfunction. Am J Cardiol 1994;73:527-33.
2.   Dreyfus GD, Duboc D, Blasco A *et al*. Myocardial viability assessment in ischemic cardiomyopathy: benefits of coronary revascularization. Ann Thorac Surg 1994;57:1402-8.

3. Eitzman D, Al-Aouar Z, Kanter HL *et al*. Clinical outcome of patients with advanced coronary artery disease after viability studies with positron emission tomography. J Am Coll Cardiol 1992;20:559-65.

4. Haas F, Haehnel CJ, Picker W *et al*. Preoperative positron emission tomographic viability assessment and perioperative and postoperative risk in patients with advanced ischemic heart disease. J Am Coll Cardiol 1997;30:1693-700.

5. Beanlands RS, deKemp RA, Smith S, Johansen H, Ruddy TD. F-18-fluorodeoxyglucose PET imaging alters clinical decision making in patients with impaired ventricular function. Am J Cardiol 1997;79:1092-5.

6. Louie HW, Laks H, Milgalter E *et al*. Ischemic cardiomyopathy: criteria for coronary revascularization and cardiac transplantation. Circulation 1991;84(5 Suppl):III-290-5.

7. Blitz A, Laks H. The role of coronary revascularization in the management of heart failure: identification of candidates and review of results. Curr Opin Cardiol 1996;11:276-90.

8. Rahimtoola SH. A perspective on the three large multicenter randomized clinical trials of coronary bypass surgery for chronic stable angina. Circulation 1987;72:V123-35.

9. Braunwald E, Rutherford JD. Reversible ischemic left ventricular dysfunction: Evidence for "hibernating myocardium". J Am Coll Cardiol 1986;8:1467-70.

10. Heyndrickx GR, Baig H, Nellens P, Leusen I, Fishbein MC, Vatner SF. Depression of regional blood flow and wall thickening after brief coronary occlusions. Am J Physiol 1978;234:H653-9.

11. Braunwald E, Kloner RA. The stunned myocardium: prolonged, postischemic ventricular dysfunction. Circulation 1982;66:1146-9.

12. Gewirtz H, Fischman AJ, Abraham S, Gilson M, Strauss HW, Alpert N. Positron emission tomographic measurements of absolute regional myocardial blood flow permits identification of nonviable myocardium in patients with chronic myocardial infarction. J Am Coll Cardiol 1994;23:851-9.

13. Ng C, Huang SC, Schelbert H, Buxton D. Validation of a model for [1-11C] acetate as a tracer of cardiac oxidative metabolism. Am J Physiol 1994;266:H1304-15.

14. Brown M, Marshall DR, Burton BS, Sobel BE, Bergmann SR. Delineation of myocardial oxygen utilization with carbon-11-labeled acetate. Circulation 1987;76:687-96.

15. Buxton DB, Schwaiger M, Nguyen A, Phelps ME, Schelbert HR. Radiolabeled acetate as a tracer of myocardial tricarboxylic acid cycle flux. Circ Res 1988;63:628-34.

16. Buxton DB, Nienaber CA, Luxen A *et al*. Noninvasive quantitation of regional myocardial oxygen consumption in vivo with [1-^{11}C] acetate and dynamic positron emission tomography. Circulation 1989;79:134-42.

17. Henes CG, Bergmann SR, Walsh MN, Geltman E. Recovery of myocardial perfusion and oxygen consumption after htombolysis delineated with positron emission tomography (PET) [abstract]. Circulation 1989;80(4 Suppl):II312.

18. Armbrecht JJ, Buxton DB, Schelbert HR. Validation of [1-^{11}C] acetate as a tracer for noninvasive assessment of oxidative metabolism with positron emission tomography in normal, ischemic, post-ischemic and hyperemic canine myocardium. Circulation 1991;81:1594-605.

19. Gropler RJ, Siegel BA, Sampathkumaran K *et al*. Dependence of recovery of contractile function on maintenance of oxidative metabolism after myocardial infarction. J Am Coll Cardiol 1992;19:989-97.

20. Gropler RJ, Geltman EM, Sampathkumaran K *et al*. Functional recovery after coronary revascularization for chronic coronary artery disease is dependent on maintenance of oxidative metabolism. J Am Coll Cardiol 1992;20:569-77.

21. Feigl EO, Neat GW, Huang AH. Interrelations between coronary artery pressure, myocardial metabolism and coronary blood flow. J Mol Cell Cardiol 1990;22:375-90.

22. Czernin J, Porenta G, Brunken R et al. Regional blood flow, oxidative metabolism, and glucose utilization in patients with recent myocardial infarction. Circulation 1993;88:884-95.
23. Wolpers HG, Burchert W, van den Hoff J, Weinhardt R, Meyer GJ, Lichtlen PR. Assessment of myocardial viability by use of ^{11}C-acetate and positron emission tomography. Circulation 1997;95:1417-24.
24. Hata T, Nohara R, Fujita M et al. Noninvasive assessment of myocardial viability by positron emission tomography with ^{11}C acetate in patients with old myocardial infarction. Usefulness of low-dose dobutamine infusion. Circulation 1996;94:1834-41.
25. Hicks RJ, Melon P, Kalff V et al. Metabolic imaging by positron emission tomography early after myocardial infarction as a predictor of recovery of myocardial function after reperfusion. J Nucl Cardiol 1994;1:124-37.
26. Phelps ME, Hoffman EJ, Selin CE et al. Investigation of [18F] 2-fluoro-2-deoxyglucose for the measure of myocardial glucose metabolism. J Nucl Med 1978;19:1311-9.
27. Ratib O, Phelps ME, Huang SC, Henze E, Selin CE, Schelbert HR. Positron tomography with deoxyglucose for estimating local myocardial glucose metabolism. J Nucl Med 1982;23:577-86.
28. Krivokapich J, Huang SC, Phelps ME et al. Estimation of rabbit myocardial metabolic rate for glucose using fluorodeoxyglucose. Am J Physiol 1982;243:H884-95.
29. Schelbert HR, Phelps ME, Selin C, Marshall RC, Hoffman EJ, Kuhl DE. Regional myocardial ischemia assessed by [18]Fluoro-2-deoxyglucose and positron emission computed tomography. In: Kreuzer H, Parmley WW, Rentrop P, Heiss HW, editors. Quantification of myocardial ischemia. New York: Gehard Witzstrock Publishing House; 1980. p. 437-47.
30. Marshall RC, Tillisch JH, Phelps ME et al. Identification and differentiation of resting myocardial ischemia and infarction in man with positron computed tomography 18F-labeled fluorodeoxyglucose and N-13 ammonia. Circulation 1983;67:766-78.
31. Tillisch J, Brunken R, Marshall R et al. Reversibility of cardiac wall motion abnormalities predicted by positron tomography. N Engl J Med 1986;314:884-8.
32. Vanoverschelde JL, Wijns W, Depré C et al. Mechanisms of chronic regional postischemic dysfunction in humans. New insights from the study of noninfarcted collateral-dependent myocardium. Circulation 1993;87:1513-23.
33. Rahimtoola SH. Hibernating myocardium has reduced blood flow at rest that increases with low-dose dobutamine. Circulation 1996;94:3055-61.
34. Marinho NV, Keogh BE, Costa DC, Lammerstma AA, Ell PJ, Camici PG. Pathophysiology of chronic left ventricular dysfunction. New insights from the measurement of absolute myocardial blood flow and glucose utilization. Circulation 1996;93:737-44.
35. Gerber BL, Melin JA, Bol A, Labar D, Cogneau M, Michel C, Vanoverschelde JJ. Nitrogen-13-ammonia and oxygen-15-water estimates of absolute myocardial perfusion in left ventricular ischemic dysfunction. J Nucl Med 1998;39:1655-62.
36. Sun KT, Czernin J, Krivokapich J et al. Effects of dobutamine stimulation on myocardial blood flow, glucose metabolism and wall motion in normal and dysfunctional myocardium. Circulation 1996;94:3146-54.
37. Depré C, Vanoverschelde JLJ, Melin JA et al. Structural and metabolic correlates of the reversibility of chronic left ventricular ischemic dysfunction in humans. Am J Physiol 1995;268:H1265-H75.
38. Grandin C, Wijns W, Melin JA et al. Delineation of myocardial viability with PET. J Nucl Med 1995;36:1543-52.
39. Shivalkar B, Maes A, Borgers M et al. Only hibernating myocardium invariably shows early recovery after coronary revascularization. Circulation 1996;94:308-15.

40. Elsässer A, Schlepper M, Klövekorn WP *et al.* Hibernating myocardium: an incomplete adaptation to ischemia. Circulation 1997;96:2920-31.
41. Iida H, Rhodes CG, de Silva R *et al.* Myocardial tissue fraction - correction for partial volume effects and measure of tissue viability. J Nucl Med 1991;32:2169-75.
42. Yamamoto Y, De Silva R, Rhodes CG *et al.* A new strategy for the assessment of viable myocardium and regional myocardial blood flow using ^{15}O-water and dynamic positron emission tomography. Circulation 1992;86:167-78.
43. de Silva R, Yamamoto Y, Rhodes CG *et al.* Preoperative prediction of the outcome of coronary revascularization using positron emission tomography. Circulation 1992;86:1738-42.
44. Tamaki N, Yonekura Y, Yamashita K *et al.* Positron emission tomography using fluorine-18 deoxyglucose in evaluation of coronary artery bypass grafting. Am J Cardiol 1989;64:860-5.
45. Tamaki N, Ohtani H, Yamashita K *et al.* Metabolic activity in the areas of new fill-in after thallium-201 reinjection: comparison with positron emission tomography using fluorine-18-deoxyglucose. J Nucl Med 1991;32:673-8.
46. Marwick TH, MacIntyre WJ, Lafont A, Nemec JJ, Salcedo EE. Metabolic responses of hibernating and infarcted myocardium to revascularization. A follow-up study of regional perfusion, function, and metabolism. Circulation 1992;85:1347-53.
47. Lucignani G, Paolini G, Landoni C *et al.* Presurgical identification of hibernating myocardium by combined use of technetium-99m hexakis 2-methoxyisobutylisonitrile single photon emission tomography and fluorine-18 fluoro-2-deoxy-D-glucose positron emission tomography in patients with coronary artery disease. Eur J Nucl Med 1992;19:874-81.
48. Carrel T, Jenni R, Haubold-Reuter S, Von Schulthess G, Pasic M, Turina M. Improvement of severely reduced left ventricular function after surgical revascularization in patients with preoperative myocardial infarction. Eur J Cardiothorac Surg 1992;6:479-84.
49. Gropler RJ, Geltman EM, Sampathkumaran K *et al.* Comparison of carbon-11-acetate with fluorine-18-fluorodeoxyglucose for delineating viable myocardium by positron emission tomography. J Am Coll Cardiol 1993;22:1587-97.
50. Knuuti M, Saraste M, Nuutila P *et al.* Myocardial viability: fluorine-18-deoxyglucose positron emission tomography in prediction of wall motion recovery after revascularization. Am Heart J 1994;127:785-96.
51. vom Dahl J, Eitzman DT, Al-Aouar ZR *et al.* Relation of regional function, perfusion, and metabolism in patients with advanced coronary artery disease undergoing surgical revascularization. Circulation 1994;90:2356-66.
52. Tamaki N, Kawamoto M, Tadamura E *et al.* Prediction of reversible ischemia after revascularization. Perfusion and metabolic studies using positron emission tomography. Circulation 1995;91:1697-705.
53. Maes A, Flameng W, Nuyts J *et al.* Histological alterations in chronically hypoperfused myocardium. Correlation with PET findings. Circulation 1994;90:735-45.
54. Bonow RO, Dilsizian V, Cuocolo A, Bacharach SL. Identification of viable myocardium in patients with chronic coronary artery disease and left ventricular dysfunction. Comparison of thallium scintigraphy with reinjection and PET imaging with 18F-fluorodeoxyglucose. Circulation 1991;83:26-37.
55. Fath-Ordoubadi F, Pagano D, Marinho NV, Keogh BE, Bonser RS, Camici PG. Coronary revascularization in the treatment of moderate and severe postischemic left ventricular dysfunction. Am J Cardiol 1998;82:26-31.
56. Choi Y, Brunken RC, Hawkins RA *et al.* Factors affecting myocardial 2-[F-18]fluoro-2-deoxy-D-glucose uptake in positron emission tomography studies of normal humans. Eur J Nucl Med 1993;20:308-18.

57. Chan A, Czernin J, Brunken R, Choi Y, Krivokapich J, Schelbert HR. Effects of fasting on the incidence of blood flow metabolism mismatches in chronic CAD patients [abstract]. J Am Coll Cardiol 1993;21(2 Suppl A):129A.
58. Maki M, Luotolahti M, Nuutila P et al. Glucose uptake in the chronically dysfunctional but viable myocardium. Circulation 1996;93:1658-66.
59. Berry JJ, Baker JA, Pieper KS, Hanson MW, Hoffman JM, Coleman RE. The effect of metabolic milieu on cardiac PET imaging using fluorine-18-deoxyglucose and nitrogen-13- ammonia in normal volunteers. J Nucl Med 1991;32:1518-25.
60. Schöder H, Campisi R, Ohtake T et al. Predictive accuracy of PET flow/F-18 FDG mismatch is maintained in type II diabetes mellitus patients [abstract]. J Nucl Med 1997;38(5 Suppl):55P.
61. DeFronzo RA, Tobin JD, Andres R. Glucose clamp technique: a method for quantifying insulin secretion and resistance. Am J Physiol 1979;237:E214-23.
62. Knuuti MJ, Nuutila P, Ruotsalainen U et al. Euglycemic hyperinsulinemic clamp and oral glucose load in stimulating myocardial glucose utilization during positron emission tomography. J Nucl Med 1992;33:1255-62.
63. Ohtake T, Yokoyama I, Watanabe T et al. Myocardial glucose metabolism in noninsulin-dependent diabetes mellitus patients evaluated by FDG-PET. J Nucl Med 1995;36:456-63.
64. Nienaber CA, Brunken RC, Sherman CT et al. Metabolic and functional recovery of ischemic human myocardium after coronary angioplasty. J Am Coll Cardiol 1991;18:966-78.
65. Haas F, Haehnel N, Augustin N et al. Prevalence and time-course of functional improvements in stunned and hibernating myocardium in patients with coronary artery disease (CAD) and congestive heart failure (CHF) [abstract]. J Am Coll Cardiol 1997;29(2 Suppl A):376A.
66. Vanoverschelde JL, Melin JA, Depré C, Borgers M, Dion R, Wijns W. Time-course of functional recovery of hibernating myocardium after coronary revascularization [abstract]. Circulation 1994;90(4 Suppl):I378.
67. Luu M, Stevenson LW, Brunken RC, Drinkwater DM, Schelbert HR, Tillisch JH. Delayed recovery of revascularized myocardium after referral for cardiac transplantation. Am Heart J 1990;119:668-70.
68. Flameng W, Suy R, Schwarz F et al. Ultrastructural correlates of left ventricular contraction abnormalities in patients with chronic ischemic heart disease: determinants of reversible segmental asynergy post-revascularization surgery. Am Heart J 1981;102:846-57.
69. Borgers M, Ausma J. Structural aspects of the chronic hibernating myocardium in man. Basic Res Cardiol 1995;90:44-6.
70. Ausma J, Wijffels M, Thonae F, Wouters L, Allessie M, Borgers M. Structural changes of atrial myocardium due to sustained atrial fibrillation in the goat. Circulation 1997;96:3157-63.
71. Ausma J, Wijffels M, van Eys G et al. Dedifferentiation of atrial cardiomyocytes as a result of chronic atrial fibrillation. Am J Pathol 1997;151:985-97.
72. Schwarz ER, Schaper J, vom Dahl J et al. Myocyte degeneration and cell death in hibernating human myocardium. J Am Coll Cardiol 1996;27:1577-85.
73. Schwaiger M, Sun D, Deeb GM et al. Expression of myocardial glucose transporter (GLUT) mRNAs in patients with advanced coronary artery disease (CAD) [abstract]. Circulation 1994;90(4 Suppl):I113.
74. Young LH, Renfu Y, Russell R et al. Low-flow ischemia leads to translocation of canine heart GLUT-4 and GLUT-1 glucose transporters to the sarcolemma in vivo. Circulation 1997;95:415-22.
75. Lopaschuk GD, Stanley WC. Glucose metabolism in the ischemic heart. Circulation 1997;95:313-5.

76. Narula J, Haider N, Virmani R *et al*. Apoptosis in myocytes in end-stage heart failure. N Engl J Med 1996;335:1182-9.
77. Haunstetter A, Izumo S. Apoptosis: basic mechanisms and implications for cardiovascular disease. Circ Res 1998;82:1111-29.
78. Stevenson WG, Stevenson LW, Middlekauff HR *et al*. Improving survival for patients with advanced heart failure: A study of 737 consecutive patients. J Am Coll Cardiol 1995;26:1417-23.
79. Alderman EL, Fisher LD, Litwin P *et al*. Results of coronary artery surgery in patients with poor left ventricular function (CASS). Circulation 1983;68:785-95.
80. Passamani E, Davis KB, Gillespie MJ, Killip T. A randomized trial of coronary artery bypass surgery. Survival of patients with low ejection fraction. N Engl J Med 1985;312:1665-71.
81. Maes A, Flameng W, Borgers M *et al*. Regional myocardial blood flow, glucose utilization and contractile function before and after revascularization and ultrastructural findings in patients with chronic coronary artery disease. Eur J Nucl Med 1995;22:1299-305.
82. Paolini G, Lucignani G, Zuccari M *et al*. Identification and revascularization of hibernating myocardium in angina-free patients with left ventricular dysfunction. Eur J Cardiothorac Surg 1994;8:139-44.
83. vom Dahl J, Altehoefer C, Büchin P *et al*. Einfluss von Myokardvitalitat und Koronarrevaskularisation auf klinische Entwicklung und Prognose: Eine Verlaufsbeobachtung bei 161 Patienten mit kononarer Herzkrankheid. Kardiol 1996;85:868-81.
84. Pagano D, Bonser RS, Townend JN, Ordoubadi F, Lorenzoni R, Camici PG. Predictive value of dobutamine echocardiography and positron emission tomography in identifying hibernating myocardium in patients with postischaemic heart failure. Heart 1998;79:281-8.
85. Beanlands RS, Hendry PJ, Masters RG, deKemp RA, Woodend K, Ruddy TD. Delay in revascularization is associated with increased mortality in patients with severe left ventricular dysfunction and viable myocardium on fluorine-18-fluorodeoxyglucose positron emission tomographic imaging. Circulation 1998;98(19 Suppl):II51-6.
86. Pagano D, Townend JN, Littler WA, Horton R, Camici PG, Bonser RS. Coronary artery bypass surgery as treatment for ischemic heart failure: the predictive value of viability assessment with quantitative positron emission tomography for symptomatic and functional outcome. J Thorac Cardiovasc Surg 1998;115:791-9.
87. Yoshida K, Gould KL. Quantitative relation of myocardial infarct size and myocardial viability by positron emission tomography to left ventricular ejection fraction and 3-year mortality with and without revascularization. J Am Coll Cardiol 1993;22:984-97.
88. Goldman L, Hashimoto B, Cook EF, Loscalzo A. Comparative reproducibility and validity of systems for assessing cardiovascular functional class: advantages of a new specific activity scale. Circulation 1981;64:1227-34.
89. Di Carli MF, Asgarzadie F, Schelbert HR *et al*. Quantitative relation between myocardial viability and improvement in heart failure symptoms after revascularization in patients with ischemic cardiomyopathy. Circulation 1995;92:3436-44.
90. Pagley PR, Beller GA, Watson DD, Gimple LW, Ragosta M. Improved outcome after coronary bypass surgery in patients with ischemic cardiomyopathy and residual myocardial viability. Circulation 1997;96:793-800.
91. Tamaki N, Kawamoto M, Takahashi N *et al*. Prognostic value of an increase in fluorine-18 deoxyglucose uptake in patients with myocardial infarction: Comparison with stress thallium imaging. J Am Coll Cardiol 1993;22:1621-7.
92. Lee KS, Marwick TH, Cook SA *et al*. Prognosis of patients with left ventricular dysfunction, with and without viable myocardium after myocardial infarction. Circulation 1994;90:2687-94.

93. Duong TH, Hendi P, Fonarow G *et al.* Role of positron emission tomographic assessment of myocardial viability in the management of patients who are referred for cardiac transplantation [abstract]. Circulation 1995;92(8 Suppl):I123.

94. Auerbach MA, Yagoubi S, Gambhir S *et al.* The prevalence of viable myocardium in 288 patients with congestive heart failure [abstract]. J Am Coll Cardiol 1998;31(25 Suppl A):375A.

95. Miller TR, Wallis JW, Landy BR, Gropler RJ, Sabharwal CL. Measurement of global and regional left ventricular function by cardiac PET. J Nucl Med 1994;35:999-1005.

96. Boyd HL, Gunn RN, Marinho NV *et al.* Non-invasive measurement of left ventricular volumes and function by gated positron emission tomography. Eur J Nucl Med 1996;23:1594-602.

97. Brunken RC, Kottou S, Nienaber CA *et al.* PET detection of viable tissue in myocardial segments with persistent defects at Tl-201 SPECT. Radiology 1989;172:65-73.

98. Burt RW, Perkins OW, Oppenheim BE *et al.* Direct comparison of fluorine-18-FDG SPECT, fluorine-18-FDG PET and rest thallium-201 SPECT for detection of myocardial viability. J Nucl Med 1995;36:176-9.

99. Sandler MP, Patton JA. Fluorine 18-labeled fluorodeoxyglucose myocardial single-photon emission computed tomography: An alternative for determining myocardial viability. J Nucl Cardiol 1996;3:342-9.

100. Bax JJ, Visser FC, van Lingen A *et al.* Feasibility of assessing regional myocardial uptake of ^{18}F-fluorodeoxyglucose using single photon emission computed tomography. Eur Heart J 1993;14:1675-82.

101. Bax JJ, Cornel JH, Visser FC *et al.* Prediction of recovery of myocardial dysfunction after revascularization comparison of fluorine-18 fluorodeoxyglucose/thallium-201 SPECT, thallium-201 stress-reinjection SPECT and dobutamine echocardiography. J Am Coll Cardiol 1996;28:558-64.

102. Sawada S, Elsner G, Segar DS *et al.* Evaluation of patterns of perfusion and metabolism in dobutamine-responsive myocardium. J Am Coll Cardiol 1997;29:55-61.

103. Matsunari I, Beoning G, Ziegler SI *et al.* Attenuation-corrected 99mTc-tetrofosmin single-photon emission computed tomography in the detection of viable myocardium: comparison with positron emission tomography using 18F-fluorodeoxyglucose. J Am Coll Cardiol 1998;32:927-35.

4. Assessment of myocardial viability by thallium-201

JEROEN J BAX, JEAN-LOUIS J VANOVERSCHELDE &
ERNST E VAN DER WALL

Introduction

Over the past 20 years it has become evident that left ventricular (LV) dysfunction in patients with chronic coronary artery disease is not necessarily an irreversible process, but that improvement of LV function following revascularization may occur [1]. This improvement of function can be observed in patients with substantial dysfunctional but viable myocardium. In contrast, when the dysfunction is based upon scar tissue, no improvement after revascularization can be anticipated. Hence, in patients with viable tissue, the improvement of LV function (translating in survival benefit) after revascularization may outweigh the increased risk of revascularization procedures in these patients. Accordingly, much energy has been invested in the development of noninvasive techniques that are capable of identifying patients with dysfunctional but viable myocardium. These techniques are based upon the characteristics of viable myocardium, including cell membrane integrity, intact mitochondria, preserved glucose and (possibly) fatty acid metabolism, and inotropic reserve [2]. Thallium-201 has been used for the assessment of cell membrane integrity [3], mitochondrial activity can be explored with technetium-99m sestamibi [4], glucose and fatty acid metabolism have been evaluated with F18-fluorodeoxyglucose (FDG) [5] and different radioiodinated fatty acids [6], and inotropic reserve can be probed by dobutamine echocardiography [7]. In this chapter, the use of thallium-201 to detect viable myocardium is discussed. Following the paragraphs on the rationale of thallium-201 imaging, the different protocols and the different viability criteria, the available studies using thallium-201 in patients with chronic coronary artery disease are discussed. These include comparative studies (comparing thallium-201 imaging to other "viability techniques"), studies focusing on prediction of functional outcome after revascularization, and studies evaluating the prognostic value of thallium-201 imaging.

Rationale of thallium-201 imaging, different protocols

Thallium-201 has been used extensively to assess myocardial perfusion, both at rest and following pharmacological or physical stress [3]. Following

A. E. Iskandrian and E. E. van der Wall (eds.), Myocardial Viability, 73-89.
© 2000 *Kluwer Academic Publishers. Printed in the Netherlands.*

intravenous administration, the initial uptake of thallium-201 into the myocardium parallels regional blood flow [3]. Subsequent retention of the tracer is dependent on cell membrane integrity; scar tissue is not able to retain thallium-201. These properties form the basis for viability assessment by thallium-201.

Various protocols have been developed over the past years for the assessment of viability with thallium-201. A large part of the development and validation of these protocols has been performed at the Cardiology Branch of National Heart, Lung, and Blood Institute of the National Institutes of Health in Bethesda, USA [8].

Stress-redistribution imaging

The first protocol existed of a post-stress image and a 3-4 hour delayed image (stress-redistribution imaging). Defects on the post-stress image could either represent areas of hypoperfusion or scar tissue. If fill-in of these defects ("redistribution") was observed, the tissue was considered viable. In contrast, persistence of the defects ("fixed or irreversible defects") was thought to indicate scar tissue [8]. However, Gibson *et al.* [9] pointed out that fixed defects on stress-redistribution imaging were not always irreversibly injured. In patients undergoing revascularization, the authors demonstrated that 45% of the fixed defects in fact exhibited an improvement in thallium-201 uptake post-revascularization. Other studies demonstrated that up to 50% of the fixed defects on stress-redistribution thallium-201 imaging, revealed metabolic activity (evidenced by preserved FDG uptake) [10] or demonstrated improvement of function after revascularization [11]. It was thus concluded that stress-redistribution imaging underestimated myocardial viability [8].

It was hypothesized that some fixed defects were subtended by severely stenotic coronary arteries and that a longer period than the 3-4 hour redistribution period may be needed for adequate uptake of thallium-201 in these regions. Accordingly Gutman *et al.* [12] demonstrated the superiority of a 18-24 hour delayed image over the conventional 3-4 hour delayed image for the detection of viable myocardium. More than 20% of the fixed defects on stress-(3-4 hour) redistribution imaging demonstrated fill-in on the 18-24 hour redistribution image. However, over 35% of the segments that were classified irreversible on delayed redistribution imaging improved after revascularization [13]. In addition, up to 50% of the irreversible defects on delayed redistribution imaging demonstrated preserved FDG uptake [14]. Thus, delayed redistribution imaging still underestimated viability [8]. The failure of some segments to demonstrate reversibility was thought to be related to the concentrations of thallium-201 in the blood. In severely hypoperfused regions, the circulating thallium-201 levels may be too low to allow enough extraction by the myocardium to result in fill-in of the defects.

To circumvent this problem, thallium-201 reinjection imaging has been introduced.

Stress-redistribution-reinjection imaging

In 1990, Dilsizian *et al.* [15] first reported on the use of stress-redistribution-reinjection imaging. The authors studied 100 patients with this protocol. Following the conventional stress and 3-4 hour delayed imaging, a second dose of thallium-201 (1 mCi, 37 MBq) was injected intravenously and 10-15 minutes thereafter the reinjection images were acquired. The authors demonstrated that nearly 50% of the fixed defects on the 3-4 hour redistribution images demonstrated reversibility on the reinjection images. Similar findings were reported in other studies [16]. More recent studies have tried to shorten this protocol; Van Eck-Smit *et al.* [17] developed an immediate reinjection protocol. In this protocol, the reinjection of thallium-201 is performed immediately following the acquisition of the stress images, followed by acquisition of the reinjection images 1 hour thereafter. Hence, the protocol is shortened substantially and the redistribution image is omitted. This protocol awaits further validation in terms of prediction of functional outcome after revascularization.

Rest-redistribution imaging

Another protocol that has gained substantial popularity is the rest-redistribution protocol. While the stress-redistribution-reinjection protocol provides information on viability and stress-induced ischemia, the rest-redistribution protocol provides only information on resting perfusion and viability. The rest-redistribution protocol is a simple protocol, in which the resting image is performed immediately following tracer injection (which provides an estimate of resting perfusion) and the redistribution image is acquired 3-4 hours later (reflecting the amount of viable tissue). An example of a rest-redistribution thallium-201 study is demonstrated in Figure 1. In patients with chronic coronary artery disease and severely depressed LV function a rest-redistribution protocol may be sufficient to answer the clinical question if revascularization needs to be considered or whether conservative (medical) treatment may be favored. This protocol may be of particular interest in patients with ischemic cardiomyopathy in whom exercise testing may not be feasible. However, more recent data have demonstrated that the combination of information on viability and ischemia may provide a more optimal means for the prediction of functional recovery post-revascularization [18,19].

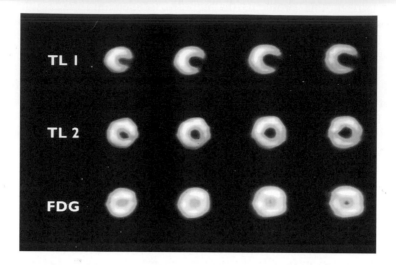

Figure 1. Comparison between rest-redistribution thallium-201 SPECT and FDG SPECT. The top row shows the short axis thallium-201 slices obtained immediately following injection at rest (TL 1). A defect is visible in the lateral wall. The middle row demonstrates the 3-4 hour redistribution thallium-201 images (TL 2) and shows reversibility of the defect in the lateral wall, indicating viable tissue in this region. The bottom row shows the FDG SPECT images, confirming the presence of viable tissue in the lateral wall as indicated by the preserved FDG uptake in this region (from Bax *et al* [39], J Nucl Med 1998;39:1481-6, with permission).

Viability criteria on thallium-201 imaging

Different viability criteria have been used with thallium-201 imaging. In the conventional stress-redistribution studies, defect-reversibility was used as the criterium for viable myocardium. Indeed segments with reversibility demonstrated improved or normalized thallium-201 uptake after revascularization associated with improvement in regional contraction. However, as pointed out in the previous paragraph, defect-reversibility on thallium-201 stress-redistribution underestimated viability as defined by improvement of function post-revascularization [11]. In the initial thallium-201 reinjection studies [15], defect-reversibility on either the 3-4 hour images or on the reinjection images was considered to represent viability. Moreover, these criteria were both sensitive and specific for the prediction of improvement of regional contractile function post-revascularization [15].

From further studies [20,21] it became evident that the quantitation of thallium-201 activity is also important for the differentiation between viable and nonviable tissue. Bonow *et al.* [20] compared the value of thallium-201 stress-redistribution-reinjection imaging with FDG positron emission tomography (PET); 16 patients with chronic coronary artery disease and LV dysfunction (LVEF 27±9%) were evaluated by the two techniques. These patients were selected on the basis of irreversible defects on stress-(3-4) hour redistribution imaging. A total of 166 irreversible segments were identified on the 3-4 hour redistribution images, representing 38% of all segments. These irreversible defects were subsequently divided into mild (60-85% of peak activity), moderate (50-59% of peak activity) and severe defects (<50% of peak activity). FDG uptake was present in 91% of the mild fixed defects and in 84% of the moderate fixed defects. In the severe fixed defects, only 51% of the segments exhibited FDG uptake (indicating viable tissue). Similarly, reinjection of thallium-201 resulted in reversibility in 51% of the defects. Hence, these data indicated that segments with ≥50% thallium-201 activity on the redistribution images can be considered as viable and that in the segments with <50% thallium-201 activity on the redistribution images the presence or absence of reversibility following reinjection will distinguish between viable and scar tissue.

On rest-redistribution imaging the same criteria have been applied, including the presence of significant redistribution (5% or 10% increase in activity) on the late image, ≥50% thallium-201 activity on the late image or the combination of both criteria [22].

A last criterium that may be useful in the identification of viable myocardium is reverse redistribution. The pattern of reverse redistribution is defined as the appearence or worsening of a defect on the delayed images (either the (3-4 hour) redistribution images with stress-(3-4 hour) redistribution imaging or the (3-4 hour) delayed images with rest-redistribution imaging) as compared to the initial images [23]. Marin-Neto *et al.* [24] have demonstrated that 82% of the segments demonstrating reverse redistribution during stress-(3-4 hour) redistribution imaging were classified viable following reinjection of thallium-201. Data by Sciagra *et al.* [25] however demonstrated limited value of reverse redistribution in the prediction of functional recovery following revascularization.

Comparison between thallium-201 imaging and other viability techniques

A large number of studies has been reported comparing thallium-201 imaging to other viability techniques. The shortcoming of the majority of these studies is the lack of assessment of functional outcome following revascularization.

Comparison to FDG imaging

As stated before, stress-(3-4 hour) redistribution imaging underestimated viability, which also became evident in direct comparisons with FDG PET. Brunken *et al.* [10] demonstrated that a substantial number of fixed defects (47%) on stress-(3-4 hour) redistribution imaging, revealed preserved FDG uptake on PET. In a second study, Brunken *et al.* [14] demonstrated underestimation of viability by 24 hour delayed imaging as compared to FDG PET. More recently, Bonow *et al.* [20] showed an excellent agreement between thallium-201 reinjection imaging and FDG PET. These findings were confirmed by Tamaki *et al.* [26], showing an agreement of 85% between FDG PET and thallium-201 reinjection for the detection of viable myocardium.

Dilsizian *et al.* [27] have also performed a comparative study between FDG PET and thallium-201 rest-redistribution imaging. In 20 patients, a total of 594 segments were evaluated. FDG PET classified 59 segments as nonviable; 49 (83%) of these segments were classified as nonviable by thallium-201 rest-redistribution. Conversely, FDG PET identified 535 segments as viable; 486 (91%) of these segments were classified viable on thallium-201 rest-redistribution. Accordingly, the agreement between the two techniques was 90%.

Comparison to technetium-99m sestamibi imaging

Dilsizian *et al.* [28] have performed a head-to-head comparison between thallium-201 reinjection imaging and technetium-99m sestamibi imaging. A study cohort of 54 patients were studied; all had depressed LV function (LVEF $34 \pm 14\%$). They underwent both a stress (3-4 hour) redistribution-reinjection study and a same-day rest-stress technetium-99m sestamibi SPECT. The concordance between absence or presence of reversibility was 75% between the two studies; when the data were analyzed quantitatively and the viability criteria were extended to reversibility and the 50% cutoff level, the agreement between the two techniques increased to 93%. Additional studies by Cuocolo *et al.* and Dondi *et al.* [29-31] however, demonstrated significant underestimation of viability by technetium-99m sestamibi imaging as compared to thallium-201 reinjection and thallium-201 rest-redistribution imaging.

Comparison to dobutamine echocardiography

A substantial number of studies have compared thallium-201 imaging with dobutamine echocardiography [32-35]. Panza *et al.* [34] have performed a direct comparison between dobutamine echocardiography and thallium-201 reinjection imaging. In this study, a total of 311 segments were analyzed by both techniques (Figure 2). Thallium-201 reinjection imaging classified 262 (84%) of the segments as viable, and 49 (16%) as nonviable. The majority of the scintigraphically nonviable segments did not show a contractile reserve on dobutamine echocardiography and were thus concordantly classified as nonviable, yielding an agreement of 88% for assessing nonviability. However, a substantial number (36%) of the scintigraphically viable segments, did not show a contractile reserve, yielding an agreement of only 64% for the detection of viable myocardium. Thus, thallium-201 imaging tended to overestimate viability, or dobutamine echocardiography tended to underestimate viability. This observation has been consistently observed throughout the different studies comparing dobutamine echocardiography and thallium-201 imaging [32-35]. Similar observations have also been described in direct comparisons between FDG SPECT and dobutamine echocardiography [36]. It has been suggested that nuclear imaging may be more susceptible to identify viable tissue; some segments may be more damaged on the ultrastructural level that inotropic reserve is no longer present, while cell membrane integrity (assessed by thallium-201) and glucose utilization (assessed by FDG) are still intact [37]. Preliminary data suggest that some of these segments may need longer time to recover in function post-operatively [38].

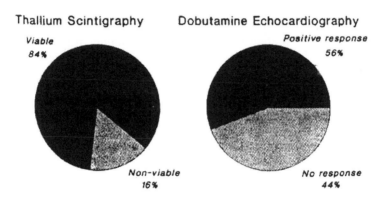

Figure 2. Pie chart comparing thallium-201 results to dobutamine echocardiography results. A significantly higher percentage of segments was classified viable by thallium-201 imaging as compared to dobutamine echocardiography (from Panza *et al* [34], Circulation 1995;91:990-8, with permission).

Prediction of functional outcome post-revascularization

The most frequently used "gold standard" for the detection of viable myocardium, has been the prediction of improvement of function following revascularization. Most studies have focused on the prediction of improvement of regional LV function, whereas, from a clinical point-of-view, improvement of global LV function may be more relevant. The available data in the literature concerning the prediction of functional outcome after revascularization will be summarized briefly in the following paragraphs.

Thallium-201 reinjection imaging

Currently, 11 studies (301 patients) employing a reinjection protocol to predict improvement of regional LV function after revascularization have been reported [Table 1]. The first study was performed by the NIH-group and included 20 patients. The authors presented a highly positive (95%) and negative predictive value (80%). More recent studies have been consistent in demonstrating an excellent negative predictive value but they also demonstrated a decline in the positive predictive value. The mean negative predictive value was 83% (ranging from 71% to 100%) and the mean positive predictive value was 57% (ranging from 29% to 95%). The differences in predictive values between the individual studies are possibly related to differences in equipment, protocols and analyses, but may also relate to differences in study populations [2]. Still, thallium-201 reinjection appears to have a low positive predictive value, indicating that a substantial amount of segments that are classified as viable may not recover in function after revascularization. This finding may be altered if a longer follow-up is used (almost all studies used a 3-month follow-up period). In addition, some segments with an intact cell membrane (and thus classified viable on thallium-201 imaging) may be too severely damaged to recover in function.

Table 1. Positive and negative predictive value (PPV, NPV) of thallium-201 reinjection imaging to detect improvement in regional contractile function after revascularization (301 patients, 11 studies)

Author	nr pts	PPV (%) (segments)	NPV (%) (segments)
1. Vanoverschelde [32]	73	48 (213/440)	79 (198/252)
2. Ohtani [11]	24	73 (33/45)	75 (12/16)
3. Arnese [35]	38	30 (34/113)	94 (63/67)
4. Bax [55]	17	40 (25/62)	93 (28/30)
5. Tamaki [26]	11	79 (38/48)	75 (6/8)
6. Dilsizian [15]	20	95 (35/37)	80 (8/10)
7. Haque [56]	26	85 (33/39)	100 (4/4)
8. Taki [57]	34	29 (2/7)	76 (13/17)
9. Lipiecki [58]	15	61 (37/61)	78 (46/59)
10. Gürsürer [59]	12	83 (80/96)	75 (3/4)
11. Kostopoulos [60]	31	71 (67/95)	90 (62/69)
Weighted mean		57 (597/1043)	83 (443/536)

Thallium-201 rest-redistribution

Twenty-two studies (557 patients) using a rest-redistribution protocol to predict improvement of regional LV function after revascularization have been published thusfar [Table 2]. The negative predictive value was excellent (mean 80%, ranging from 62% to 100%) and the positive predictive value was somewhat lower (mean 69%, ranging from 45% to 95%). Again, the differences in equipment, differences in analyses (different normalization procedures, different viability criteria) and differences in study populations may be responsible for the inter-study variation in predictive values. Bax *et al.* [39] demonstrated that the use of cutoff values (percentage uptake at the redistribution images) to identify viable myocardium resulted in high negative predictive values with lower positive predictive values. Conversely, when redistribution was used as a marker of viable myocardium, higher positive predictive values were obtained, but at the expense of lower negative predictive values. Similar findings were observed by Gunning *et al.* [40].

Table 2. Positive and negative predictive value (PPV, NPV) of thallium-201 rest-redistribution imaging to detect improvement in regional contractile function after revascularization (557 patients, 22 studies)

Author	nr pts	PPV (%) (segments)	NPV (%) (segments)
1.Mori [61]	17	79 (11/14)	62 (23/37)
2.Marzullo [62]	14	95 (42/44)	77 (24/31)
3.Udelson [4]	18	75 (15/20)	92 (24/26)
4.Qureshi [33]	34	45 (38/85)	94 (59/63)
5.Ragosta [22]	21	57 (81/141)	77 (27/35)
6.Alfieri [63]	13	92 (92/100)	70 (14/20)
7.Charney [64]	14	90 (19/21)	92 (11/12)
8.Perrone [65]	18	72 (73/101)	100 (8/8)
9.Nagueh [66]	19	54 (42/78)	87 (27/31)
10.Matsunari [67]	25	69 (45/65)	71 (10/14)
11.Cuocolo [68]	38	75 (116/154)	81 (35/43)
12.Bax [69]	32	49 (51/105)	90 (55/61)
13.Sciagra [70]	35	70 (NA)	65 (NA)
14.Marzullo [71]	22	79 (50/63)	88 (37/42)
15.Matsunari [72]	14	69 (25/36)	87 (13/15)
16.Sciagra [73]	29	68 (90/132)	70 (57/82)
17.Bax [39]	24	62 (24/39)	82 (55/67)
18.Pace [74]	46	74 (35/47)	76 (34/45)
19.Senior [75]	22	91 (108/119)	80 (39/49)
20.Gunning [40]	30	53 (59/111)	76 (73/96)
21.Gunning [76]	15	58 (39/67)	75 (49/65)
22.Sicari [77]	57	74 (110/149)	79 (60/76)
Weighted mean		69 (1165/1700)	80 (734/918)

NA: not available

The earlier studies used 50% thallium-201 activity as the cutoff level to discriminate between viable and nonviable myocardium [22]. These studies showed a high negative predictive value, with a lower positive predictive value. More recent studies demonstrated that higher cutoff levels improved the positive predictive value, but at the cost of lowering the negative predictive value [33]. The currently available data suggest that the optimal cutoff value is probably between 60% and 70% [33,39,41]. Besides optimalization of the viability criteria, several studies have indicated that nitroglycerin-augmented thallium-201 reinjection imaging [42] may enhance detection of viable tissue; this technique needs further testing and validation against functional outcome following revascularization.

Prediction of improvement of global LV function

Vanoverschelde *et al.* [32] studied 73 patients with severely depressed LV function with thallium-201 reinjection SPECT and demonstrated a negative predictive value of 65% with a positive predictive value of 80% for the prediction of improvement in LVEF. Iskandrian *et al.* [43] used a rest-redistribution protocol and demonstrated that 12 of 14 (86%) patients with scintigraphic evidence of viability improved in LVEF, whereas only 2 of 10 (20%) patients without viability did improve in LVEF. Ragosta *et al.* [22] furthermore demonstrated that the change in LVEF was related to pre-operative thallium uptake (Figure 3).

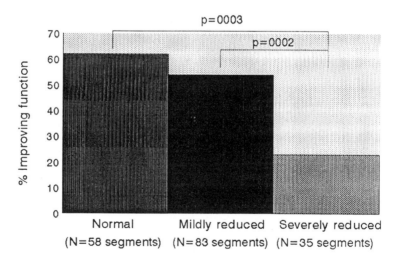

Figure 3. Scatter plot illustrating the relation between pre-operative tracer uptake on thallium-201 rest-redistribution imaging and the magnitude in change in LVEF post-revascularization (from Ragosta *et al* [22], Circulation 1993;87:1630-41, with permission).

Prognostic value of thallium-201 imaging

Five retrospective FDG PET studies [44-48] have evaluated the prognostic value of this technique. The patients were divided into four groups, according to the treatment (revascularization or medical treatment) and the presence/absence of viable myocardium. The results indicated that patients with viable myocardium who were treated medically were at the highest risk for future events (Figure 4).

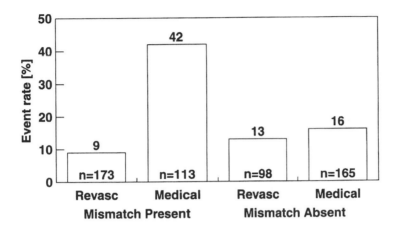

Figure 4. Bar graph demonstrating the relation between the event rate, viability on FDG PET and treatment (revascularization or medical therapy) (from Bax and Wijns [34], J Nucl Med 1999; in press, with permission).

Similar results have been demonstrated in various studies employing thallium-201 scintigraphy. Gioia *et al.* [49] evaluated 85 patients with thallium-201 rest-redistribution imaging; 38 patients underwent revascularization and 47 were treated conservatively. These patients did not differ in baseline characteristics, including LVEF (29±10% vs 31±10%). The percentages of normal images, fixed defects and reversible defects were also comparable between the 2 groups. The mean follow-up was 31 months; the annual mortality was 13% in the medically treated patients as compared to 6% in the revascularized patients. Another study from the same group evaluated 81 patients who were treated medically [50]; the patients with viability (as evidenced by the presence of redistribution) had a significantly higher event rate during the 31±24 months follow-up period (Figure 5), indicating the adverse prognosis of patients with viable myocardium who are treated conservatively. Similar data have been reported by Cuocolo *et al.* [51]. The most carefully conducted study was reported by Pagley *et al.* [52]. The authors clearly demonstrated that patients with ischemic cardiomyopathy undergoing revascularization had a superior outcome as compared to patients without viability.

Finally, Pasquet *et al.* [53] have recently demonstrated that ischemia and/or viability on thallium-201 reinjection imaging is associated with a favorable prognosis when these patients were revascularized.

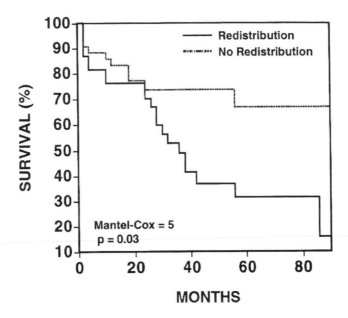

Figure 5. Survival curves in patients with and without viability as evidenced by the presence or absence of redistribution on thallium-201 rest-redistribution imaging (from Gioia *et al* [50], J Nucl Cardiol 1996;3:150-6, with permission).

Conclusions

The currently available data demonstrate clearly the usefulness of thallium-201 for the assessment of viable myocardium. Both thallium-201 reinjection and rest-redistribution imaging are capable of predicting functional recovery post-revascularization and these techniques provide important prognostic information. Despite the potential of technetium labeled agents to assess myocardial viability (see Chapter by Sciagra) thallium-201 retains its place in the clinical arena.

References

1. Rahimtoola SH. Importance of diagnosing hibernating myocardium: How and in whom? J Am Coll Cardiol 1997;30:1701-6.
2. Bax JJ, Wijns W, Cornel JH, Visser FC, Fioretti PM. Accuracy of currently available techniques for prediction of functional recovery after revascularization in patients with left ventricular dysfunction due to chronic coronary artery disease: comparison of pooled data. J Am Coll Cardiol 1997;30:1451-60.
3. Beller GA, Ragosta M, Watson DD, Gimple LW. Myocardial thallium-201 scintigraphy for assessment of viability in patients with severe left ventricular dysfunction. Am J Cardiol 1992;70:18E-22E.
4. Udelson JE, Coleman PS, Metherall J *et al.* Predicting recovery of severe regional ventricular dysfunction; Comparison of resting scintigraphy with 201Tl and 99Tc-sestamibi. Circulation 1994;89:2552-61.
5. Schelbert HR. Measurments of myocardial metabolism in patients with ischemic heart disease. Am J Cardiol 1998;82:61K-67K.
6. Knapp FF Jr, Franken P, Kropp J. Cardiac SPECT with Iodine-123-labeled fatty acids: evaluation of myocardial viability with BMIPP. J Nucl Med 1995;36:1022-30.
7. Cornel JH, Bax JJ, Fioretti PM. Assessment of myocardial viability by dobutamine stress echocardiography. Curr Opin Cardiol 1996;11:621-6.
8. Dilsizian V, Bonow RO. Current diagnostic techniques of assessing myocardial viability in hibernating and stunned myocardium. Circulation 1993; 87:1-20.
9. Gibson RS, Watson DD, Taylor GJ *et al.* Prospective assessment of regional myocardial perfusion before and after coronary revascularization surgery by quantitative thallium-201 scintigraphy. J Am Coll Cardiol 1983;1:804-15.
10. Brunken R, Schwaiger M, Grover-McKay M, Phelps ME, Tillisch J, Schelbert HR. Positron emission tomography detects tissue metabolic activity in myocardial segments with persistent thallium perfusion defects. J Am Coll Cardiol 1987;10:557-67.
11. Ohtani H, Tamaki N, Yonekura Y *et al.* Value of thallium-201 reinjection after delayed SPECT imaging for predicting reversible ischemia after coronary artery bypass grafting. Am J Cardiol 1990;66:394-9.
12. Gutman J, Berman DS, Freeman M *et al.* Time to completed redistribution of thallium-201 in exercise myocardial scintigraphy: Relationship to the degree of coronary artery stenosis. Am Heart J 1983;106:989-95.
13. Kiat H, Berman DS, Maddahi J *et al.* Late reversibility of tomographic myocardial thallium-201 defects: An accurate marker of myocardial viability. J Am Coll Cardiol 1988;12:1456-63.
14. Brunken RC, Mody F, Hawkins RA, Nienaber CA, Phelps ME, Schelbert HR. Positron emission tomography detects metabolic viability in myocardium with persistent 24-hour single-photon emission computed tomography 201Tl defects. Circulation 1992;86:1357-69.
15. Dilsizian V, Rocco TP, Freedman NMT, Leon MB, Bonow RO. Enhanced detection of ischemic but viable myocardium by the reinjection of thallium after stress-redistribution imaging. N Engl J Med 1990;323:141-6.
16. Tamaki N, Ohtani H, Yonekura Y *et al.* Significance of fill-in after thallium-201 reinjection following delayed imaging: Comparison with regional wall motion and angiographic findings. J Nucl Med 1990;31:1617-24.
17. Van Eck-Smit BLF, van der Wall EE, Kuijper AFM, Zwinderman AH, Pauwels EKJ. Immediate thallium-201 reinjection following stress imaging: A time-saving approach for detection of myocardial viability. J Nucl Med 1993;34:737-43.
18. Kitsiou AN, Srinivasan G, Quyyumi AA, Summers RM, Bacharach SL, Dilsizian V. Stress-induced reversible and mild-to-moderate irreversible thallium defects: Are they equally accurate for predicting recovery of regional left ventricular function after revascularization? Circulation 1998;98:501 8.

19. Bax JJ, Vanoverschelde JLJ, Cornel JH *et al.* Optimal viability criteria on thallium-201 reinjection SPECT to predict improvement of function after revascularization [abstract]. J Am Coll Cardiol 1999;33(Suppl A):416A.
20. Bonow RO, Dilsizian V, Cuocolo A, Bacharach SL. Identification of viable myocardium in patients with chronic coronary artery disease and left ventricular dysfunction. Comparison of thallium scintigraphy with reinjection and PET imaging with 18-F-fluorodeoxyglucose. Circulation 1991;83:26-37.
21. Dilsizian V, Freedman NMT, Bacharach SL, Perrone-Filardi P, Bonow RO. Regional thallium uptake in irreversible defects magnitude of change in thallium activity after reinjection distinguishes viable from nonviable myocardium. Circulation 1992;85:627-34.
22. Ragosta M, Beller GA, Watson DD, Kaul S, Gimple LW. Quantitative planar rest-redistribution Tl-201 imaging in detection of myocardial viability and prediction of improvement in left ventricular function after coronary artery bypass surgery in patients with severely depressed left ventricular function. Circulation 1993;87:1630-41.
23. Maddahi J, Berman DS. Reverse redistribution of thallium-201. J Nucl Med 1995;36:1019-21.
24. Marin-Neto JA, Dilsizian V, Arrighi JA *et al.* Thallium reinjection demonstrates viable myocardium in regions with reverse redistribution. Circulation 1993;88:1736-45.
25. Sciagra R, Pupi A, Pellegri M *et al.* Prediction of post-revascularization functional recovery of asynergic myocardium using quantitative thallium-201 rest-redistribution tomography: Has the reverse redistribution pattern an independent significance? Eur J Nucl Med 1998;25:594-600.
26. Tamaki N, Ohtani H, Yamashita K *et al.* Metabolic activity in the areas of new fill-in after thallium-201 reinjection: Comparison with positron emission tomography using fluorine-18-deoxyglucose. J Nucl Med 1991;32:673-8.
27. Dilsizian V, Perrone-Filardi P, Arrighi JA *et al.* Concordance and discordance between stress-redistribution-reinjection and rest-redistribution thallium imaging for assessing viable myocardium. Comparison with metabolic activity by positron emission tomography. Circulation 1993;88:941-52.
28. Dilsizian V, Arrighi JA, Diodati JG *et al.* Myocardial viability in patients with chronic coronary artery disease. Comparison of 99mTc-Sestamibi with thallium reinjection and [18F]fluorodeoxyglucose. Circulation 1994;89:578-87.
29. Cuocolo A, Pace L, Ricciardelli B, Ciariello M, Trimarco B, Salvatore M. Identification of viable myocardium in patients with chronic coronary artery disease: Comparison of thallium-201 scintigraphy with reinjection and technetium-99m-methoxyisobutyl isonitrile. J Nucl Med 1992;33:505-11.
30. Cuocolo A, Maurea S, Pace L *et al.* Resting technetium-99m methoxyisobutylisonitrile cardiac imaging in chronic coronary artery disease: Comparison with rest-redistribution thallium-201 scintigraphy. Eur J Nucl Med 1993;20:1186-92.
31. Dondi M, Tartagni F, Fallani F *et al.* A comparison of rest sestamibi and rest-redistribution single photon emission tomography: possible implications for myocardial viability detection in infarcted patients. Eur J Nucl Med 1993;20:26-31.
32. Vanoverschelde JLJ, D'Hondt AM, Marwick T *et al.* Head-to-head comparison of exercise-redistribution-reinjection thallium single-photon emission computed tomography and low dose dobutamine echocardiography for prediction of reversibility of chronic left ventricular ischemic dysfunction. J Am Coll Cardiol 1996;28:432-42.
33. Qureshi U, Nagueh SF, Afridi I *et al.* Dobutamine echocardiography and quantitative rest-redistribution ^{201}Tl tomography in myocardial hibernation. Relation of contractile reserve to ^{201}Tl uptake and comparative prediction of recovery of function. Circulation 1997;95:626-35.
34. Panza JA, Dilsizian V, Laurienzo JM, Curiel RV, Katsiyiannis PT. Relation between thallium uptake and contractile response to dobutamine. Implications regarding

myocardial viability in patients with chronic coronary artery disease and left ventricular dysfunction. Circulation 1995;91:990-8.

35. Arnese M, Cornel JH, Salustri A *et al*. Prediction of improvement of regional left ventricular function after surgical revascularization: A comparison of low-dose dobutamine echocardiography with 201-TL SPECT. Circulation 1995;91:2748-52.

36. Cornel JH, Bax JJ, Elhendy A *et al*. Agreement and disagreement between "metabolic viability" and "contractile reserve" in akinetic myocardium. J Nucl Cardiol 1999;6:383-8.

37. Baumgartner H, Porenta G, Lau Y *et al*. Assessment of myocardial viability by dobutamine echocardiography, positron emission tomography and thallium-201 SPECT. Correlation with explanted hearts. J Am Coll Cardiol 1998;32:1701-8.

38. Bax JJ, Poldermans D, Visser FC *et al*. Delayed recovery of hibernating myocardium after surgical revascularization: Implications for discrepancy between metabolic imaging and dobutamine echocardiography for assessment of myocardial viability. J Nucl Cardiol. In press 1999.

39. Bax JJ, Cornel JH, Visser FC *et al*. Comparison of fluorine-18-FDG with rest-redistribution thallium-201 SPECT to delineate viable myocardium and predict functional recovery after revascularization. J Nucl Med 1998;39:1481-6.

40. Gunning MG, Anagnostopoulos C, Knight CJ *et al*. Comparison of ^{201}Tl, ^{99m}Tc-tetrofosmin, and dobutamine magnetic resonance imaging for identifying hibernating myocardium. Circulation 1998;98:1869-74.

41. Pace L, Perrone-Filardi P, Mainenti P *et al*. Identification of viable myocardium in patients with chronic coronary artery disease using rest-redistribution thallium-201 scintigraphy: Optimal image analysis. J Nucl Med 1998;39:1869-74.

42. He ZX, Darcourt J, Guignier A *et al*. Nitrates improve detection of ischemic but viable myocardium by thallium-201 reinjection SPECT. J Nucl Med 1993;34:1472-7.

43. Iskandrian AS, Hakki A, Kane SA *et al*. Rest and redistribution thallium-201 myocardial scintigraphy to predict improvement in left ventricular function after coronary arterial bypass grafting. Am J Cardiol 1983;51:1312-6.

44. Eitzman D, Al-Aouar ZR, Kanter HL *et al*. Clinical outcome of patients with advanced coronary artery disease after viability studies with positron emission tomography. J Am Coll Cardiol 1992;20:559-65.

45. Di Carli M, Davidson M, Little R *et al*. Value of metabolic imaging with positron emission tomography for evaluating prognosis in patients with coronary artery disease and left ventricular dysfunction. Am J Cardiol 1994;73:527-33.

46. Vom Dahl J, Altehoefer C, Sheehan FH *et al*. Effect of myocardial viability assessed by technetium-99m-sestamibi SPECT and fluorine-18-FDG PET on clinical outcome in coronary artery disease. J Nucl Med 1997;38:742-8.

47. Tamaki N, Kawamoto M, Takahashi N *et al*. Prognostic value of an increase in fluorine-18 deoxyglucose uptake in patients with myocardial infarction: comparison with stress thallium imaging. J Am Coll Cardiol 1993;22:1621-7.

48. Lee KS, Marwick TH, Cook SA *et al*. Prognosis of patients with left ventricular dysfunction, with and without viable myocardium after myocardial infarction. Relative efficacy of medical therapy and revascularization. Circulation 1994;90:2687-94.

49. Gioia G, Powers J, Heo J, Iskandrian AS. Prognostic value of rest-redistribution tomographic thallium-201 imaging in ischemic cardiomyopathy. Am J Cardiol 1995;75:759-62.

50. Gioia G, Milan E, Giubbini R, DePace N, Heo J, Iskandrian AS. Prognostic value of tomographic rest-redistribution thallium-201 imaging in medically treated patients with coronary artery disease and left ventricular dysfunction. J Nucl Cardiol 1996;3:150-6.

51. Cuocolo A, Petretta M, Nicolai E, Pace L, Bonaduce D, Salvatore M, Trimarco B. Successful coronary revascularization improves prognosis in patients with previous myocardial infarction and evidence of viable myocardium at thallium-201 imaging. Eur J Nucl Med 1998;25:60-8.

52. Pagley PR, Beller GA, Watson DD, Gimple LW, Ragosta M. Improved outcome after coronary bypass surgery in patients with ischemic cardiomyopathy and residual myocardial viability. Circulation 1997;96:793-800.
53. Pasquet A, Robert A, D'Hondt AM, Dion R, Melin JA, Vanoverschelde JLJ. Prognostic value of myocardial ischemia and viability in patients with chronic left ventricular ischemic dysfunction. Circulation 1999;100:141-8.
54. Bax JJ, Wijns W. FDG imaging to assess myocardial viability: PET, SPECT or gamma camera coincidence imaging? J Nucl Med. In press 1999.
55. Bax JJ, Cornel JH, Visser FC et al. Prediction of recovery of myocardial dysfunction following revascularization; Comparison of F18-fluorodeoxyglucose/thallium-201 single photon emission computed tomography, thallium-201 stress-reinjection single photon emission computed tomography and dobutamine echocardiography. J Am Coll Cardiol 1996;28:558-64.
56. Haque T, Furukawa T, Takahashi M, Kinoshita M. Identification of hibernating myocardium by dobutamine stress echocardiography: Comparison with thallium-201 reinjection imaging. Am Heart J 1995;130:553-63.
57. Taki J, Nakajima K, Matsunari I et al. Assessment of improvement of myocardial fatty acid uptake and function after revascularization using iodine-123-BMIPP. J Nucl Med 1997;38:1503-10.
58. Lipiecki J, Maublant JC, Citron B et al. Comparable uptake of thallium-201 and technetium-99m MIBI in hibernating and "maimed" myocardium. Am J Cardiol 1997;79:940-3.
59. Gürsürer M, Pinarli AE, Aksoy M et al. Assessment of viable myocardium and prediction of postoperative improvement of left ventricular function in patients with severe left ventricular dysfunction by quantitative planar stress-redistribution-reinjection 201-Tl imaging. Int J Cardiol 1997;58:179-84.
60. Kostopoulos KG, Kranidis AI, Bouki KP et al. Detection of myocardial viability in the prediction of improvement in left ventricular function after successful coronary revascularization by using the dobutamine stress echocardiography and quantitative SPECT rest-redistribution-reinjection ^{201}Tl imaging after dipyridamole infusion. Angiology 1996;47:1039-46.
61. Mori T, Minamiji K, Kurogane H, Ogawa K, Yoshida Y. Rest-injected thallium-201 imaging for assessing viability of severe asynergic regions. J Nucl Med 1991;32:1718-24.
62. Marzullo P, Parodi O, Reisenhofer B et al. Value of rest thallium-201/technetium-99m Sestamibi and dobutamine echocardiography for detecting myocardial viability. Am J Cardiol 1993;71:166-72.
63. Alfieri O, La Canna G, Giubinni R, Pardini A, Zogno M, Fucci C. Recovery of myocardial function. Eur J Cardiothorac Surg 1993;7:325-30.
64. Charney R, Schwinger ME, Chun J et al. Dobutamine echocardiography and resting-redistribution thallium-201 scintigraphy predicts recovery of hibernating myocardium after coronary revascularization. Am Heart J 1994;128:864-9.
65. Perrone-Filardi P, Pace L, Prastaro M et al. Assessment of myocardial viability in patients with chronic coronary artery disease. Rest-4-hour-24-hour ^{201}Tl tomography versus dobutamine echocardiography. Circulation 1996;94:2712-9.
66. Nagueh SF, Vaduganathan P, Ali N et al. Identification of hibernating myocardium: Comparative accuracy of myocardial contrast echocardiography, rest-redistribution thallium-201 tomography and dobutamine echocardiography. J Am Coll Cardiol 1997;29:985-93.
67. Matsunari I, Fujino S, Taki J et al. Quantitative rest technetium-99m tetrofosmin imaging in predicting functional recovery after revascularization: Comparison with rest-redistribution thallium-201. J Am Coll Cardiol 1997;29:1226-33.

68. Cuocolo A, Nicolai E, Petretta M *et al.* One-year effect of myocardial revascularization on resting left ventricular function and regional thallium uptake in chronic CAD. J Nucl Med 1997;38:1684-92.

69. Bax JJ, Visser FC, Van Lingen A, Sloof GW, Cornel JH, Visser CA. Comparison between 360° and 180° data sampling in thallium-201 rest-redistribution single-photon emission tomography to predict functional recovery after revascularization. Eur J Nucl Med 1997;24:516-22.

70. Sciagra R, Bisi G, Santoro GM *et al.* Comparison of baseline-nitrate technetium-99m sestamibi with rest-redistribution thallium-201 tomography in detecting viable hibernating myocardium and predicting postrevascularization recovery. J Am Coll Cardiol 1997;30:384-91.

71. Marzullo P, Sambucetti G, Parodi O *et al.* Regional concordance and discordance between rest thallium 201 and sestamibi imaging for assessing tissue viability: Comparison with postrevascularization functional recovery. J Nucl Cardiol 1995;2:309-16.

72. Matsunari I, Fujino S, Taki J *et al.* Significance of late redistribution thallium-201 imaging after rest injection for detection of viable myocardium. J Nucl Med 1997;38:1073-8.

73. Sciagra R, Santoro GM, Bisi G, Pedenovi P, Fazzini PF, Pupi A. Rest-redistribution thallium-201 SPECT to detect myocardial viability. J Nucl Med 1998;39:384-90.

74. Pace L, Perrone-Filardi P, Mainenti P *et al.* Combined evaluation of rest-redistribution thallium-201 tomography and low-dose dobutamine echocardiography enhances the identification of viable myocardium in patients with chronic coronary artery disease. Eur J Nucl Med 1998;25:744-50.

75. Senior R, Glenville B, Basu S *et al.* Dobutamine echocardiography and thallium-201 imaging predict functional improvement after revascularization in severe ischaemic left ventricular dysfunction. Br Heart J 1995;74:358-64.

76. Gunning MG, Anagnostopoulos C, Davies G *et al.* Simultaneous assessment of myocardial viability and function for the detection of hibernating myocardium using ECG-gated $^{99}Tc^m$-tetrofosmin emission tomography: A comparison with ^{201}Tl emission tomography combined with cine magnetic resonance imaging. Nucl Med Commun 1999;20:209-14.

77. Sicari R, Varga A, Picano E, Borges AC, Gimelli A, Marzullo P. Comparison of combination of dipyridamole and dobutamine during echocardiography with thallium scintigraphy to improve viability detection. Am J Cardiol 1999;83:6-10.

5. Technetium-99m-labeled perfusion tracers for the detection of myocardial viability

ROBERTO SCIAGRÀ

Introduction

Technetium-99m(Tc-99m)-labeled myocardial perfusion tracers offer several advantages over thallium-201 for the diagnosis and evaluation of coronary artery disease. However, because of the results of some early human studies, concerns were advanced about their usefulness and reliability for the detection of viable hibernating myocardium. The majority of the experimental data and the more recent clinical reports have greatly reduced these concerns, so that the use of Tc-99m-labeled myocardial perfusion tracers for the issue of viability detection should be probably considered a reasonable alternative to the other established methods. The largest experience has been collected about Tc-99m-sestamibi and will be thoroughly examined in the following sections. Promising data, which are briefly reported as well, are now becoming available about the other currently used Tc-99m-labeled perfusion tracer, Tc-99m-tetrofosmin.

Tc-99m-sestamibi

Experimental basis

Tc-99m-sestamibi uptake in the myocells is proportional to coronary blood flow [1,2]. The uptake mechanism of this lipophilic cationic tracer is mainly passive and related to the presence of negative potentials across the sarcolemmal and mitochondrial membranes [3]. This phenomenon is also the basis of tracer retention within the cell [3]. Since cellular viability is necessary for the maintenance of trans-membrane electrochemical gradients, an intuitive relationship exists between Tc-99m-sestamibi uptake and retention and preserved cellular integrity. A quite large body of experimental evidence supports this conclusion. In cultured chick embryo myocites, Piwnica-Worms *et al.* [4] demonstrated that thallium-201 uptake declined progressively with increasing cell ATP depletion; conversely, Tc-99m-sestamibi uptake transiently increased and then declined to very low values when cell damage became most severe. The authors even

A. E. Iskandrian and È. E. van der Wall (eds.), Myocardial Viability, 91-112.
© 2000 *Kluwer Academic Publishers. Printed in the Netherlands.*

hypothesized that at moderate levels of cell damage Tc-99m-sestamibi would still show cellular viability, whilst thallium-201 would already demonstrate irreversible damage. In an isolated rat heart model, Beanlands *et al.* [5] demonstrated that various compounds that induce irreversible cellular damage also affected Tc-99m-sestamibi uptake and retention. Furthermore, they found a relationship between the severity of cellular damage and the decrease in Tc-99m-sestamibi activity, even after correcting for the changes in blood flow (Figure 1).

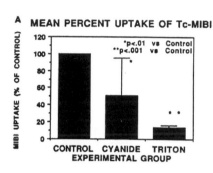 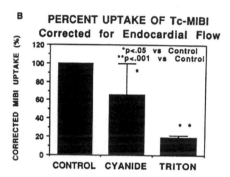

Figure 1. Bar graph showing the mean peak uptake of Tc-99m-sestamibi (MIBI) for each group of rat hearts, divided according to the absence of cell damage (controls), to the presence of cyanide-induced cell injury (seven-fold increase in CK release compared to controls), and to the presence of Triton-induced cell injury (45-fold increase in CK release compared to controls, seven-fold increase compared to cyanide-injured cells). Panel A shows the values without flow correction, panel B the percent uptake values corrected for variations in endocardial flow assessed by microspheres. A relationship between the severity of cell damage and Tc-99m-sestamibi uptake is demonstrated. Reprinted with permission from Beanlands *et al.*, Circulation 1990;82:1802-14.

Canby *et al.* [6] submitted experimental animals to the prolonged occlusion of a coronary artery injecting both thallium-201 and Tc-99m-sestamibi at the end of the occlusion period or after vessel reopening. They observed a substantial agreement between microsphere-measured coronary blood flow and both thallium-201 and Tc-99m-sestamibi uptake at the various time points. They registered a slight overestimation of flow by the two tracers for flow values between 10% and 40% of normal, overestimation which was no longer observed, particularly using Tc-99m-sestamibi, for flow levels under 10%, suggesting the inability of necrotic myocardium to take up the two tracers (Figure 2). A discrepancy between coronary blood flow determined using microspheres and Tc-99m-sestamibi uptake was registered also by Sinusas *et al.* [7], who injected both tracers during prolonged (3 hours) coronary occlusion and 90 minutes after reperfusion; they observed that in the latter instance Tc-99m-sestamibi activity was

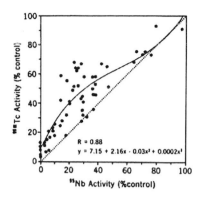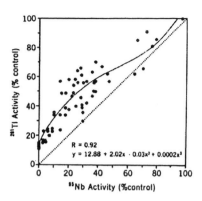

Figure 2. Scatterplots showing the relationship between blood flow assessed with Nb-95-microspheres and Tc-99m-sestamibi (left panel) or thallium-201 (right panel) uptake, expressed in percentage of control values, in myocardial samples from dogs injected 5 minutes before the end of coronary occlusion and killed 35 minutes thereafter. A third-degree polynomial fitting curve is depicted in each panel, while the dotted lines represent the line of identity. An overestimation of flow is registered with both tracers, particularly at flow levels ranging from 10 to 40% of control. At very low flow values (10%), the overestimation seems reduced, particularly with Tc-99m-sestamibi. Reprinted with permission from Canby *et al.*, Circulation 1990;81:289-96.

significantly lower than microsphere activity, thus indicating that other factors over blood flow influenced Tc-99m-sestamibi uptake, which therefore probably reflected also cellular viability (Figure 3). Freeman *et al.* reported similar results [8]. Sansoy *et al.* [9] demonstrated very close values for thallium-201 and Tc-99m-sestamibi uptake in a model of prolonged occlusion and reperfusion, although the redistribution images with thallium-201 achieved a slightly but significantly higher activity than the Tc-99m-sestamibi redistribution images.

In summary, all these data suggest that Tc-99m-sestamibi is not a pure flow tracer, but it tracks also the cell membrane integrity and therefore has a potential value as viability tracer, although some differences in tracer kinetics could lead to diverse results compared to thallium-201.

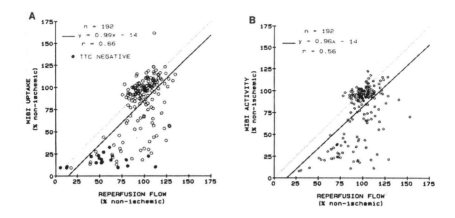

Figure 3. Scatterplots showing Tc-99m-sestamibi (MIBI) uptake versus microsphere-measured flow during reperfusion (both expressed in percent of nonischemic values) in experimental animals injected with Tc-99m-sestamibi 90 minutes after the end of coronary occlusion. Panel A shows the values at endocardial level, panel B shows the transmural values. In both cases, Tc-99m-sestamibi uptake is clearly lower than reperfusion flow; the difference is more marked in the nonviable segments, identified by the lack of triphenyltetrazolium staining (TTC negative). Reprinted with permission from Sinusas *et al.*, Circulation 1990;82:1424-37.

Clinical studies

There are no doubts that Tc-99m-sestamibi achieves excellent results for coronary artery disease detection, evaluation and prognostication, and that these results are very well comparable with those obtained using thallium-201 [10,11], with some potential advantage in particular settings and for the evaluation of left ventricular function using gated single-photon emission computed tomography (SPECT). In the context of the first studies about the use of Tc-99m-sestamibi for coronary artery disease detection, however, some data emerged that suggested a potential underestimation of myocardial viability. For instance, Parodi *et al.* [12] registered Tc-99m-sestamibi resting uptake defects in patients without known history of prior myocardial infarction. A major limit to this observation is that it was obtained using qualitative planar imaging in patients who were not evaluated for the specific issue of myocardial viability. In another study performed using planar imaging, Rocco *et al.* [13] identified the absence of Tc-99m-sestamibi uptake at visual assessment in seven of 37 segments with normal wall motion. However, quantitative Tc-99m-sestamibi uptake was significantly higher (62 ± 15%) in these segments than in the other segments with visually absent uptake and akinesia (39 ± 16%, p = 0.02).

Furthermore, these results are not directly applicable to the issue of myocardial viability because segments with preserved wall motion are by definition viable. The concerns about the reliability of Tc-99m-sestamibi as viability tracer were reinforced by other studies that compared resting imaging with this agent with reinjection or rest-redistribution thallium-201 scintigraphy. Cuocolo *et al.* [14] demonstrated a significant under-estimation of stress defect reversibility using stress-rest Tc-99m-sestamibi planar scintigraphy (18%) than using stress-redistribution-reinjection thallium-201 images (47%, $p < 0.001$). However, the segments were examined independently of their wall motion status and only visual analysis was used. The same group studied a similar patient population [15], performing rest-redistribution thallium-201 planar images and divided the segments according to the degree of defect reversibility: they observed a lower resting Tc-99m-sestamibi uptake score in 26 of 285 examined segments, which had a normal or only moderately reduced delayed thallium-201 uptake score. Using quantitative analysis of planar thallium-201 rest-redistribution and resting Tc-99m-sestamibi images, Maurea *et al.* [16] demonstrated a significantly lower Tc-99m-sestamibi uptake in segments supplied by totally occluded coronary vessels with good collaterals; furthermore, a significantly lower Tc-99m-sestamibi uptake compared to delayed thallium-201 was also registered in the segments with hypokinesia or a-dyskinesia, but not in those segments with normal wall motion. However, in the two groups of dysfunctional segments, the mean values of Tc-99m-sestamibi uptake appeared quite high, being 86% and 69% of maximum, respectively. Using resting qualitative SPECT, Dondi *et al.* [17] demonstrated in 8 of 104 severe stress defects the lack of reversibility in resting Tc-99m-sestamibi compared to thallium-201 rest-redistribution imaging, but functional parameters of these segments were not examined. On the other hand, Diliszian *et al.* [18] found that the underestimation of stress defect reversibility in resting Tc-99m-sestamibi SPECT compared to thallium-201 reinjection involved only 4 of 37 akinetic or dyskinetic regions, in which viability was a relevant diagnostic issue. Different results were reported by Kaufmann *et al.* [19] using quantitative analysis of SPECT data and comparing Tc-99m-sestamibi and thallium-201 uptake in patients with clear left ventricular dysfunction due to chronic coronary artery disease. They registered very close levels of resting Tc-99m-sestamibi and resting and redistribution thallium-201 activity (Figure 4). In summary, these comparative studies suggest that the discrepancy between Tc-99m-sestamibi and thallium-201 uptake is at best a modest one, with questionable clinical consequences. Furthermore, more recent reports have clearly shown that thallium-201 imaging in general [20], and defect reversibility in particular [21], are quite poor reference standards for myocardial viability (see also Chapter 4 by Bax *et al.*).

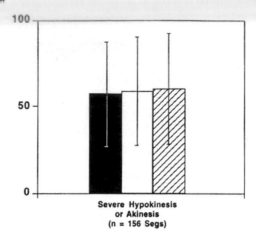

Figure 4. Bar graph showing thallium-201 uptake early after resting injection (solid bar), three hours after injection (open bar) and resting Tc-99m-sestamibi uptake (hatched bar) in segments with severe wall motion abnormality. Values are expressed in percent of normal as the mean ± standard deviation. The substantial overlap of the results is readily appreciable. Reprinted with permission from Kauffman *et al.*, J Am Coll Cardiol 1996;27: 592-7.

Among the noninvasive methods for viability detection, myocardial metabolic imaging using fluorine-18 deoxyglucose (FDG) and positron emission tomography (PET) is considered one of the most reliable and accurate [20]. Therefore, the studies comparing Tc-99m-sestamibi imaging with FDG PET data have given a major contribution to define the value of Tc-99m-sestamibi imaging for the assessment of viability. First, it must be remembered that it was proposed with good results to use Tc-99m-sestamibi instead of nitrogen-13 (N-13)-ammonia or of oxygen-15 (O-15)-water to achieve the perfusion data to be compared with FDG metabolism [22]. Other authors, however, starting from this approach, tried also to analyze the relationship between resting Tc-99m-sestamibi uptake and FDG signs of preserved metabolism. Altehoefer *et al.* [23], studying 46 patients, demonstrated FDG uptake in 23% of the segments with reduced Tc-99m-sestamibi uptake; however, FDG uptake was never observed in segments with Tc-99m-sestamibi activity < 30% of maximum; furthermore, 80% of segments with very low Tc-99m-sestamibi activity showed no signs of viability in PET. The same authors extended these observations in another study to a much larger patient population, with similar results [24]. A disagreement between Tc-99m-sestamibi and FDG data was observed in 39 of 111 patients, but 47 of 57 segments with Tc-99m-sestamibi activity < 30% of maximum were found nonviable also by FDG PET (Figure 5); an overall relationship was demonstrated (r = 0.61, p < 0.001) between Tc-99m-sestamibi uptake and FDG PET viability.

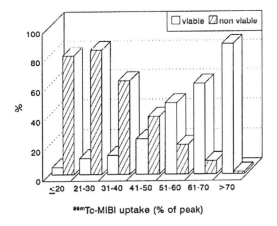

Figure 5. Bar graph showing the relationship between the percentage of viable (normalized FDG uptake > 70%) or nonviable (normalized FDG uptake < 50%) segments according to PET imaging and the level of Tc-99m-sestamibi (MIBI) activity. Reprinted with permission from Altehoefer *et al.* J Nucl Med 1994;35:569-74.

These results were partly contradicted in a report by Sawada *et al.* [25], who detected FDG signs of preserved viability in 5 of 18 patients with perfusion defects in Tc-99m-sestamibi SPECT and did not demonstrate a difference in the rate of FDG uptake in the segments with <50% Tc-99m-sestamibi uptake versus the segments with Tc-99m-sestamibi activity > 50% and < 60%. However, it has to be noted that defect overestimation by Tc-99m-sestamibi was mainly observed in inferior wall defects, where the lack of attenuation correction in SPECT compared to PET images could have played a major role. Also in the study by Soufer *et al.* [26] the defect location was very important for determining a disagreement between FDG PET and Tc-99m-sestamibi data. The authors demonstrated a good agreement between Tc-99m-sestamibi and PET data in 131 of 185 regions, PET viability in 39 regions negative for Tc-99m-sestamibi and preserved Tc-99m-sestamibi uptake in 15 regions without FDG signs of viability. Inferior segments contributed to more than 50% of discordant segments with FDG viability and Tc-99m-sestamibi uptake defect. Another factor that could partly explain the underestimation of viability using Tc-99m-sestamibi could be the degree of left ventricular impairment. According to Arrighi *et al.* [27], a Tc-99m-sestamibi/FDG mismatch was more frequently observed in patients with severe left ventricular ejection fraction decrease (< 25%) than in those with more moderate functional reduction. In a subgroup of patients of their already mentioned study, Dilsizian *et al.* [18] compared the results of stress-redistribution-reinjection thallium-201

SPECT and stress-rest Tc-99m-sestamibi SPECT with FDG PET. In this group, FDG uptake was detected in 17 of 22 regions in which reversibility was discordantly demonstrated by either Tc-99m-sestamibi (4 regions) or thallium-201 (18 regions). Seventeen of those 22 regions, however, had only a mild-to-moderate decrease in Tc-99m-sestamibi activity when SPECT quantification was performed. Thus, considering also the quantitative data, the underestimation of viability by Tc-99m-sestamibi compared to thallium-201 and to PET involved only four regions. In summary, these studies confirm the possibility of some underestimation of viability using Tc-99m-sestamibi as compared to PET, but also suggest that an appropriate evaluation of Tc-99m-sestamibi data, including quantification of tracer activity and use of proper thresholds, clearly limits the degree of underestimation. It is also important to emphasize that also thallium-201 is known to underestimate viability as compared to PET and that even this latter method is not devoid of limitations when compared with the other gold standards, such as the demonstration of functional recovery of an asynergic region after successful revascularization [20].

The first studies that evaluated the capability of Tc-99m-sestamibi imaging to recognize viable hibernating myocardium having as reference the post-revascularization outcome were published by Marzullo *et al.* who used the quantitative analysis of planar imaging [28], and extended in one report the comparison to thallium-201 and low-dose dobutamine echocardiography [29]. Although the authors concluded in both studies that Tc-99m-sestamibi is not a reliable viability tracer, their results do not completely support this conclusion. In the first report, the predictive values of Tc-99m-sestamibi imaging were indeed quite good, registering a 79% positive and a 76% negative predictive value [28]. In the second study, sensitivity and specificity of Tc-99m-sestamibi (75% and 84%, respectively) were close to what was obtained using thallium-201 (86% and 92%, respectively) or low-dose dobutamine echocardiography (82% and 92%, respectively) [29]. More convincing and even statistically significant was the underestimation of viability using Tc-99m-sestamibi compared to thallium in a later report by the same group [30]. A major limitation of this and of the two other mentioned studies is related to the use of planar imaging, which is no longer considered appropriate for Tc-99m-sestamibi scintigraphy. Furthermore, the results were analyzed on a segment basis only, with relatively few segments wrongly classified and no data were reported about the potential impact of these incorrect evaluations on patient management. On the other hand, the potential value of Tc-99m-sestamibi SPECT to predict post-revascularization recovery was demonstrated in two studies performed using SPECT. Maublant *et al.* [31], using a qualitative scoring of Tc-99m-sestamibi uptake were able to identify a normal, mildly reduced or moderately reduced activity in 15 of 21 regions with subsequent recovery and in none of the regions which showed unchanged asynergy after coronary artery bypass grafting. Udelson *et al.* [32] compared the quantitative uptake of resting Tc-99m-sestamibi SPECT and of rest-redistribution thallium-201 and were able to correctly classify most asynergic regions as either viable or nonviable using the same activity cut off value of 60% of maximum, with positive predictive values of 80% and 75%, respectively for Tc-99m-sestamibi and thallium-201, and negative predictive values of 96% and 92%, respectively (Figure 6). Two other studies used as reference standard both the post-revascularization recovery and the analysis of the histologic changes in bioptic samples obtained within asynergic regions. In patients with severe wall motion abnormalities in the territory of the left anterior descending artery, Dakik *et al.* [33] observed a good correlation between quantified Tc-99m-sestamibi uptake and amount of viable tissue in the bioptic specimens (Figure 7). Furthermore, a significantly higher Tc-99m-sestamibi activity was demonstrated in the segments with post-revascularization recovery than in the others. Maes *et al.* [34] studied 30 patients with similar features, and submitted them to Tc-99m-sestamibi SPECT, perfusion/metabolism PET, transmural biopsy and post-operative control of wall motion outcome after revascularization. They observed significantly higher Tc-99m-sestamibi activity in patients with PET viability and with post-revascularization recovery than in the remaining patients. Moreover, they demonstrated an inverse linear relation between Tc-99m-sestamibi uptake and percent fibrosis in the biopsy specimen.

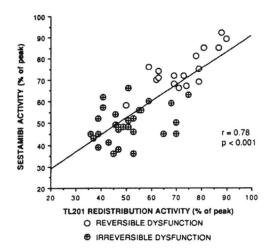

Figure 6. Scatterplot showing the relationship between thallium-201 (Tl-201) redistribution and Tc-99m-sestamibi activity in segments with regional dysfunction of patients submitted to coronary revascularization. The open circles represent the segments with reversible dysfunction, the circles with the cross those with unchanged dysfunction. Reprinted with permission from Udelson *et al. Circulation* 1994;89:2552-61.

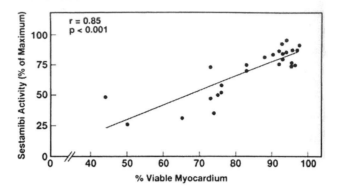

Figure 7. Correlation between Tc-99m-sestamibi activity and percent of viable myocardium in biopsy specimens of the anterior wall. Reprinted with permission from Dakik *et al.* Circulation 1997;96:2892-8.

Taking into account the major role which dedicated scintigraphic protocols, such as late redistribution, reinjection and rest-redistribution imaging play for viability detection using thallium-201, attempts have been made to introduce modifications to the standard resting Tc-99m-sestamibi image in order to improve the tracer ability to recognize viable myocardium. With respect to the very limited redistribution of Tc-99m-sestamibi, Dilsizian *et al.* [18] demonstrated in redistribution images a significant increase in Tc-99m-sestamibi activity in 6 of 16 regions in which viability was underestimated compared with thallium-201. Maurea *et al.* [35] demonstrated Tc-99m-sestamibi redistribution in 24% of segments with severe uptake defects; in the subgroup of patients submitted to coronary revascularization, the finding of Tc-99m-sestamibi redistribution appeared to be very sensitive and specific for predicting functional recovery.
An alternative approach to increase the value of Tc-99m-sestamibi imaging for viability detection was proposed by Worsley *et al.* [36], who administered the tracer using a slow intravenous infusion and demonstrated an increase in tracer uptake in segments with reduced activity in standard images.

Gated SPECT imaging

Since the acquisition of Tc-99m-sestamibi SPECT images with electrocardiographic gating gives the opportunity to combine perfusion data with functional information, other authors examined the possible role of gated SPECT for improving the recognition of myocardial viability with

Tc-99m-sestamibi. González *et al.* [37] performed a visual analysis of Tc-99m-sestamibi uptake in stress and rest images and classified the asynergic segments as viable based on the presence of either normal uptake or of stress defect reversibility. Then, they also considered the gated resting images and classified as viable the segments with preserved wall motion or thickening according to the visual evaluation of systolic and diastolic frames. Their results were rather disappointing (overall accuracy = 53%) and were not significantly influenced by the addition of gated data (overall accuracy = 59%). The authors also examined the relation between post-revascularization outcome and quantitative data derived from polar map displays obtained from both gated and ungated SPECT studies. There was a significant relationship between changes in defect extent and severity and post-revascularization recovery, and the relationship was slightly more significant using the gated than the ungated polar maps. Unfortunately, no data are reported about the sensitivity and specificity achievable with the use of quantitative analysis. A most important limitation of this study is that the patient population included a majority of patients with preserved left ventricular function, and that the value of resting Tc-99m-sestamibi uptake in stress defects without reversibility was disregarded. In a most recent study, Levine *et al.* [38] also tried to estimate the possible advantage of obtaining functional data with gated SPECT over the sole evaluation of perfusion images. Using a scoring scheme for both perfusion and gated SPECT wall motion, they achieved a good sensitivity (79%) but a poor specificity (55%) with the perfusion score and a further increase in sensitivity (95%), without specificity changes (50%) and a significant improvement in overall accuracy (91% versus 85%) when the persistence of some degree of wall motion (thus excluding akinetic and dyskinetic segments only) was added as an additional viability criterion. These promising results must be cautiously evaluated because of the study limitations. First, all revascularized segments, independently of their pre-revascularization wall motion status, were included in the analysis; second, a segment was defined viable according to post-revascularization follow up not only in the presence of functional recovery but also in the case of perfusion improvement.

Tc-99-sestamibi nitrate imaging

The most interesting dedicated protocol for the detection of viable myocardium using Tc-99m-sestamibi is based on the injection of the tracer in combination with the short-term administration of nitrates. It is well known that among the anti-ischemic actions of this category of drugs there is the capability to dilate epicardial coronary artery stenoses and to improve collateral flow in the coronary vessels [39]. These actions do not play a major role in the chronic therapy with these agents, but can be probably elicited during the short-term administration of relatively high dose of nitrates. Preliminary experiences had already demonstrated a possible role of nitrate administration for the detection of hibernating myocardium. Helfant *et al.* [40] had shown a relationship between transient recovery of regional wall motion in contrast ventriculography performed during nitrate administration and subsequent recovery after coronary artery bypass grafting. On the other hand, various studies had demonstrated that perfusion tracer uptake was increased under nitrate administration and suggested a relationship with the presence of collateral circulation [41]. As regards redistribution thallium-201 imaging, He *et al.* [42] had shown an increase in stress defect reversibility after sublingual nitrates; a similar observation was made in rest Tc-99m-teboroxime imaging by Bisi *et al.* [43]. In patients with recent myocardial infarction, Galli *et al.* [44] found that resting Tc-99m-sestamibi defects that improved under nitrates were related with better regional wall motion and more severe coronary obstruction than defects that did not show any change.

The first demonstration that nitrate Tc-99m-sestamibi imaging could be a valuable approach to the detection of viable hibernating myocardium was reported by Bisi *et al.* [45]. In their first study, they submitted to both baseline resting and nitrate Tc-99m-sestamibi SPECT 19 patients with left ventricular dysfunction due to chronic coronary artery disease and who later underwent either bypass surgery or coronary angioplasty. The extent of the perfusion defects under baseline conditions and under nitrate infusion was evaluated using a reference database of normal controls and expressed in terms of percentage of left ventricular wall. The authors observed a close relationship between the finding of a reduction in defect extent under nitrates compared to baseline and the finding of post-revascularization recovery of regional wall motion in the involved coronary artery territory (Figure 8). The same group explored the possibility that the increase in Tc-99m-sestamibi activity in nitrate SPECT were not caused by a real increase in tracer uptake but were just apparent and related through the partial volume effect to the wall motion or wall thickening improvement produced by the general hemodynamic action of nitrates [46]. They compared the predictive value of nitrate-induced perfusion versus regional wall motion changes, with the latter assessed using first pass angiocardiography performed during Tc-99m-sestamibi injection both at rest and under nitrate infusion. The results of this study showed that there was only a poor relationship between nitrate-induced wall motion changes and post-revascularization recovery, with only 25 of 44 asynergic regions correctly classified as either viable or nonviable, while the relationship was significantly higher when nitrate-induced perfusion changes were examined, with 40 of 44 regions assigned to the true category.

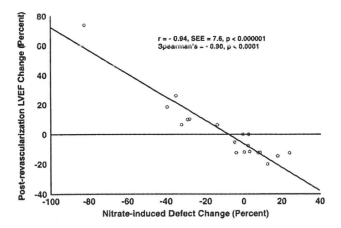

Figure 8. Correlation between the change in extent of perfusion defects induced by nitrate infusion (expressed as percent of the baseline resting value) and the change in left ventricular ejection fraction (LVEF) detected after coronary revascularization (expressed as percent of the prerevascularization LVEF). Reprinted with permission from Bisi *et al.* J Am Coll Cardiol 1994;24:1282-9.

Other groups [47-49], who were able to reproduce the above-described results, although with minor modifications of the imaging protocol, independently demonstrated the value of nitrate Tc-99m-sestamibi imaging. The gain over baseline imaging achieved using nitrate SPECT was assessed by Sciagrà *et al.* [50] in a study in which they compared the receiver operating characteristic (ROC) curves of baseline and nitrate defect extent for the detection of viable hibernating myocardium, demonstrating a significantly larger area under the nitrate curve. The same authors also compared baseline-nitrate Tc-99m-sestamibi results with thallium-201 rest-redistribution SPECT [51], demonstrating a substantial equivalence in overall accuracy and predictive value, with slightly (but not significantly) better results using Tc-99m-sestamibi. Furthermore, these data suggest that nitrate induced changes in tracer uptake give important information and therefore that the direct quantification of nitrate Tc-99m-sestamibi activity without comparison with the baseline value could be less effective (Figure 9). Other authors, however, achieved very good results using nitrate enhanced Tc-99m-sestamibi imaging alone [52].

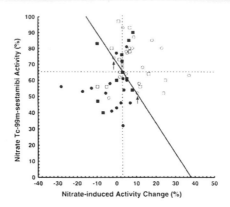

Figure 9. Scatterplot showing the relationship between nitrate-induced activity change and nitrate Tc-99m-sestamibi activity. The squares represent the coronary territories with less severe pre-revascularization wall motion abnormality, the circles those with severe dysfunction. The open symbols represent the territories with post-revascularization functional recovery, the solid ones those with unchanged regional dysfunction. The vertical and horizontal dotted lines indicate the threshold value of each variable which best differentiate viable from nonviable coronary territories. The solid line depicts the discriminant function including both variables that appears to differentiate optimally viable from nonviable territories. The arrows indicate two territories reclassified as nonviable after the jack-knife cross-validation procedure. Reprinted with permission from Sciagrà *et al.* J Am Coll Cardiol 1997;30:384-91.

Tc-99m-tetrofosmin

Tc-99m-tetrofosmin is currently regarded as alternative to Tc-99m-sestamibi for myocardial perfusion scintigraphy using a technetium-99m-labeled tracer [53]. This compound is a lipophilic phosphine ethane cation, with uptake and retention kinetics quite similar to those of Tc-99m-sestamibi, including a postulated major role played by sarcolemmal and mitochondrial trans-membrane potentials [54,55]. Minor differences are present in net extraction, redistribution (which seems completely lacking), lung, and liver clearance, but have no major consequences on clinical utilization. Because of the more recent introduction, both experimental and clinical studies about the use of Tc-99m-tetrofosmin for the issue of viability detection are much more limited than those available for Tc-99m-sestamibi.

Koplan *et al.* [56] compared thallium-201 and Tc-99m-tetrofosmin uptake in a canine model of prolonged low coronary flow with resulting severe ventricular dysfunction. The mean ischemic to normal uptake ratio of Tc-99m-tetrofosmin was similar to initial thallium-201 ratio but significantly lower than delayed thallium-201 ratio. However, there was preserved Tc-99m-tetrofosmin uptake in segments with clearly reduced coronary flow.

As regards the clinical studies, Matsunari *et al.* [57] performed a comparison of the evolution of stress-induced defects in stress-rest Tc-99m-tetrofosmin SPECT and thallium-201 stress-redistribution-reinjection SPECT. Of 209 stress defects identified by both tracers, 73 were found to be reversible using thallium-201 but not reversible using Tc-99m-tetrofosmin, with a final apparent underestimation of viability in 35% of exercise abnormal segments. Tc-99m-tetrofosmin uptake quantification allowed the reduction of viability underestimation in several segments, with a final agreement in 90% of segments. Conversely, redistribution imaging did not give any contribution to the containment of viability underestimation. In another study from the same group [58], resting Tc-99m-tetrofosmin SPECT was compared with rest-redistribution thallium-201 SPECT, having as reference the post-revascularization outcome of regional asynergy. Using ROC analysis and a different optimal threshold of activity for each tracer, the authors reported the same positive predictive value (69%) and a slightly higher negative predictive value (82%) for Tc-99m-tetrofosmin compared to thallium-201 (71%) (Figure 10).

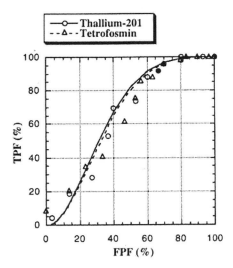

Figure 10. ROC curves of resting Tc-99m-tetrofosmin and rest-redistribution thallium-201 activity in segments undergoing revascularization. Measured points (symbols) have been obtained for every 5% change in threshold activity, and have been fitted with the appropriate curve. The closed symbols indicate the optimal threshold value for thallium-201 (circle, 55% of peak activity) and for Tc-99m-tetrofosmin (triangle, 50% of peak activity), respectively. FPF = false positive fraction (100 - specificity); TPF = true positive fraction (sensitivity). Reprinted with permission from Matsunari *et al.* J Am Coll Cardiol 1997;29:1226-33.

Taking into account the lack of redistribution of Tc-99m-tetrofosmin, some groups tried to combine resting imaging with the administration of nitrates. Thorley *et al.* [59] demonstrated reversibility in 12 of 23 stress induced defects, which did not improve in standard resting images. Derebek *et al.* [60] submitted patients to thallium-201 stress-redistribution-reinjection and to 24 hour late redistribution imaging and to stress-rest Tc-99m-tetrofosmin imaging followed the subsequent day by resting 1-hour Tc-99m-tetrofosmin infusion after sublingual administration of nitrates. Of 100 fixed defects in standard Tc-99m-tetrofosmin imaging, 15 showed improvement after nitrates and infusion, with a final agreement regarding reversibility in 91% of stress induced defects. However, wall motion data were not considered in this population, so that no conclusion can be derived for the specific issue of viability detection. In a study group consisting of patients with left ventricular dysfunction, Flotats *et al.* [61] compared rest-reinjection-redistribution thallium-201 SPECT with resting and post-nitrate imaging with Tc-99m-tetrofosmin using a double-day protocol. They could demonstrated after nitrates an increase in Tc-99m-tetrofosmin uptake over the 50% activity threshold in 11 of 73 segments, with a final overall agreement in viability classification between thallium-201 and Tc-99m-tetrofosmin in 90% of the examined segments. Similar results, but in a mixed population of patients with and without left ventricular dysfunction, were more recently reported by Peix *et al.* [62]. In summary, these results seem to suggest that also Tc-99m-tetrofosmin could have a potential role as viability tracer, but further studies are needed before the same reliability of Tc-99m-sestamibi can be achieved.

Conclusions

The definitive role of Tc-99m-sestamibi or Tc-99m-tetrofosmin imaging in the context of the various methods currently available for the noninvasive detection of viable hibernating myocardium and the prediction of post-revascularization outcome of patients with left ventricular dysfunction because of chronic coronary artery disease is still debated. Table 1 tries to summarize the available data. The total number of patients submitted to perfusion imaging with a Tc-99m-labeled tracer in published studies is already quite large, with over 350 patients evaluated, although some overlap certainly exists between reports from the same authors. Unfortunately, the published studies differ in many respects, including the selection of the patient population, the imaging protocol, and the approach to data analysis. Therefore, no attempt has been made to calculate mean values for the estimated diagnostic parameters: in general, the achieved reliability appears quite satisfactory. Interestingly, the diagnostic performance of Tc-99m-sestamibi (the data for Tc-99m-tetrofosmin are still

Table 1. Sensitivity, specificity, overall accuracy and predictive values of Tc-99-sestamibi for the detection of myocardial viability in studies having as reference the post-revascularization outcome.

Reference	Imaging protocol	Data analysis	Patients (segs.)	LVEF (%)	Sens. (%)	Spec. (%)	Acc. (%)	PPV (%)	NPV (%)
Marzullo 1992	Planar resting	Quantitative	14 (73)	43±9	83	68	77	78	75
Marzullo 1993	Planar resting	Quantitative	14 (75)	39±7	75	84	76	88	62
Udelson 1994	SPECT resting	Quantitative	18 (46)	34±10	94	86	89	80	96
Bisi 1994	SPECT nitrate-resting	Quantitative	19 (45)	35±10	91	88	89	71	97
Maublant 1995	SPECT resting	Qualitative	25 (27)	52±15	100	67	93	91	100
Bisi 1995	SPECT nitrate-resting	Quantitative	28 (44)	36±10	95	88	91	86	96
Marzullo 1995	Planar resting	Quantitative	22 (105)	44±13	71	53	63	63	63
Maurea 1995	SPECT nitrate-resting	Quantitative	8 (52)	36±9	88	89	88	88	89
Sciagrà 1996	SPECT resting	Quantitative	40 (66)	35±9	75	66	70	62	78
Sciagrà 1996	SPECT nitrate	Quantitative	40 (66)	35±9	96	66	79	68	96
Gonzalez 1996	SPECT resting	Qualitative	36 (90)	52±15	79	35	53	48	67
Gonzalez 1996	Gated SPECT	Qualitative	36 (80)	52±15	77	44	59	52	71
Li 1996	SPECT nitrate-resting	Quantitative	27 (198)	35±13	83	81	82	81	84
Greco 1996	SPECT nitrate-resting	Qualitative	23	43±4	75	71	74	86	56
Maes 1997	SPECT resting	Quantitative	23	47±13	92	60	78	75	86
Dakik 1997	SPECT resting	Quantitative	21 (85)	41±13	82	50	71	75	60
Sciagrà 1997	SPECT nitrate-resting	Qualitative	35 (56)	36±8	77	77	77	79	74
Schneider 1998	SPECT nitrate	Quantitative	31	54±12	95	83	90	90	91
Matsunari[a] 1997	SPECT resting	Quantitative	21 (79)	42±8	96	30	71	69	82

[a] = this study was performed using Tc-99m-tetrofosmin.
Legend: LVEF = left ventricular ejection fraction; Segs. = segments; Sens. = sensitivity; Spec. = specificity; Acc. = overall accuracy; PPV = positive predictive value; NPV = negative predictive value.

scanty) seems to be maintained in the study cohorts including patients with more severe left ventricular dysfunction. With respect to the technical issues, the best data are apparently obtained using quantitative SPECT and the addition of nitrate-enhanced imaging. Thus, it could be suggested that Tc-99m-labeled perfusion tracers are a reliable approach to viability detection if a dedicated protocol and appropriate imaging modalities are employed. Various points still need to be addressed: for instance, the relationship with post-revascularization global left ventricular function evolution and with long-term prognosis. Preliminary data suggest that Tc-99m-sestamibi SPECT can predict global left ventricular ejection fraction changes and that nitrate imaging is more effective than baseline imaging also in this regard [63]. Other preliminary data indicate that a relationship between detection of myocardial viability, subsequent treatment and prognosis can be found using nitrate-enhanced Tc-99m-sestamibi SPECT with results comparable to those reported using FDG PET or thallium-201 imaging [64]. Another issue that deserves further studies is the potential role of gated SPECT for the detection of myocardial viability. Although limited and conflicting data have been so far published [37,38], the lack of major additional costs using gated SPECT imaging and the perspective of combining this approach with other modifications of the standard protocol (like nitrate enhanced imaging), or with inotropic stimulations to assess the contractile reserve of asynergic segments [65], indicate that further substantial developments have to be expected regarding the role of Tc-99m-labeled perfusion tracers for detection of viability.

References

1. Okada RD, Glover D, Gaffney T, Williams S. Myocardial kinetics of technetium-99m-hexakis-2-methoxy-2-methylpropyl-isonitrile. Circulation 1988;77:491-8.
2. Leppo JA, Meerdink DJ. Comparison of the myocardial uptake of a technetium-labeled isonitrile and thallium. Circ Res 1989;65:632-9.
3. Piwnica-Worms D, Kronauge JF, Chiu ML. Uptake and retention of hexakis (2-methoxyisobutyl isonitrile) technetium (I) in cultured chick myocardial cells. Mitochondrial and plasma membrane potential dependence. Circulation 1990;82:1826-38.
4. Piwnica-Worms D, Chiu ML, Kronauge JF. Divergent kinetics of 201Tl and 99mTc-sestamibi in cultured chick ventricular myocites during ATP depletion. Circulation 1992;85:1531-41.
5. Beanlands RSB, Dawood F, Wen WH et al. Are the kinetics of technetium-99m methoxyisobutyl isonitrile affected by cell metabolism and viability? Circulation 1990;82:1802-14.
6. Canby RC, Silber S, Pohost GM. Relations of the myocardial imaging agents 99mTc-MIBI and 201Tl to myocardial blood flow in a canine model of myocardial ischemic insult. Circulation 1990;81:289-96.
7. Sinusas AJ, Trautman KA, Bergin JD et al. Quantification of area at risk during coronary occlusion and degree of myocardial salvage after reperfusion with technetium-99m methoxyisobutyl isonitrile. Circulation 1990;82:1424-37.

8. Freeman I, Grunwald AM, Hoory S, Bodenheimer MM. Effect of coronary occlusion and myocardial viability on myocardial activity of technetium-99m-sestamibi. J Nucl Med 1991;32:292-8.

9. Sansoy V, Glover DK, Watson DD *et al*. Comparison of thallium-201 resting redistribution with technetium-99m-sestamibi uptake and functional response to dobutamine for assessment of myocardial viability. Circulation 1995;92:994-1004.

10. Wackers F, Berman D, Maddahi J *et al*. Technetium-99m hexakis 2-methoxyisobutyl isonitrile: human biodistribution, dosimetry, safety and preliminary comparison to thallium-201 for myocardial perfusion imaging. J Nucl Med 1989;30:301-11.

11. Kiat H, Maddahi J, Roy LT *et al*. Comparison of technetium 99m methoxy isobutyl isonitrile and thallium-201 for evaluation of coronary artery disease by planar and tomographic methods. Am Heart J 1989;117:1-11.

12. Parodi O, Marcassa C, Casucci R *et al*. Accuracy and safety of Technetium-99m hexakis 2-methoxy-2-isobutyl isonitrile (sestamibi) myocardial scintigraphy with high dose dipyridamole test in patients with effort angina pectoris: a multicenter study. J Am Coll Cardiol 1991;18:1439-44.

13. Rocco TP, Dilsizian V, Strauss HW, Boucher CA. Technetium-99m isonitrile myocardial uptake at rest. II. Relation to clinical markers of potential viability. J Am Coll Cardiol 1989;14:1678-84.

14. Cuocolo A, Pace L, Ricciardelli B, Chiariello M, Trimarco B, Salvatore M. Identification of viable myocardium in patients with chronic coronary artery disease: comparison of thallium-201 scintigraphy with reinjection and technetium-99m-methoxyisobutyl isonitrile. J Nucl Med 1992;33:505-11.

15. Cuocolo A, Maurea S, Pace L *et al*. Resting technetium-99m methoxyisobutylisonitrile cardiac imaging in chronic coronary artery disease: comparison with rest-redistribution thallium-201 scintigraphy. Eur J Nucl Med 1993;20:1186-92.

16. Maurea S, Cuocolo A, Pace L *et al*. Rest-injected thallium-201 redistribution and resting technetium-99m methoxyisobutylisonitrile uptake in coronary artery disease: relation to the severity of coronary artery stenosis. Eur J Nucl Med 1993;20:502-10.

17. Dondi M, Tartagni F, Fallani F *et al*. A comparison of rest sestamibi and rest-redistribution thallium single photon emission tomography: possible implications for myocardial viability detection in infarcted patients. Eur J Nucl Med 1993;20:26-31.

18. Dilsizian V, Arrighi JA, Diodati JG *et al*. Myocardial viability in patients with chronic coronary artery disease. Comparison of 99mTc-sestamibi with thallium reinjection and [18F] fluorodeoxyglucose. Circulation 1994;89:578-87.

19. Kauffman GJ, Boyne TS, Watson DD, Smith WH, Beller GA. Comparison of rest thallium-201 imaging and rest technetium-99m sestamibi imaging for assessment of myocardial viability in patients with coronary artery disease and severe left ventricular dysfunction. J Am Coll Cardiol 1996;27:1592-7.

20. Bax JJ, Wijns W, Cornel JH, Visser FC, Boersma E, Fioretti PM. Accuracy of the currently available techniques for prediction of functional recovery after revascularization in patients with left ventricular dysfunction due to chronic coronary artery disease: comparison of pooled data. J Am Coll Cardiol 1997;30:1451-60.

21. Sciagrà R, Santoro GM, Bisi G, Pedenovi P, Fazzini PF, Pupi A. Rest-redistribution thallium-201 SPECT to detect myocardial viability. J Nucl Med 1998;39:384-90.

22. Lucignani G, Paolini G, Landoni C *et al*. Presurgical identification of hibernating myocardium by combined use of technetium-99m hexakis 2-methoxyisobutylisonitrile single photon emission tomography and fluorine-18-fluoro-2-deoxy-D-glucose positron emission tomography in patients with coronary artery disease. Eur J Nucl Med 1992;19:874-81.

23. Altehoefer C, Kaiser HJ, Dörr R *et al*. Fluorine-18 deoxyglucose PET for the assessment of viable myocardium in perfusion defects in 99mTc-MIBI SPET: a comparative study in patients with coronary artery disease. Eur J Nucl Med 1992;19:334-42.

24. Altehoefer C, von Dahl J, Biedermann M *et al*. Significance of defect severity in technetium-99m-MIBI SPECT at rest to assess myocardial viability: comparison with fluorine-18-FDG PET. J Nucl Med 1994;35:569-74.
25. Sawada SG, Allman KC, Muzik O *et al*. Positron emission tomography detects evidence of viability in rest technetium-99m sestamibi defects. J Am Coll Cardiol 1994;23:92-8.
26. Soufer R, Dey HM, Ng CK, Zaret BL. Comparison of sestamibi single-photon emission computed tomography with positron emission tomography for estimating left ventricular myocardial viability. Am J Cardiol 1995;75:1214-19.
27. Arrighi JA, Ng CK, Dey HM, Wackers FJT, Soufer R. Effect of left ventricular function on the assessment of myocardial viability by technetium-99m sestamibi and correlation with positron emission tomography in patients with healed myocardial infarcts or stable angina pectoris or both. Am J Cardiol 1997;80:1007-13.
28. Marzullo P, Sambuceti G, Parodi O. The role of sestamibi scintigraphy in the radio-isotopic assessment of myocardial viability. J Nucl Med 1992;33:1925-30.
29. Marzullo P, Parodi O, Reisenhofer B *et al*. Value of rest thallium-201/technetium-99m sestamibi scans and dobutamine echocardiography for detecting myocardial viability. Am J Cardiol 1993;71:166-72.
30. Marzullo P, Sambuceti G, Parodi O *et al*. Regional concordance and discordance between rest thallium 201 and sestamibi imaging for assessing tissue viability: comparison with postrevascularization functional recovery. J Nucl Cardiol 1995;2:309-16.
31. Maublant JC, Citron B, Lipiecki J *et al*. Rest technetium 99m-sestamibi tomoscintigraphy in hibernating myocardium. Am Heart J 1995;129:306-14.
32. Udelson JE, Coleman PS, Metherall J *et al*. Predicting recovery of severe regional ventricular dysfunction: comparison of resting scintigraphy with 201Tl and 99mTc-sestamibi. Circulation 1994;89:2552-61.
33. Dakik HA, Howell JF, Lawrie GM *et al*. Assessment of myocardial viability with 99mTc-sestamibi tomography before coronary bypass graft surgery: correlation with histopathology and postoperative improvement in cardiac function. Circulation 1997;96:2892-8.
34. Maes AF, Borgers M, Flameng W *et al*. Assessment of myocardial viability in chronic coronary artery disease using technetium-99m sestamibi SPECT. Correlation with histologic and positron emission tomographic studies and functional follow up. J Am Coll Cardiol 1997;29:62-8.
35. Maurea S, Cuocolo A, Soricelli A *et al*. Myocardial viability index in chronic coronary artery disease : technetium-99m-methoxy isobutyl isonitrile redistribution. J Nucl Med 1995;36:1953-60.
36. Worsley DF, Fung AY, Jue J, Burns RJ. Identification of viable myocardium with technetium-99m-MIBI infusion. J Nucl Med 1995;36:1037-9.
37. González P, Massardo T, Muñoz A *et al*. Is the addition of ECG gating to technetium-99m sestamibi SPET of value in the assessment of myocardial viability? An evaluation based on two-dimensional echocardiography following revascularization. Eur J Nucl Med 1996;23:1315-22.
38. Levine MG, McGill CC, Ahlberg AW *et al*. Functional assessment with electrocardiographic gated single-photon emission computed tomography improves the ability of technetium-99m sestamibi myocardial perfusion imaging to predict myocardial viability in patients undergoing revascularization. Am J Cardiol 1999;83:1-5.
39. Abrams J. Mechanisms of action of the organic nitrates in the treatment of myocardial ischemia. Am J Cardiol 1992;70:30B-42B.
40. Helfant RH, Pine R, Meister SG, Feldman MS, Trout RG, Banka VS. Nitroglyserin to unmask reversible asynergy. Correlation with post coronary bypass ventriculography. Circulation 1974;50:108-33.

41. Aoki M, Sakai K, Koyanagi S, Takeshita A, Nakamura M. Effect of nitroglycerin on coronary collateral function during exercise evaluated by quantitative analysis of thallium-201 single photon emission computed tomography. Am Heart J 1991;121:1361-6.
42. He Z-X, Darcourt J, Guigner A *et al.* Nitrates improve detection of ischemic but viable myocardium by thallium-201 reinjection SPECT. J Nucl Med 1993;34:1472-7.
43. Bisi G, Sciagrà R, Santoro GM, Zerauschek F, Fazzini PF. Sublingual isosorbide dinitrate to improve Tc-99m-teboroxime perfusion defect reversibility. J Nucl Med 1994;35:1274-8.
44. Galli M, Marcassa C, Imparato A, Campini R, Orrego PS, Giannuzzi P. Effects of nitroglycerin by Technetium-99m sestamibi tomoscintigraphy on resting regional myocardial hypoperfusion in stable patients with healed myocardial infarction. Am J Cardiol 1994;74:843-8.
45. Bisi G, Sciagrà R, Santoro GM, Fazzini PF. Rest technetium-99m sestamibi tomography in combination with short-term administration of nitrates: feasibility and reliability for prediction of postrevascularization outcome of asynergic territories. J Am Coll Cardiol 1994;24:1282-9.
46. Bisi G, Sciagrà R, Santoro GM, Rossi V, Fazzini PF. Techentium-99m-sestamibi imaging with nitrate infusion to detect viable hibernating myocardium and predict postrevascularization recovery. J Nucl Med 1995;36:1994-2000.
47. Maurea S, Cuocolo A, Soricelli A *et al.* Enhanced detection of viable myocardium by technetium-99m-MIBI imaging after nitrate administration in chronic coronary artery disease. J Nucl Med 1995;36:1945-52.
48. Li ST, Liu XJ, Lu ZL *et al.* Quantitative analysis of technetium 99m 2-methoxyisobutyl isonitrile single-photon emission computed tomography and isosorbide dinitrate infusion in assessment of myocardial viability before and after revascularization. J Nucl Cardiol 1996;3:457-63.
49. Greco C, Tanzilli G, Ciavolella M *et al.* Nitroglycerin-induced changes in myocardial sestamibi uptake to detect tissue viability: radionuclide comparison before and after revascularization. Coronary Artery Disease 1996;7:877-84.
50. Sciagrà R, Bisi G, Santoro GM, Agnolucci M, Zoccarato O, Fazzini PF. Influence of the assessment of defect severity and intravenous nitrate administration during tracer injection on the detection of viable hibernating myocardium with data-based quantitative technetium 99m-labeled sestamibi single photon emission computed tomography. J Nucl Cardiol 1996;3:221-30.
51. Sciagrà R, Bisi G, Santoro GM *et al.* Comparison of baseline-nitrate technetium-99m-sestamibi with rest-redistribution thallium-201 tomography in detecting viable hibernating myocardium and predicting postrevascularization recovery. J Am Coll Cardiol 1997;30:384-91.
52. Schneider CA, Voth E, Gawlich S *et al.* Significance of rest technetium-99m sestamibi imaging for the prediction of improvement of left ventricular dysfunction after Q wave myocardial infarction: importance of infarct location adjusted thresholds. J Am Coll Cardiol 1998;32:648-54.
53. Zaret BL, Rigo P, Wackers FJTh *et al.* Myocardial perfusion imaging with 99mTc-tetrofosmin. Comparison to 201Tl imaging and coronary angiography in a phase III multicentre trial. Circulation 1995;91:313-9.
54. Platts EA, North TL, Picket RD, Kelley JD. Mechanism of uptake of technetium-tetrofosmin. I: Uptake into isolated adult rat ventricular myocites and subcellular localization. J Nucl Cardiol 1995;2:317-26.
55. Younes A, Songadele JA; Maublant J *et al.* Mechanism of uptake of technetium-tetrofosmin. II: uptake into isolated adult rat heart mitochondria. J Nucl Cardiol 1995;2:327-33.

56. Koplan BA, Beller GA, Ruiz M *et al*. Comparison between thallium-201 and technetium-99m-tetrofosmin uptake with sustained low flow and profound systolic dysfunction. J Nucl Med 1996;37:1398-402.
57. Matsunari I, Fujino S, Taki J *et al*. Myocardial viability assessment with technetium-99m-tetrofosmin and thallium-201 reinjection in coronary artery disease. J Nucl Med 1995;36:1961-7.
58. Matsunari I, Fujino S, Taki J *et al*. Quantitative rest technetium-99m tetrofosmin imaging in predicting functional recovery after revascularization: comparison with rest-redistribution thallium-201. J Am Coll Cardiol 1997;29:1226-33.
59. Thorley PJ, Bloomer TN, Sheard KL *et al*. The use of GTN to improve the detection of ischaemic myocardium using 99mTc-tetrofosmin. Nucl Med Commun 1996;17:669-74.
60. Derebek E, Kozan O, Durak H *et al*. Sublingual nitrate plus 99Tcm-tetrofosmin infusion in the detection of severely ischaemic but viable myocardium: a comparative study with stress, redistribution, reinjection and late redistribution 201Tl imaging. Nucl Med Commun 1996;17:864-71.
61. Flotats A, Carrió I, Estorch M *et al*. Nitrate administration to enhance detection of myocardial viability by technetium-99m tetrofosmin single-photon emission tomography. Eur J Nucl Med 1997;24:767-73.
62. Peix A, López A, Ponce F *et al*. Enhanced detection of reversible myocardial hypoperfusion by technetium 99m-tetrofosmin imaging and first-pass radionuclide angiography after nitroglycerin administration. J Nucl Cardiol 1998;5:469-76.
63. Sciagrà R, Pupi A, Pellegri M, Santoro GM, Casolo GC, Sestini S. Prediction of global left ventricular (LV) ejection fraction (EF) improvement after coronary revascularization (rev) using Tc-99m-Sestamibi SPECT [abstract]. J Nucl Med 1999;40(5 Suppl):49P.
64. Sciagrà R, Pellegri M,. Santoro GM, Sestini F, Zerauschek F, Fazzini PF. Prognostic implications of viability detection with baseline-nitrate Tc-99m-Sestamibi SPECT in patients with LV dysfunction [abstract]. Eur J Nucl Med 1998;25:851.
65. Iskandrian AS, Acio E. Methodology of a novel myocardial viability protocol. J Nucl Cardiol 1998;5:206-9.

6. Fatty-acid SPECT imaging for assessment of myocardial viability

MARIO S. VERANI

Introduction

Because fatty acids are the preferred source of energy substrate by the contracting myocardium, fatty-acid imaging has been viewed with interest in the last four decades as a potential noninvasive means to explore the myocardial metabolism [1,2]. Over the years, a large number of iodine-labeled fatty acids have been tried either experimentally or clinically (Table 1). Yet, the clinical utilization of fatty-acid imaging in the United States has been hampered by the lack of a commercially available product as well as by uncertainties about the intrinsic mechanisms of uptake, concentration and release of different fatty acids by the myocytes. In Japan, the branched fatty acid iodine-123 methyl-pentadecanoic acid (BMIPP) is commercially available and has been used with some frequency.

Table 1. Labeled fatty acids tested as myocardial imaging agents

[17-^{123}I] iodoheptadecanoic acid (^{123}I-17-H^{O}A)
^{131}I iodo-9-hexadecanoic acid (^{131}I-HA)
^{123}I heptadecanoic acid (^{123}-I-H^{O}A)
^{125}I hexadecanoic acid (^{125}I-HA)
^{131}I heptadecanoic acid (^{131}I-H^{O}A)
^{123}I hexadecanoic acid (^{123}I-16-HA)
9-[^{123m}Te] telluraheptadecanoic acid (^{123}Te HAD)
15-(p-iodophenyl)-6-tellurapentadecanoic acid
[^{131}I]-12-N-(p-iodophenylsulfonamide) decanoic acid
[^{131}I]-11-N-(p-iodophenylsufonamide) decanoic acid
^{123}I-15-(p-iodophenyl) pentadecanoic acid (p-IPPA), also called
^{123}I phenylpentadecanoic acid (^{123}IPPA)
^{123}I methylpentadecanoic acid (BMIPP)
^{123}I dimethylpentadecanoic acid (DMIPP)

The compounds that have been tested can generally be divided into two groups: the straight-chain fatty acids (such as iodine-123 phenylpentadecanoic acid-IPPA) and the branch-chain-fatty acids (such as iodine-123 beta methyl-pentadecanoic acid or BMIPP). The straight-chain

A. E. Iskandrian and E. E. van der Wall (eds.), Myocardial Viability, 113-129.
© 2000 *Kluwer Academic Publishers. Printed in the Netherlands.*

fatty acids are taken up by the myocardium in proportion to the myocardial blood flow, following which the compound either undergoes beta-oxidation or is incorporated in the triglyceride cellular pool. With some of the fatty acids, such as heptadecanoic acid (H^OA), the elimination rate from the cells reflects iodide efflux from the myocyte into the blood [3].   Despite a respectable early clinical experience [4-6] with H^OA, this agent is no longer used. The branch-chain fatty acids are retained for a much longer period of time into the myocytes because of their predominant incorporation into the triglyceride pool with little beta-oxidation or iodide efflux (Figure 1).

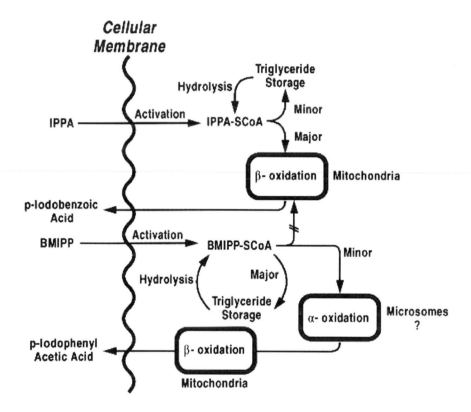

Figure 1. Scheme comparing the relative intracellular metabolism of IPPA and BMIPP ("Cardiodine"). While IPPA can undergo immediate β-oxidation, the apparent obligatory initial α-oxidation of BMIPP (i.e. loss of carboxyl carbon) is required before the resulting α-methyl product can undergo subsequent cyles of β-oxidation. Although not understood, the sensitivity of cellular uptake of BMIPP may be a factor in explaining the unique regional "mismatch" often observed between relative regional uptake of flow tracers and BMIPP. Such a mismatch apparently has not been reported for IPPA. Reproduced with permission from Knapp et al [24].

To a certain extent, the metabolic pathways followed by fatty acids once inside the myocytes depends on the chain length. Otto *et al.* [7] studied the myocardial uptake of six different species of fatty acids, with different numbers of CII2 radicals. Myocardial extraction was highest for fatty acids with 18-21 CH2 radicals. Compounds with less than 15 CH2 radicals underwent predominantly beta-oxidation whereas compounds with 18 or more CH2 radicals underwent predominantly triglyceride pool storage. Fatty acids stored in the triglyceride pool were also characterized by providing a higher heart-to-blood count ratio. Thus, a chain length of 15 to 17 carbon atoms may be more suitable for probing beta-oxidation whereas a longer carbon-chain length has more potential for probing the storage pools. Most of the recent investigations with fatty acids have explored either I-123 IPPA or I-123 BMIPP. Thus, this chapter will focus predominantly on these two compounds.

IPPA metabolic imaging

In 1980, Machulla and co-workers [8, 9] first synthesized and investigated the use of para (p) IPPA as a myocardial imaging agent. Kulkarni and Parkey [10] in 1982 reported on an improved radiodination method to synthesize PPA using organometallic intermediates. These investigators first demonstrated that I-123 IPPA had a fast blood clearance with a half-time of 2.5 minutes, rapid myocardial extraction and biexponential clearance with a fast component, which had a half-time of 3.5 minutes, and a slow component, with a half-time of 130 minutes.
I-123 IPPA is characterized by a high cardiac extraction (4.4% of the injected dose per gram of myocardium) than that of carbon 14-labeled palmitic acid (2.8 % of the injected dose per gram of myocardium). These investigators also noticed that the fast washout component (due to beta oxidation) accounted for approximately 75% of the total washout in 10 minutes) [11]. Reske and associates [12] also investigated the uptake and turnover rate of IPPA in rodents. After a rest IPPA injection, cardiac uptake reached its peak of 4.4% of the injected dose per gram. This was followed by rapid clearance which was completed by 10 minutes.
Rellas and co-workers [13] investigated the potential use of IPPA SPECT to identify myocardial injury following temporary or permanent coronary arterial occlusion. They studied dogs with left anterior descending coronary artery occlusion for 90-120 minutes. Dogs with fixed coronary occlusion for this period of time showed decreased uptake and washout of IPPA in the infarcted areas with a slower washout in those regions (9% increase) than the normal regions (15% decrease), whereas dogs submitted to coronary occlusion for 90 minutes followed by reperfusion, had a decreased uptake of IPPA and decreased clearance in the infarction regions.

The clearances, however, could not distinguish reperfused or non-reperfused regions. While interesting, this study did not directly support or deny the possible use of IPPA for myocardial viability since in dogs with 90 minutes occlusion with or without reperfusion, there is always a mixture of infarcted and viable tissue.

Dudczak and colleagues [14] may have been the first to suggest the potential use of IPPA to assess myocardial viability. In 1983 these investigators reported on 50 patients imaged with I-123 IPPA, 40 of whom had coronary artery disease and 10 had a dilated cardiomyopathy. Images were acquired in dynamic mode for 15 minutes after the intravenous injection of IPPA. They observed reduced accumulation of IPPA in infarcted as well as non-infarcted regions perfused by vessels with coronary stenosis. The myocardial clearance time was prolonged in regions with myocardial infarction (66.5 minutes) and in regions supplied by stenosed arteries without infarction (54.4 minutes). Patients with cardiomyopathy in general also had a prolonged washout (69 minutes). Several other studies on the use of IPPA in patients have been reported. In some of them IPPA was injected during exercise stress. Wolfe *et al.* [15] studied 10 patients with hypertensive left ventricular hypertrophy and 14 normal volunteers. These authors observed a greater heterogeneity in IPPA uptake in patients with left ventricular hypertrophy than normal controls, although both had similar clearance. Kropp and colleagues [16] studied 29 patients with and 13 without evidence of coronary disease using IPPA SPECT imaging, with the tracer injected during submaximal exercise. Sensitivity and specificity for detection of coronary disease were high (ranging from 77 to 95%). In this study, 19 patients had a repeat study after coronary bypass graft surgery; 90% of the revascularized segments had enhanced uptake of IPPA (which usually was accompanied by a faster washout postoperatively). Kennedy *et al.* [17] assessed the uptake and washout of IPPA in 15 normal volunteers and 18 patients with coronary artery disease. In this study, IPPA was also injected during exercise. A relatively uniform IPPA uptake and clearance was observed from 4 to 20 minutes after exercise in the normal volunteers. In the coronary disease patients, the authors observed enhanced myocardial IPPA activity accompanied by delayed clearance in the segments perfused by coronary arteries with stenosis. This study, however, did not address the issue of viability per se.

Hansen *et al.* [18] compared IPPA SPECT imaging to thallium-201 SPECT in a group of 33 patients with stable coronary artery disease and 14 normal volunteers. The tracers were injected at peak exercise and the IPPA images acquired at 9 minutes and repeated at 40 minutes post-injection. A resting study was performed in selected patients at a later date. Either the initial distribution or the clearance of IPPA were considered abnormal in 27 of 33 patients (82%). Among 25 patients with both an IPPA and a thallium-SPECT study available for comparison, 21 had abnormal IPPA studies whereas 18 had an abnormal thallium SPECT. Although abnormalities in uptake and washout were frequent, the authors did not specifically address the issue of viability. Schad and co-workers [19] investigated 38 patients with IPPA injected during bicycle exercise, utilizing a multicrystal gamma camera. In this study, there were 26 patients with coronary artery disease, 9 with dilated cardiomyopathy and 3 with prior heart transplant. Dynamic images were obtained from which they generated curves representing the first-pass of the bolus and the myocardial uptake and washout (the latter representing the metabolic component of the study). The authors observed a good agreement between the regional metabolic rates by IPPA and coronary angiography.

Ugolini and co-workers [20] performed IPPA SPECT imaging in 9 normal volunteers and 19 patients with dilated cardiomyopathy, with the injections done at rest. The patients with dilated cardiomyopathy had greater heterogeneity of IPPA uptake and faster clearance than normal subjects.

Murray and co-investigators [21] attempted to study myocardial viability with IPPA imaging. They studied 15 patients with coronary artery disease and left ventricular dysfunction (left ventricular injection fraction < 35%). In this study, IPPA was injected at rest and dynamic images obtained with a multicrystal gamma camera. On the basis of these images, the authors generated parametric images of regional IPPA uptake and clearance. These new images were then compared to the results of transmural myocardial biopsies obtained at the time of surgery. All patients also underwent echocardiography and exercise radionuclide angiography. The scintigraphic criteria of viability in this study was the presence of "16% or greater washout in at least 50% of a given vessel territory". Nonviable segments had <15% of washout, "unless they had substantial IPPA uptake in at least 50% of the involved vascular territory." Pathologically, the criteria for viability was <50% myocardial fibrosis present in the samples examined – an unorthodox criteria. The authors observed a mean IPPA clearance of 17.8% in biopsy-viable segments, compared to 21% in healthy volunteers and 13.4% in biopsy-nonviable segments. Systolic wall motion at rest and/or exercise improved in 75% of the segments that were viable by IPPA and failed to improve in 67% of segments that were nonviable by IPPA. Perhaps because of the unorthodox viability criteria, only 16% of the biopsied segments were considered nonviable. The narrow difference in washout between normal and abnormal segments, the need for a multicrystal camera and the fact that these results have not been reproduced by other groups limit the conclusions of this investigation.

Iskandrian *et al.* [22] more recently assessed myocardial viability by dynamic tomographic I-123 IPPA imaging and compared it to rest/redistribution thallium-201 imaging in 21 patients with substantial left ventricular dysfunction (mean ejection fraction 34±11%). Five serial 180-degree SPECT images of 8 minutes duration each were obtained starting 4 minutes after the injection of IPPA. Although there was a good agreement between IPPA and thallium for the presence or absence of perfusion defects (kappa = 0.78) and their nature (reversible, mild-fixed, or severe-fixed) (kappa = 0.54), there were more reversible defects by IPPA than by thallium imaging (7 vs 3 segments per patient). The number of reversible IPPA defects was higher in the patients who had improvement in left ventricular ejection fraction after coronary bypass grafting than in the patients without improvement. The authors concluded that I-123 IPPA SPECT imaging was a promising technique for assessment of viability.

A prospective, multicenter trial was designed to evaluate the potential use of I-123 IPPA for detection of myocardial viability and prediction of improved ventricular function after coronary artery bypass graft (CABG). The endpoint of this trial was an increase of 10 points or more in left ventricular ejection fraction after coronary revascularization. One hundred-nineteen patients with a left ventricular ejection fraction of less than 40% underwent I-123 IPPA SPECT and blood pool radionuclide angiography before CABG. The latter was repeated 6 to 8 weeks after CABG to assess the changes in ejection fraction. The study endpoint was achieved in 19% of the patients. By multivariate analysis, the number of segments which were IPPA-viable was the most significant predictor of an improvement in ejection fraction among several clinical and angiographic characteristics. It also had a statistically significant incremental value to the best possible statistical model generated using only clinical and angiographic variables. The overall sensitivity and specificity of IPPA-viable segments to achieve the study endpoint, however, were relatively low (48% and 79%) [23].

In summary, I-123 IPPA is an interesting compound which potentially could be used for assessing both myocardial perfusion (on the early images after administration) and metabolism (on the late images which reflect the rate of beta-oxidation). The ultimate role of I-123 IPPA in the diagnosis of myocardial viability and prediction of post-revascularization improvement in regional contraction remains unsettled. Although IPPA is an excellent marker of beta-oxidation, the rapid clearance from the myocardium during tomographic imaging remains a very substantial impediment to its widespread clinical use.

I-123 BMIPP

The introduction of a variety of radicals on the chemical structure of the long-chain fatty acids leads to inhibition of beta-oxidation. With this in mind, BMIPP (15-p-iodophenyl)-3-RS-methylpentadecanoic acid, which has a chemistry structure similar to IPPA with the addition of a methyl radical in the beta position, was synthesized at the Oakridge National Laboratory in Oakridge, Tennessee. In this compound, the iodine-123 attaches to the para position of the terminal phenol ring. After it is taken up by the myocyte, BMIPP undergoes cytosolic activation to BMIPP-CoA, followed by slow storage in the triglyceride pool. A similar compound has been synthesized by Mallinkrodt, Inc. which has a methyl radical introduced into the 9-position and identified as 9-BMIPP, in contrast to the insertion into the 3-position as in BMIPP [24]. Another related compound is 3-DMIPP (dimethyl iodophenylpentadecanoic acid), which contains 2 methyl radicals instead of only one. The introduction of a second methyl radical confers to the fatty acid an even tighter retention than that of BMIPP. Similar to the para-and ortho-IPPA compounds, an excessive myocardial retention may be disadvantageous to the extent that it precludes assessing the clearance kinetics, which represents metabolic properties, although it may enhance the assessment of myocardial perfusion.

Assessment of myocardial viability with I-123 BMIPP was evaluated in a canine model by Nohara *et al.* [25]. They used an occlusion/reperfusion model of left anterior descending artery with concomitant permanent occlusion of its first diagonal branch. Two hours after occlusion, blood flow decreased to 20% in the infarct area and to 64% in the previously reperfused vascular territory, despite comparable wall motion reduction in both areas. BMIPP activity was reduced to 40% in the infarct area and to 75% in the previously ischemic area, which paralleled a reduction in ATP of 32% and 69% (Figure 2). Thus, the authors concluded BMIPP uptake correlated with tissue ATP levels and hence might be a useful marker of viability. Previous evidence of the metabolic activity of IPPA was provided by Fujibayashi *et al.* [26] in a mouse model treated with an electron transport uncoupler. Under those conditions, they observed reduced BMIPP uptake which was correlated with reduced ATP levels. The reduction in BMIPP uptake was inversely related to the severity of blood flow reduction.

The kinetics of I-123 BMIPP after regional ischemia and reperfusion were further investigated by Hosokawa *et al.* [27] in a canine model. These investigators demonstrated that although the extraction and retention of BMIPP were well-preserved during mild or even severe ischemia, the percent washout at 8 minutes increased from a control of 50% to 61% during severe ischemia. Back diffusion of non-metabolized BMIPP seems to be significantly increased in the early phase of severe ischemia.

Dormehl *et al.* [28] compared the kinetics of I-123 pIPPA, I-123 oIPPA and BMIPP in normal baboons before and after administration of carnitine palmitoyl transferase-1 inhibitor. These authors concluded that beta-oxidation accounted for 47-50% of the clearance of the IPPA fatty acids but for only 10% of that of BMIPP.

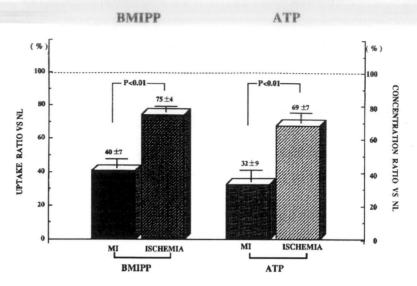

Figure 2. Uptake ratio of ^{123}I-BMIPP and ATP content compared to normal region is shown. BMIPP and ATP content both at infarct (MI:diagonal) and ischemic area (ISCHEMIA:LAD) showed comparable change after procedure. ATP content was slightly lower in relative uptake than BMIPP at both area. NL=normal. Reproduced with permission from Nohara et al [25].

The influence of blood substrate levels on myocardial kinetics of I-123 BMIPP has been investigated by Kurata *et al.* [29]. These authors concluded that there is limited influence of blood substrate levels on myocardial BMIPP uptake, although high serum free fatty acid levels may be associated with slow clearance of BMIPP from the myocardium. Patients with coronary artery disease without myocardial infarction may also have abnormal findings on BMIPP. Tateno *et al.* [30] studied 31 such patients, 19 of whom had unstable angina and 12 stable angina. The studies were compared to rest-stress thallium SPECT and coronary angiography. Decrease in BMIPP uptake was more often seen in the unstable angina (79%) than in the stable angina group (38%). Frequency and severity of BMIPP abnormalities increased with the severity of stress-induced ischemia and the severity of coronary artery stenosis.

Fujiwara *et al.* [31] assessed the effect of oral glucose loading on I-123 BMIPP imaging in patients with coronary artery disease. BMIPP was performed in the fasting state and repeated after oral glucose loading in 29 patients, and SPECT images obtained 20 minutes and 4 hours after the injection of the tracer. In the fasting state, clearance was minimal (11% on the average) but after glucose loading it increased to 27% and was faster in the ischemic myocardium than in nonischemic myocardium. The sensitivity of glucose loaded BMIPP for detection of high-grade coronary stenosis (>90%) was higher than that without glucose loading, although both were relatively low (75% versus 55%). The ultimate value of glucose loading during BMIPP imaging has yet to be defined.

Patients with unstable angina are quite likely to have abnormal resting BMIPP scans. In the study by Takeishi *et al.* [32], 11 of 20 patients with unstable angina had abnormal BMIPP images. These patients were characterized by having more severe coronary stenosis and collateral circulation than patients with normal images. The clinical implications of these findings are not clear. The changes in myocardial fatty uptake and function after revascularization were studied by Taki *et al.* using I-123-BMIPP [33]. These authors investigated 34 patients who underwent rest BMIPP and stress reinjection thallium-201 before and 2-5 weeks after PTCA (n=23) or bypass grafting (n=11). Cardiac function was assessed by blood pool radionuclide angiography (n=26) or 2D echocardiography (n=8) before and after revascularization. Of 32 patients with reduced BMIPP uptake before revascularization, 28 patients had improved perfusion by thallium-201 and 20 patients had improved BMIPP uptake after revascularization. Wall motion abnormality was present in 16 of the above 20 patients before revascularization and improved in 15 of them after revascularization. The improvement in the ejection fraction after revascularization correlated with the area of improved BMIPP (r=0.84, p<0.0005). Although improvement in ejection fraction and thallium uptake were significantly correlated, the correlations were weaker (r=0.48). The discordant area between BMIPP and thallium reinjection before revascularization was moderately correlated to EF improvement (r=0.58).

Iodine-123 BMIPP was compared to myocardial perfusion in patients with acute coronary syndromes by Kobayashi *et al.* [34]. These authors studied 30 patients with unstable angina and 15 patients with acute myocardial infarction. BMIPP imaging was performed using dynamic SPECT, beginning 2 minutes after the injection and obtaining images every 3 minutes for 15 minutes with a triple-headed gamma camera. These images were compared to conventional BMIPP SPECT performed 30 minutes after the injection. The premise was that the early images reflect myocardial perfusion whereas the delayed images reflect metabolic events. A mismatch between the 30-minute BMIPP images and the resting thallium-201 images occurred in 27 of 30 patients in the unstable angina group (Figure 3) and 8 of 15 patients in the myocardial infarction group (Figure 4). Early BMIPP uptake and resting thallium-201 uptake agreed well, with a kappa value of 0.823. Thus, this study suggested that myocardial perfusion and fatty acid metabolism can be potentially evaluated using a single injection of BMIPP and obtaining early (2-5 minutes) and late (30 minutes) images after the injection in patients with acute coronary syndromes.

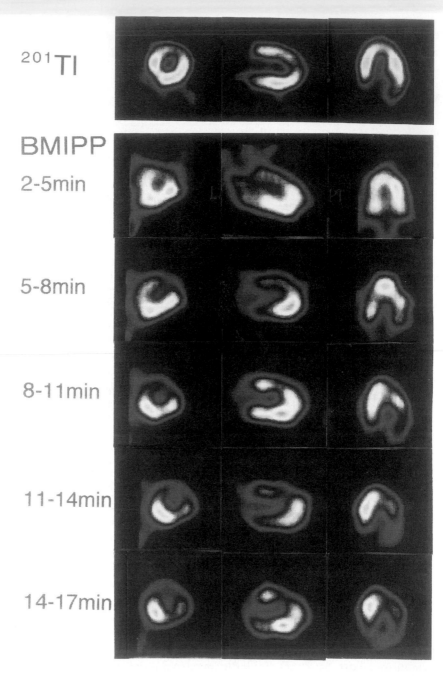

Figure 3. Resting ^{201}Tl and serial BMIPP images from patient with unstable angina pectoris. Coronary angiography showed significant coronary stenosis in left anterior descending and left circumflex artery. Mildly reduced uptake in anterolateral area was observed in both 2-5 min BMIPP and resting ^{201}Tl images. BMIPP accumulation in anterolateral area was gradually decreased in serial BMIPP images. Initial distribution of BMIPP accurately reflected myocardial perfusion imaging. Reproduced with permission from Kobayashi et al [34].

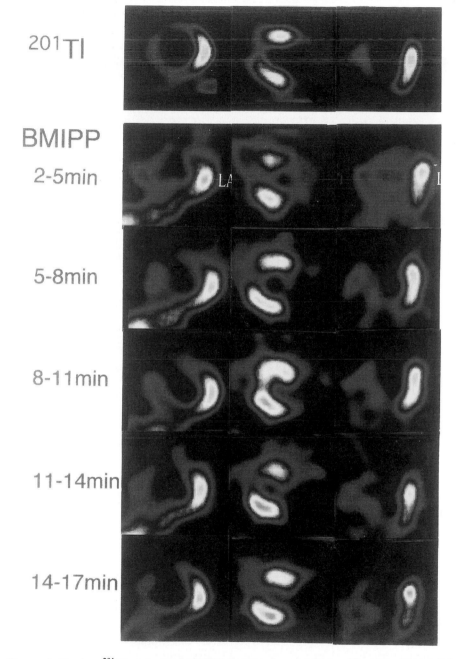

Figure 4. Resting ^{201}Tl and serial BMIPP images from patient with acute myocardial infarction. Large anteroseptal defect was observed in both serial BMIPP and resting ^{201}Tl images. Reproduced with permission from Kobayashi et al [34].

The relationship between blood flow and BMIPP fatty acid metabolism in patients with "subacute" myocardial infarction was reported by De Geeter *et al.* [35]. These investigators studied 26 patients within 2 weeks after myocardial infarction by performing Tc-99m sestamibi and BMIPP SPECT imaging. Myocardial segments associated with acute thrombolysis and/or PTCA had higher sestamibi than BMIPP uptake, supporting the premise that a more prominent reduction of BMIPP was due to the late recovery of fatty acid metabolism after reperfusion.

According to Ito *et al.* [36], the recovery of left ventricular dysfunction in patients with acute myocardial infarction can be predicted by the discordance in defect size between I-123 BMIPP and thallium-201 SPECT images. The severity score in these patients was usually larger by BMIPP than by thallium-201. The extent of discordance and severity scores between BMIPP and thallium-201 during the acute stage correlated well with the improvement in wall motion and in ejection fraction. Tamaki *et al.* [37] confirmed the above findings and reported that the number of discordant segments by BMIPP and thallium-201 imaging in patients with recent myocardial infarction was the best predictor of future cardiac events (Figure 5). The presence of discordant BMIPP/thallium-201 uptake was an independent predictor of future cardiac events and was more powerful than the number of coronary stenosis by angiography.

A comparison between thallium-201 and I-123 BMIPP uptakes was performed by Taki *et al.* [38] in 45 patients with chronic coronary artery disease. In patients with reversible thallium-201 defects, the uptake of BMIPP was more severely decreased than that of thallium reinjection images in 50% of the segments, equally decreased in 39% and more severely decreased in 11% of segments. Resting fatty acid uptake was often more reduced than thallium-201 uptake in segments with stress-induced ischemia, while in segments with fixed thallium defects BMIPP and thallium-201 uptake during reinjection agreed well.

In patients with chronic ischemic heart disease, an increased BMIPP uptake relative to perfusion by thallium-201 has been reported [39]. Such a "reversed" BMIPP/thallium mismatch was found in 74% of myocardial segments that were FDG viable. The frequency of this reversed BMIPP/thallium mismatch was higher in segments with "older" than with "subacute" myocardial infarction (65% versus 24%).

The prediction of reversibility of regional left ventricular dysfunction after coronary angioplasty using BMIPP imaging was reported by Haque *et al.* [40]. Akinetic segments with preserved wall thickness by echocardiography, as well as thinned, akinetic segments with preserved fatty acid uptake, often improved after angioplasty, whereas thinned segments with less than 50% of normal fatty acid uptake failed to improve. Thus, uptake of BMIPP was helpful to predict improvement of regional function.

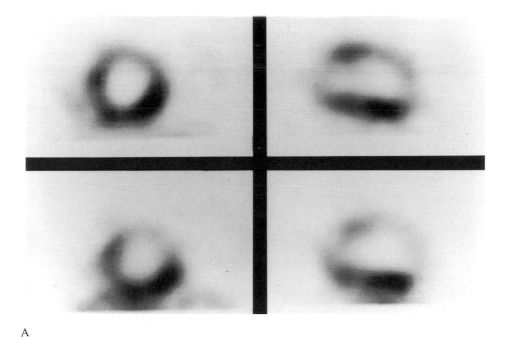

A

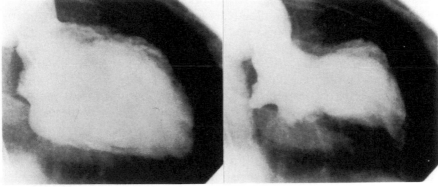

B

*Figure 5*A. Representative short-axis (left) and vertical long-axis (right) thallium images at rest on top and corresponding BMIPP images on bottom taken 30 minutes after tracer administration of patient with acute anterior myocardial infarction. Decreased perfusion on thallium scan in anterior region with further decrease in BMIPP uptake (discordant BMIPP uptake) in same region is noted. *B.* Contrast ventriculograms at end-diastolic (left) and end-systolic (right) phase of same patient show severe hypokinesis in anterior region corresponding to the areas of discordant BMIPP uptake (arrows). Reproduced with permission from Tamaki et al from "Radionuclide assessment of myocardial fatty acid metabolism by PET and SPECT". J Nucl Cardiol 1995;2:256-66.

The outcome significance of thallium-201 and I-123 BMIPP perfusion-metabolism mismatch has been investigated in patients with pre-infarction angina by Nakata *et al.* [41]. Thirty-two patients with a first acute myocardial infarction treated with primary coronary angioplasty underwent BMIPP and thallium-201 tomographic imaging. Both tracers were injected a mean of 10-15 days after the acute infarction. Twenty patients had pre-existing angina ("pre-infarction angina") and 12 patients had no angina before the infarction. Patients with angina preceding myocardial infarction had a lower thallium severity index (less extensive perfusion abnormalities) than that by BMIPP, whereas patients with no history of angina preceding the infarction had no such difference. The mismatch between thallium-201 and BMIPP was significantly related to improved wall motion during follow-up.

Although the majority of investigators have used BMIPP imaging following rest injections, Mori *et al.* [42] injected BMIPP during exercise and compared it to rest-delayed thallium-201 SPECT. Most areas perfused by stenotic vessels had abnormal uptake of BMIPP and discordance between BMIPP and thallium-201 defect extents were encountered often, although its significance in terms of functional recovery was not assessed.

The impairment of BMIPP uptake which has been described in patients with hypertrophic cardiomyopathy appears to precede abnormalities in oxidative and glucose metabolism. The BMIPP uptake is often impaired in these patients, whereas abnormalities of FDG uptake and carbon-11 (C-11) acetate are less frequent [43]. Thus, abnormalities in BMIPP were found in approximately two-thirds of patients with hypertrophic cardiomyopathy, whereas abnormalities in FDG uptake were found in 26% and of acetate metabolism in 45% of patients.

Metabolic abnormalities in BMIPP handling have also been described in hypertrophic cardiomyopathy patients by Matsuo *et al.* [44]. In these patients, disparity between BMIPP and thallium-201 uptake was more often observed in segments with reversible exercise thallium-201 defects. The changes in BMIPP metabolism in patients with hypertrophic cardiomyopathy were further studied by Shimizu *et al.* [45]. The authors described abnormality in BMIPP scintigraphy in 12 of 17 such patients. thallium-201 scintigraphic abnormalities were found in 15 of 30 segments showing decreased accumulation of BMIPP. The authors concluded that abnormalities of fatty acid metabolism occur more often than perfusion abnormalities in these patients.

A curious finding of absent I-123-BMIPP uptake has been occasionally found (0.9% frequency among 1,258 patients studied in Japan) [46]. A study of such patients in comparison with C-11-palmitate, F18-FDG and C-11 acetate showed these patients had a global decrease of palmitate extraction, often accompanied by increased FDG accumulation. Oxidative metabolism assessed by C-11-acetate did not differ from that in control patients.

In summary, BMIPP appears to be an interesting agent. Whether it is superior to the various thallium-201 or sestamibi protocols designed to test myocardial viability (including the pre-injection use of nitroglycerin) should be a fertile subject for future investigations.

Acknowledgements

The authors wish to thank Ms. JoAnn Rabb for her expert secretarial assistance.

References

1. Evans JR, Gunton RW, Baker RG *et al*. Use of radioiodinated fatty acid for photoscans of the heart . Circ Res 1965;16:1-10.
2. Gunton RW, Evans JR, Baker RG, Spears JC, Beanlands DS. Demonstration of myocardial infarction by photoscans of the heart in man. Am J Cardiol 1965;16:482-7.
3. Visser FC, Westera G, Van Eenige MJ, Van der Wall EE, Den Hollander W, Roos JP. The myocardial elimination rate of radioiodinated heptadecanoic acid. Eur J Nucl Med 1985;10:118-22.
4. Van der Wall EE, Heidendal GA, den Hollander W, Westera G, Roos JP. I-123 labeled hexadecanoic acid in comparison with thallium-201 for myocardial imaging in coronary heart disease. Eur J Nucl Med 1980:5:401-5.
5. Van der Wall EE, Heidendal GA, den Hollander W, Westera G, Roos JP. Metabolic myocardial imaging with 123-I labeled heptadecanoic acid in patients with angina pectoris. Eur J Nucl Med 1981;6:391-6.
6. Van der Wall EE, Heidendal GA, den Hollander W, Westera G, Roos JP. Myocardial scintigraphy with ^{123}I-labeled heptadecanoic acid in patients with unstable angina pectoris. Postgrad Med J 1983;59 suppl 3:38-40.
7. Otto CA, Brown LE, Wieland DM, Beierwaltes WH. Radioiodinated fatty acids for myocardial imaging: effects of chain length. J Nucl Med 1981;22:613-18.
8. Machulla HJ, Marsmann M, Dutschka K. [131]I-(phenyl)-pentadecanoic acid, a highly promising radioiodinated fatty acid for myocardial studies. I. Development of synthesis and radiophamaceutical quality. Radioaktive Isot Klin Forsch 1980;14:363-7.
9. Machulla HJ, Marsmann M, Dutschka K. Radiopharmaceuticals: synthesis of radioiodinated phynyl fatty acics for studying myocardial metabolism. J Radioanal Chem 1980;56:253-8.
10. Kulkarni PV, Parkey RW. A new radioiodination method utilizating organothalium intermediate: Radioiodination of phereynypentadecanoic acid (PPA) for potential applications in myocardial imaging. J Nucl Med 1982;23 (6 suppl):p105.
11. Reske SN, Sauer W, Machulla HJ, Winkler C. 15(p-[^{123}I]iodophenyl) pentadecanoic acid as a tracer of lipid metabolism: comparison with [1-^{14}C] palmitic/acid in murine tissues. J Nucl Med 1984;25:1335-42.
12. Reske SN, Sauer W, Machulla HJ, Knust J, Winkler C. Metabolism of 15 (p^{123}I iodophenyl)-pentadecanoic acid in heart muscle and noncardiac tissues. Eur J Nucl Med 1985;10:228-34.

13. Rellas JS, Corbett JR, Kulkarni P *et al.* Iodine-123 phenylpentadecanoic acid: detection of acute myocardial infarction and injury in dogs using an iodinated fatty acid and single-photon emission tomography. Am J Cardiol 1983;52:1326-32.

14. Dudczak R, Schmoliner R, Kletter K, Frischauf H, Angelberger P. Clinical evaluation of 123I-labeled p-phenylpentadecanoic acid (p-IPPA) for myocardial scintigraphy. J Nucl Med Allied Sci 1983;27:267-79.

15. Wolfe CL, Kennedy PL, Kulkarni P, Jansen DE, Gabliani GI, Corbett JR. Iodine-123 phenylpentadecanoic acid myocardial scintigraphy in patients with left ventricular hypertrophy: alterations in left ventricular distribution and utilization. Am Heart J 1990;119:1338-47.

16. Kropp J, Likungu J, Kirchhoff PG *et al.* Single photon emission tomography imaging of myocardial oxidative metabolism with 15{p-[123]iodophynl) pentadecanoic acid in patients with coronary artery disease and aorto-coronary bypass graft surgery. Eur J Nucl Med 1991;18:467-74.

17. Kennedy PL, Corbett JR, Kulkarni PV *et al.* Iodine 123-phenylpentadecanoic acid myocardial scintigraphy: usefulness in the identification of myocardial ischemia. Circulation 1986;74:1007-15.

18. Hansen CL, Corbett JR, Pippin JJ *et al.* Iodine-123 phenylpentadecanoic acid and single-photon emission computed tomography in identifying left ventricular regional metabolic abnormalities in patients with coronary heart disease: comparison with thallium-201 myocardial tomography. J Am Coll Cardiol 1988;12:78-87.

19. Schad N, Daus HJ, Ciavolella M, Maccio H. Noninvasive functional imaging of regional rate of myocardial fatty acids metabolism. Cardiologia 1987;32:239-47.

20. Ugolini V, Hansen CL, Kulkarni PV, Jansen DE, Akers MS, Corbett JR. Abnormal myocardial fatty acid metabolism in dilated cardiomyopathy detected by Iodine-123 phenylpentadecanoic acid and tomographic imaging. Am J Cardiol 1988;62:923-8.

21. Murray G, Schad N, Ladd W *et al.* Metabolic cardiac imaging in severe coronary disease: assessment of viability with iodine-^{123}I-Iodophenyl-pentadecanoic acid and multicrystal gamma camera, and correlation with biopsy. J Nucl Med 1992;33:1269-77.

22. Iskandrian AS, Powers J, Cave V, Wasserleben V, Cassell D, Heo J. Assessment of myocardial viability by dynamic tomographic iodine 123 iodophenylpentadecanoic acid imaging: comparison with rest-redistribution thallium 201 imaging. J Nucl Cardiol 1995;2:101-9.

23. Verani MS, Taillefer R, Iskandrian AE, Mahmarian JJ, He ZX, for the Multicenter IPPA Viability Trial Investigators. I-123 Iodophenylpentadecanoic Acid (IPPA) single photon emission tomography for the prediction of enhanced left ventricular function after coronary bypass graft surgery. Submitted for publication, 1998.

24. Knapp FF Jr, Kropp J. Iodine-123-labelled fatty acids for myocardial single-photon emission tomography: current status and future perspectives. Eur J Nucl Med 1995;22:361-81.

25. Nohara R, Okuda K, Ogino M *et al.* Evaluation of myocardial viability with iodine-123-BMIPP in a canine model. J Nucl Med 1996;37:1403-7.

26. Fujibayashi Y, Yonekura Y, Takemura Y *et al.* Myocardial accumulation of iodinated beta-methyl-branched fatty acid analogue, iodine-125-15-(p-iodophenyl)-3-(R,S) methylpentadecanoic acid (BMIPP), in relation to ATP concentration. J Nucl Med 1990;31:1818-22.

27. Hosokawa R, Nohara R, Fujibayashi Y *et al.* Myocardial kinetics of iodine-123-BMIPP in canine myocardium after regional ischemia and reperfusion: implications for clinical SPECT. J Nucl Med 1997;38:1857-63.

28. Dormehl IC, Hugo N, Rossouw D, White A, Feinendengen LE. Planar myocardial imaging in the baboon model with iodine-123-15-(iodophenyl) pentadecanoic acid (IPPA) and iodine-123-15-(P-Iodophenyl)-3-R,S-methylpentadecanoic acid (BMIPP), using time-activity curves for evaluation of metabolism. Nucl Med Biol 1995;22:837-47.

29. Kurata C, Wakabayashi Y, Shouda S *et al*. Influence of blood substrate levels on myocardial kinetics of iodine-123-BMIPP. J Nucl Med 1997;38:1079-84.
30. Tateno M, Tamaki N, Yukihiro M *et al*. Assessment of fatty acid uptake in ischemic heart disease without myocardial infarction. J Nucl Med 1996;37:1981-5.
31. Fujiwara S, Takeishi Y, Atsumi H, Takahashi K, Tomoike H. Fatty acid metabolic imaging with Iodine-123-BMIPP for the diagnosis of coronary artery disease. J Nucl Med 1997;38:175-80.
32. Takeishi Y, Fujiwara S, Atsumi H, Takahashi K, Sukekawa H, Tomoike H. Iodine-123-BMIPP imaging in unstable angina: a guide for interventional strategy. J Nucl Med 1997;38:1407-11.
33. Taki J, Nakajima K, Matsunari I *et al*. Assessment of improvement of myocardial fatty acid uptake and function after revascularization using iodine-123-BMIPP. J Nucl Med 1997;38:1503-10.
34. Kobayashi H, Kusakabe K, Momose M *et al*. Evaluation of myocardial perfusion and fatty acid uptake using a single injection of iodine-123-BMIPP in patients with acute coronary syndromes. J Nucl Med 1998;39:1117-22.
35. De Geeter F, Franken PR, Knapp FF Jr, Bossuyt A. Relationship between blood flow and fatty acid metabolism in subacute myocardial infarction: a study by means of ^{99m}Tc-Sestamibi and ^{123}I-beta-methyl-iodo-phenyl pentadecanoic acid. Eur J Nucl Med 1994;21:283-91.
36. Ito T, Tanouchi J, Kato J *et al*. Recovery of impaired left ventricular function in patients with acute myocardial infarction is predicted by the discordance in defect size on ^{123}I-BMIPP and ^{201}Tl SPET images. Eur J Nucl Med 1996;23:917-23.
37. Tamaki N, Tadamura E, Kudoh T *et al*. Prognostic value of iodine-123 labelled BMIPP fatty acid analogue imaging in patients with myocardial infarction. Eur J Nucl Med 1996;23:272-9.
38. Taki J, Nakajima K, Matsunari I, bunko H, Takada S, Tonami N. Impairment of regional fatty acid uptake in relation to wall motion and thallium-201 uptake in ischaemic but viable myocardium; assessment with iodine-123-labelled beta-methyl-branched fatty acid. Eur J Nucl Med 1995;22:1385-92.
39. Sloof GW, Visser FC, Bax JJ *et al*. Increased uptake of iodine-123-BMIPP in chronic ischemic heart disease: comparison with fluorine-18-FDG SPECT. J Nucl Med 1998;39:255-60.
40. Haque T, Furukawa T, Yoshida S *et al*. Echocardiography and fatty acid single photon emission tomography in predicting reversibility of regional left ventricular dysfunction after coronary angioplasty. Eur Heart J 1998;19:332-41.
41. Nakata T, Hashimoto A, Kobayashi H *et al*. Outcome significance of thallium-201 and iodine-123-BMIPP perfusion – metabolism mismatch in preinfarction angina. J Nucl Med 1998;39:1492-9.
42. Mori T, Hayakawa M, Hattori K *et al*. Exercise beta-methyl iodophenyl pentadecanoic acid (BMIPP) and resting thalium delayed single photon emission computed tomography (SPECT) in the assessment of ischemia and viability. Jpn Circ J 1996;60:17-26.
43. Tadamura E, Kudoh T, Hattori N *et al*. Impairment of BMIPP uptake precedes abnormalities in oxygen and glucose metabolism in hypertrophic cardiomyopathy. J Nucl Med 1998;39:390-6.
44. Matsuo S, Nakamura Y, Takahashi M, Mitsunami K, Kinoshita M. Myocardial metabolic abnormalities in hypertrophic cardiomyopathy assessed by iodine-123-labeled beta-methyl-branched fatty acid myocardial scintigraphy and its relation to exercise-induced ischemia. Jpn Circ J 1998;62:167-72.
45. Shimizu M, Yoshio H, Ino H *et al*. Myocardial scintigraphic study with ^{123}I 15-(p-iodophenyl)-3(R,S)-methylpentadecanoic acid in patients with hypertrophic cardiomyopathy. Int J Cardiol 1996;54:51-9.
46. Kudoh T, Tamaki N, Magata Y *et al*. Metabolism substrate with negative myocardial uptake of iodine-123-BMIPP. J Nucl Med 1997;38:548-53.

7. Role of FDG SPECT in viability assessment

JEROEN J. BAX, FRANS C. VISSER & ERNST E. VAN DER WALL

Introduction

Left ventricular ejection fraction (LVEF) is a major determinant of survival in patients with coronary artery disease [1]. Prognosis is particularly poor in patients with chronic coronary artery disease and severely depressed LV function (LVEF <35%) [2]. Revascularization may improve LV function in these patients when viable myocardium is present [3]. Conversely, systolic LV function does not improve in the absence of viable myocardium. Since revascularization procedures are associated with a relatively high (peri-)operative morbidity and mortality in this category of patients [4], a careful selection of patients with viable myocardium is mandatory.

Various techniques have been developed to identify viable myocardium, including scintigraphic techniques [5], low-dose dobutamine echocardiography [6] and magnetic resonance techniques [7]. Metabolic imaging with F18-fluorodeoxyglucose (FDG) and positron emission tomography (PET) is considered a very accurate technique to identify viable myocardium [8]. Many studies have indeed demonstrated that FDG PET can adequately predict functional recovery after revascularization [9]. Pooled data from 14 FDG PET studies with a total of 371 patients showed a mean sensitivity of 88% and a specificity of 73% to predict functional outcome after revascularization (Table 1) [9]. However, PET facilities are limited available and considerable efforts have been made to develop single photon emission computed tomographic (SPECT) imaging with FDG using 511 keV collimators [10-15]. In this chapter the current status of FDG SPECT imaging will be discussed.

FDG SPECT: Protocol and viability criteria

Optimal identification of jeopardized but viable myocardium requires integration of information on contractile function, perfusion and metabolic status of the myocardium. Most studies have evaluated regional contractile function with resting 2D echocardiography although radionuclide ventriculography or magnetic resonance imaging may be more ideal for this purpose [9].

A. E. Iskandrian and E. E. van der Wall (eds.), Myocardial Viability, 131-145.
© 2000 *Kluwer Academic Publishers. Printed in the Netherlands.*

Table 1. Sensitivity and specificity of FDG PET to predict improvement of regional LV function after revascularization (data based on reference 9).

Author	Pts (n)	LVEF (%)	Sens (%)	Spec (%)
Marwick *et al.*	16	NA	71	76
Gerber *et al.*	39	33	75	67
Tamaki *et al.*	20	NA	78	78
Gropler *et al.*	34	NA	83	50
Maes *et al.*	23	41	83	91
Tamaki *et al.*	43	41	88	82
Knuuti *et al.*	43	53	92	85
Baer *et al.*	42	40	92	88
Lucignani *et al.*	14	38	93	86
Carrel *et al.*	23	34	94	50
Tillisch *et al.*	17	32	95	80
Tamaki *et al.*	11	NA	100	38
Wolpers *et al.*	30	43	NA	NA
Paolini *et al.*	9	27	88	79
Weighted mean			88	73

FDG: F18-fluorodeoxyglucose; LVEF: left ventricular ejection fraction; NA: not available; PET: positron emission tomography; Sens: sensitivity; spec: specificity.

Next, resting perfusion and FDG uptake are compared in the dysfunctional regions. In the majority of the PET studies, resting perfusion has been evaluated with nitrogen-13-ammonia, although recent data by Gerber *et al.* [16] demonstrated that oxygen-15-water may provide more accurate information on perfusion in dysfunctional myocardium. In the SPECT studies either thallium-201 chloride [17] or technetium-99m-labeled agents [12,18] have been used for the assessment of myocardial perfusion. Although both tracers have been validated extensively, it should be emphasized that these agents do not permit absolute quantification of myocardial perfusion (unlike the PET tracers).

The initial FDG SPECT studies were performed during hyperinsulinemic glucose clamping. The clamping technique has several advantages over the routinely used oral glucose load [19]. Clamping permits strict regulation of the metabolic conditions, reduces heterogeneity in myocardial FDG uptake and provides excellent image quality in all patients, including diabetics [19].

Different perfusion-FDG patterns have been observed in the dysfunctional segments. The majority of the PET studies have used the classical perfusion-FDG match and mismatch patterns to differentiate between viable myocardium and scar tissue [8]. Segments with a mismatch pattern did indeed frequently improve in function after revascularization, whereas the vast majority of segments with a match did not recover in function.

Examples of a perfusion-FDG match and mismatch are shown in Figures 1 and 2. In addition, several studies demonstrated that percentage fibrosis was significantly larger in segments with a perfusion-FDG match (as compared to mismatch segments).

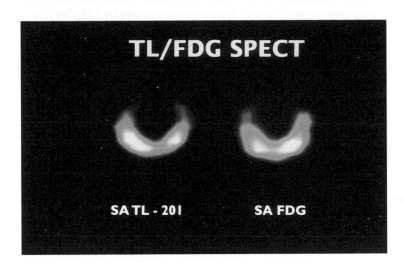

Figure 1. An example of a perfusion-FDG match. The corresponding short-axis slices show a perfusion defect in the anterior wall (left) and concordantly decreased FDG uptake (right) in this area, indicating scar tissue.

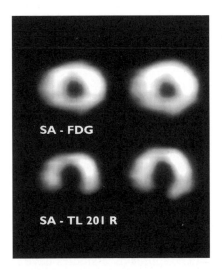

Figure 2. An example of a perfusion-FDG mismatch. The thallium-201 short axis slices (bottom) show a perfusion defect in the inferior wall with preserved FDG uptake (top), indicating viable tissue.

More recent studies have demonstrated that many segments with improvement of contractile function after revascularization had (sub-) normal perfusion [20,21]. Accordingly, the viability criteria on perfusion-FDG imaging (both PET and SPECT) should include normal perfusion and perfusion-FDG mismatch as indicators of viable tissue and perfusion-FDG match as a marker of scar tissue. Recent data from both FDG PET and FDG SPECT studies have shown that the matches can be further subdivided into mild and severe matches, representing subendocardial and transmural scars [22,23]. In a recent study, the distribution of the different patterns in 42 patients with chronic coronary artery disease and regional LV dysfunction was evaluated [23]. Approximately 50% of the segments were viable, with approximately 50% showing a mismatch pattern and 50% exhibiting normal perfusion (Figure 3).

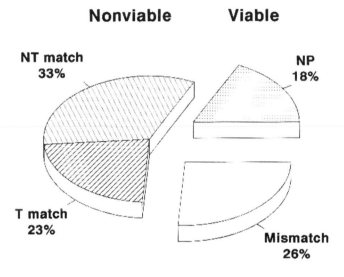

Figure 3. Distribution of different patterns on FDG SPECT in 206 dysfunctional segments in 42 patients with chronic coronary artery disease and left ventricular dysfunction. Viability (normal perfusion or perfusion-FDG mismatch pattern) was observed in 44% of the 206 dysfunctional segments; 56% of the segments were nonviable: 33% had a nontransmural perfusion-FDG match (subendocardial scar) and 23% had a transmural match (transmural scar) (data based on reference #23). NP: normal perfusion; NT match: nontransmural match; T match: transmural match.

FDG SPECT: Comparison to FDG PET

To validate the FDG SPECT approach, 5 studies have performed a head-to-head comparison between FDG SPECT and FDG PET [11,13-15,24] (Table 2). These studies were uniform in showing a good agreement between PET and SPECT in the assessment of viable myocardium. The first study was performed by Burt *et al.* [13]. Twenty patients with a defect on 4-hour delayed resting thallium-201 SPECT were studied with both FDG PET and FDG SPECT. The FDG images were obtained following an oral glucose load combined with intravenous insulin when appropriate. Sixty-one defects were observed on the delayed thallium-201 study; 11 showed preserved FDG uptake on PET and SPECT, while 45 revealed absent FDG uptake on both PET and SPECT. An agreement of 94% was obtained between the 2 approaches. Two additional studies by Martin *et al.* [24] and Chen *et al.* [14] reported comparable results. In another study, the scintigraphic data were compared with regional contractile function (assessed by 2D echocardiography) [11]. The agreement between PET and SPECT was 82% when all segments were considered and 76% when the analysis was restricted to the dysfunctional segments.

Table 2. Comparative studies between FDG PET and FDG SPECT (data based on references #11,13-15,24).

Study	pts (n)	male (%)	age (yrs)	LVEF (%)	pts with MVD (%)	pts with prev MI (%)	agreement (%)
Burt[13]	20	NA	NA	NA	NA	NA	93
Martin[24]	9	NA	NA	NA	NA	NA	100
Bax[11]	20	80	64±8	39±16	83	100	76
Chen[14]	36	NA	NA	NA	NA	NA	90
Srinivasan[15]	28	89	62±12	33±15	93	64	94

FDG: F18-fluorodeoxyglucose; LVEF: left ventricular ejection fraction; MI: myocardial infarction; MVD: multivessel disease; NA: not available; PET: positron emission tomography; prev: previous; SPECT: single photon emission computed tomography.

The most recent comparative study was performed by Srinivasan *et al.* [15]. When a 50% FDG threshold was used to differentiate between viable tissue and scar, both techniques provided equal information in 920 of 977 segments (agreement 94%). When FDG PET and FDG SPECT were compared to thallium-201 stress-redistribution-reinjection SPECT, the concordances were 92% and 90% respectively. Hence, the available data in 113 patients demonstrate the good agreement between FDG PET and FDG SPECT. Further validation of FDG SPECT was derived from studies comparing the technique to thallium-201 imaging and dobutamine echocardiography.

FDG SPECT: Comparison to thallium-201 imaging

Thallium-201 chloride has been used extensively for the detection of coronary artery disease using stress-redistribution imaging [25]. For the assessment of myocardial viability however, this protocol has been proven suboptimal [5]. Subsequently, other protocols have been developed including stress-redistribution-reinjection imaging and rest-redistribution imaging [26,27]. Both techniques have been proven useful in the prediction of recovery of function after revascularization, although some overestimation of recovery occurred [9]. Hence the sensitivity of the techniques was extremely high and the specificity was somewhat lower [9]. Currently, 3 studies have compared FDG SPECT to thallium-201 imaging [13,28,29]. The study by Burt *et al.* [13], comparing 4-hour delayed rest thallium-201 imaging to FDG SPECT has been discussed in the previous paragraph. Two other studies by Bax *et al.* [28,29] have compared thallium-201 stress-reinjection and rest-redistribution imaging with FDG SPECT.

Thallium-201 stress-reinjection imaging was compared to FDG SPECT in 17 patients with chronic coronary artery disease, depressed LV function (LVEF 36±11%) and a total of 99 dysfunctional segments on echocardiography. On thallium-201 stress-reinjection imaging 67 segments were viable, while FDG SPECT showed viability in 43 segments. The agreement between the 2 techniques was 70%. The disagreement was mainly due to segments that were classified viable by thallium-201 stress-reinjection and nonviable by FDG SPECT (Figure 4). Further analysis of the 27 segments classified viable by thallium-201 stress-reinjection and nonviable by FDG SPECT revealed that 24 of 27 (89%) segments demonstrated a "mild fixed defect" (≥50% thallium-201 uptake on the stress images without reversibility on the reinjection images) on thallium-201 imaging. As pointed out recently [30], these segments are likely to represent subendocardial scars.

Thallium-201 rest-redistribution SPECT and FDG SPECT were compared in 24 patients [29]. In this study, 92 dysfunctional segments were evaluated; the agreement of thallium-201 rest-redistribution and FDG SPECT was 70%. The disagreement between the 2 techniques was related again to 22% of the segments that were classified viable by thallium-201 rest-redistribution and nonviable by FDG SPECT (Figure 5).

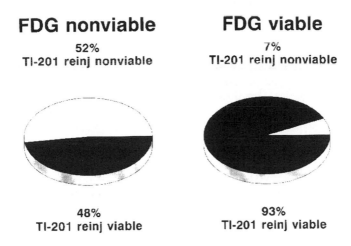

FDG nonviable

52%
Tl-201 reinj nonviable

48%
Tl-201 reinj viable

FDG viable

7%
Tl-201 reinj nonviable

93%
Tl-201 reinj viable

Figure 4. Agreement and disagreement between thallium-201 stress-reinjection imaging and FDG SPECT. While 93% of the "FDG-viable" segments were viable on thallium-201 stress-reinjection imaging, only 52% of the "FDG-nonviable" segments were also nonviable on thallium-201 stress-reinjection imaging. The disagreement was mainly caused by 48% of the "FDG-nonviable" segments that were classified viable on thallium-201 stress-reinjection imaging (data based on reference #28). Tl-201 reinj: thallium-201 stress-reinjection imaging.

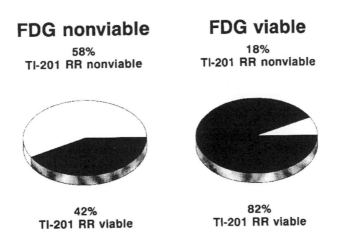

FDG nonviable

58%
Tl-201 RR nonviable

42%
Tl-201 RR viable

FDG viable

18%
Tl-201 RR nonviable

82%
Tl-201 RR viable

Figure 5. Concordance and discordance between thallium-201 rest-redistribution SPECT and FDG SPECT. The majority (82%) of the segments with viability on FDG SPECT are classified viable on thallium-201 imaging; however, a substantial percentage (42%) of "FDG-nonviable" segments are also classified viable on thallium-201 rest-redistribution SPECT (data based on reference #29). Tl-201 RR: thallium-201 rest-redistribution SPECT.

FDG SPECT: Comparison to dobutamine echocardiography

The hallmark of viability during dobutamine echocardiography is the presence of contractile reserve in dysfunctional myocardium. Comparative studies between FDG PET and low-dose dobutamine echocardiography have demonstrated a good agreement between the 2 techniques, varying from 80% to 90%, for the detection of myocardial viability [28,31-33]. Several recent studies however, comparing FDG PET to dobutamine echocardiography stressed that a substantial percentage of dysfunctional segments classified viable on FDG PET did not exhibit contractile reserve on dobutamine echocardiography [31-36]. In the study by Sun *et al.* [34] 30% of the perfusion-FDG mismatches did not have contractile reserve. Baer and coworkers [32] showed that 19% of the scintigraphically viable segments lacked recruitable contractile reserve. Sawada *et al.* [35] and Melon *et al.* [36] showed somewhat higher percentages of mismatches without contractile reserve. Similar findings were reported in a recent study comparing FDG SPECT and low-dose dobutamine echocardiography in 40 patients with chronic coronary artery disease and depressed LV function [37]; 27% of the dysfunctional segments classified viable on FDG SPECT did not exhibit contractile reserve during dobutamine echocardiography (Figure 6).

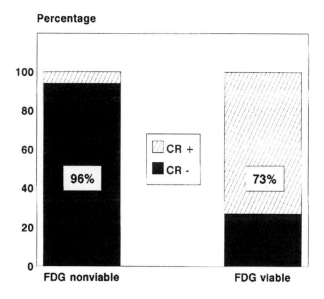

Figure 6. Agreement between low-dose dobutamine echocardiography and FDG SPECT. The majority of the "FDG-nonviable" segments did not show contractile reserve (left bar); however, a substantial percentage of the "FDG-viable" segments also lacked contractile reserve (right bar, data based on reference #37). CR: contractile reserve.

It is conceivable that different degrees of ultrastructural cell damage can cause the discrepancies between metabolic imaging with FDG and assessment of contractile reserve by dobutamine echocardiography. Preliminary data have indeed shown that segments with perfusion-metabolism mismatch without contractile reserve have more severe damage than mismatch segments with contractile reserve [38]. It is anticipated that the segments with both metabolic viability and contractile reserve will improve in function after revascularization. It is unclear whether the segments with FDG uptake but without contractile reserve will improve in function. It is plausible however, that these segments need longer time to improve in function after revascularization. This issue should be addressed in future studies.

FDG SPECT: Prediction of functional outcome following revascularization

To further validate the use of FDG SPECT for the assessment of tissue viability, 2 studies have focused on the prediction of functional recovery after revascularization [28,39]. In the largest study, 55 patients were evaluated before revascularization by FDG SPECT. The patients had an average of 2.5±0.7 stenosed vessels and significantly depressed LV function (mean LVEF 39±14%). Regional contractile function was assessed before and 3 months after revascularization by resting echocardiography. Before revascularization, 281 segments demonstrated contractile dysfunction. Recovery of function was observed in 94 (33%) segments; 80 segments were classified viable on FDG SPECT. Conversely, 187 segments did not improve in function after the revascularization; 141 of these segments were classified nonviable on FDG SPECT. Hence, the sensitivity to predict improvement of regional LV function was 85% and the specificity was 75% (Figure 7). The sensitivity/specificity were also determined in different subcategories of segments (Table 3). Specificity tended to be slightly inferior in the hypokinetic segments as compared to the akinetic segments, although not significantly different. Importantly, the sensitivity/specificity were not different in the inferior/septal regions as compared to the other regions, indicating that attenuation has a limited impact on the diagnostic accuracy of FDG SPECT. Moreover, the diagnostic accuracy of FDG SPECT to predict improvement of regional LV function after revascularization was comparable to that obtained in the FDG PET studies. Pooled analysis of the available FDG PET studies focusing on the prediction of improvement of regional LV function after revascularization, showed a mean sensitivity of 88% and a specificity of 73% [9] (Table 1).

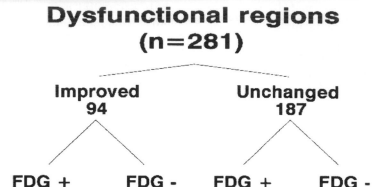

Figure 7. The sensitivity and specificity of FDG SPECT to predict improvement of regional left ventricular function after revascularization (data based on reference #39).

Table 3. Sensitivity and specificity of FDG SPECT to predict improvement of regional LV function after revascularization. Comparison of diagnostic accuracy in different subcategories of segments (data based on reference #39).

	Sens (%)	Spec (%)	DA (%)
All segments (n=281)	85	75	79
A-/Dyskinetic segments (n=153)	87	84	85
Hypokinetic segments (n=128)	82	66	71
Ant/Lat/Apical segments (n=139)	86	76	80
Inf/Sept segments (n=142)	84	75	77
Pts with LVEF ≥30% (n=109)	80	81	81
Pts with LVEF <30% (n=172)	89	72	77

Ant: anterior; DA: diagnostic accuracy; FDG: F18-fluorodeoxyglucose; Inf: inferior: Lat: lateral; LVEF: left ventricular ejection fraction; Sens: sensitivity; Sept: septal; spec: specificity; SPECT: single photon emission computed tomography.

Clinically more important is the prediction of improvement of global LV function. In the aforementioned study [39] prediction of improvement of LVEF after revascularization was also evaluated. In the 19 patients with 3 or more dysfunctional but viable segments, the LVEF improved from $28\pm8\%$ before to $35\pm9\%$ (P<0.01) 3 months after the revascularization. In contrast, in the 36 patients with 2 or less viable segments, the LVEF remained unchanged ($45\pm14\%$ versus $44\pm14\%$, ns). Similar results were obtained in the patients with a severely depressed LVEF (<30%, n=22): 14 patients with ≥3 viable segments on FDG SPECT improved in significantly in LVEF (from $25\pm6\%$ to $32\pm6\%$, P<0.01), while the LVEF remained unchanged in 8 patients with <3 viable segments ($24\pm6\%$ vs $25\pm6\%$, ns). Considering an improvement of LVEF >5% after revascularization as significant, FDG SPECT had a sensitivity of 100% and a specificity of 80%. Preliminary data demonstrated that the improvement in LVEF in patients with viable myocardium was linked to an improvement in heart failure symptoms [40]. In 18 patients with ≥3 viable segments on SPECT, the LVEF improved from $27\pm8\%$ to $34\pm9\%$ (P<0.05); 13 patients improved their NYHA status by 1 grade or more. The mean NYHA score improved from 2.9 ± 0.3 to 1.5 ± 0.7 (P<0.01). Conversely, in 14 patients with <3 viable segments the LVEF did not improve ($31\pm8\%$ versus $31\pm8\%$, ns); only 3 of these 14 patients improved in NYHA status by 1 grade or more (P<0.05 versus patients with ≥3 viable segments). The mean NYHA score remained unchanged in these patients (2.6 ± 0.5 vs 2.4 ± 0.7, ns). These preliminary data suggest that patients with substantial viable tissue improve in LVEF after revascularization and that the improvement in LVEF is accompanied by an improvement in quality of life.

FDG SPECT: Future research

1. Additional end-points.

The feasibility of FDG SPECT and its clinical value in the detection of myocardial viability have been demonstrated in the studies discussed above. Moreover, the technique allows prediction of improvement of regional and global LV function following revascularization. Although prediction of recovery is an important end-point in viability-testing, other end-points should be evaluated. First, relieve of stress-induced ischemia may not necessarily result in improvement of resting LVEF, but rather result in improvement of LVEF during exercise.

Furthermore, besides assessment of improvement of heart failure symptoms after revascularization, improvement of exercise capacity should be examined. Marwick *et al.* [41] demonstrated that patients with viable myocardium on FDG PET showed significant improvement in peak rate-pressure product, percentage of maximal heart-rate and improvement of exercise capacity (from 5.6 ± 2.7 to 7.5 ± 1.7 METS) after revascularization.

Also, several FDG PET studies have demonstrated that this technique may provide prognostic information on morbidity and mortality. Four retrospective studies [42-45] have indicated that the presence of a mismatch pattern in patients who are treated medically is associated with a high event rate. Currently, no prognostic FDG SPECT data are available and future studies are necessary to determine whether FDG SPECT yields similar prognostic information as compared to FDG PET.

2. Optimalization of the FDG SPECT protocol.

The use of FDG SPECT has gained a lot of attention since the technique is widely available and permits the use of FDG for assessment of myocardial viability on a large scale. Several modifications of the protocol have been developed recently to further simplify the technique. First, simultaneous assessment of perfusion and FDG uptake has been introduced [12,1]. The dual-isotope simultaneous acquisition protocol has important advantages including shorter imaging time and avoiding misalignment between the perfusion and FDG images. A further refinement would be gating of the images. Gating would allow assessment of function, perfusion and FDG uptake by just one technique, thereby avoiding the use of different techniques (e.g. magnetic resonance imaging or 2D echocardiography).

Furthermore, substantial efforts have been made in the development of coincidence imaging of positron emitting tracers [46]. This technique may enhance the resolution of SPECT imaging; however, with this approach attenuation correction is mandatory to obtain accurate images.

Finally, considerable effort has been invested to evaluate alternative methods to replace the hyperinsulinemic euglycemic clamp. The rationale for the clamp is as follows. Cardiac FDG uptake depends mainly on the plasma levels of free fatty acids and insulin [19]. High insulin levels promote cardiac FDG uptake, whereas high FFA levels inhibit FDG uptake. With the infusion of insulin, cardiac FDG uptake is stimulated directly and indirectly (by depression of peripheral lipolysis thereby lowering plasma FFA levels). For clinical routine however, the use of the hyperinsulinemic euglycemic clamp may be too time-consuming and laborious. Recently, the feasibility of FDG imaging following oral administration of a nicotinic acid derivative (Acipimox, Byk, The Netherlands) has been demonstrated. Acipimox inhibits peripheral lipolysis, thus reducing plasma FFA levels. Two studies have shown comparable FDG image quality with Acipimox as compared to clamping [47,48]. The use of Acipimox may further facilitate routine FDG imaging.

Conclusions

Several studies, from different centers, have indicated the feasibility of FDG SPECT. Good agreement between FDG SPECT and FDG PET was obtained. In addition, good agreement was demonstrated between FDG SPECT and other imaging techniques, including thallium-201 imaging and dobutamine echocardiography. Most important, prediction of functional recovery (regional and global) is possible with FDG SPECT and the accuracy is comparable to that of FDG PET. Preliminary data suggest that FDG SPECT can also predict improvement of quality of life, in terms of improvement of heart failure symptoms, after revascularization. Finally, new developments in technology, including dual-isotope imaging and coincidence imaging, and optimalization of protocols (simplification by the use of Acipimox) may further stimulate the use of FDG SPECT.

References

1. Harris PJ, Harrell FE Jr, Lee KL, Behar VS, Rosati RA. Survival in medically treated coronary artery disease. Circulation 1979;60:1259-69.
2. Abraham WT, Bristow MR. Specialized centers for heart failure management. Circulation 1997;96:2755-7.
3. Wijns W, Vatner SF, Camici PG. Hibernating myocardium. N Engl J Med 1998;339:173-81.
4. Mickleborough LL, Maruyama H, Takagi Y, Mohamed S, Sun Z, Ebisuzaki L. Results of revascularization in patients with severe left ventricular dysfunction. Circulation 1995;92(9 suppl):II739.
5. Dilsizian V, Bonow RO. Current diagnostic techniques of assessing myocardial viability in patients with hibernating and stunned myocardium. Circulation 1993;87:1-20.
6. Cornel JH, Bax JJ, Fioretti PM. Assessment of myocardial viability by dobutamine stress echocardiography. Curr Opin Cardiol 1996;11:621-6.
7. Van der Wall EE, Vliegen HW, De Roos A, Bruschke AVG. Magnetic resonance imaging in coronary artery disease. Circulation 1995;92:2723-39.
8. Schelbert HR. Metabolic imaging to assess myocardial viability. J Nucl Med 1994;35(4 Suppl):8S-14S.
9. Bax JJ, Wijns W, Cornel JH, Visser FC, Boersma E, Fioretti PM. Accuracy of currently available techniques for prediction of functional recovery after revascularization in patients with left ventricular dysfunction due to chronic coronary artery disease: comparison of pooled data. J Am Coll Cardiol 1997;30:1451-60.
10. Bax JJ, Visser FC, van Lingen A *et al.* Feasibility of assessing regional myocardial uptake of ^{18}F-fluorodeoxyglucose using single photon emission computed tomography. Eur Heart J 1993;14:1675-82.
11. Bax JJ, Visser FC, Blanksma PK *et al.* Comparison of myocardial uptake of fluorine-18-fluorodeoxyglucose imaged with PET and SPECT in dyssynergic myocardium. J Nucl Med 1996;37:1631-6.
12. Sandler MP, Videlefsky S, Delbeke D *et al.* Evaluation of myocardial ischemia using a rest metabolism/stress perfusion protocol with fluorine-18 deoxyglucose/technetium-99m MIBI and dual-isotope simultaneous-acquisition single-photon emission computed tomography. J Am Coll Cardiol 1995;26:870-8.
13. Burt RW, Perkins OW, Oppenheim BE *et al.* Direct comparison of fluorine-18-FDG SPECT, fluorine-18-FDG PET and rest thallium-201 SPECT for the detection of myocardial viability. J Nucl Med 1995;36:176-9.
14. Chen EQ, MacIntyre WJ, Go RT *et al.* Myocardial viability studies using fluorine-18-FDG SPECT: a comparison with fluorine-18-FDG PET. J Nucl Med 1997;38:582-6.
15. Srinivasan G, Kitsiou AN, Bacharach SL, Bartlett ML, Miller-Davis C, Dilsizian V. [18F]fluorodeoxyglucose single photon emission computed tomography: can it replace PET and thallium SPECT for the assessment of myocardial viability? Circulation 1998;97:843-50.
16. Gerber BL, Melin JA, Bol A *et al.* Nitrogen-13-ammonia and oxygen-15-water estimates of absolute myocardial perfusion in left ventricular ischemic dysfunction. J Nucl Med 1998;39:1655-62.

17. Bax JJ, Visser FC, van Lingen A *et al.* Relation between myocardial uptake of thallium-201 chloride and fluorine-18-fluorodeoxyglucose imaged with single photon emission computed tomography in normal individuals. Eur J Nucl Med 1995;22:56-60.
18. Rambaldi R, Poldermans D, Bax JJ, Fioretti PM, Krenning EP, Valkema R. Assessment of myocardial viability by dobutamine stress echo and simultaneous Tc99m-tetrofosmin/18-fluorodeoxyglucose SPECT [abstract]. J Nucl Cardiol 1997;4(suppl):S110.
19. Knuuti MJ, Nuutila P, Ruotsalainen U *et al.* Euglycemic hyperinsulinemic clamp and oral glucose load in stimulating myocardial glucose utilization during positron emission tomography. J Nucl Med 1992;33:1255-62.
20. Vanoverschelde JLJ, Wijns W, Depré C *et al.* Mechanisms of chronic regional postischemic dysfunction in humans. New insights from the study of noninfarcted collateral-dependent myocardium. Circulation 1993;87:1513-23.
21. Marinho NVS, Keogh BE, Costa DC, Lammertsma AA, Ell PJ, Camici PG. Pathophysiology of chronic left ventricular dysfunction. New insights from the measurement of absolute myocardial blood flow and glucose utilization. Circulation 1996;93:737-44.
22. Vom Dahl J, Altehoefer C, Sheehan FH *et al.* Recovery of regional left ventricular dysfunction after coronary revascularization. Impact of myocardial viability assessed by nuclear imaging and vessel patency at follow-up angiography. J Am Coll Cardiol 1996;28:948-58.
23. Bax JJ, Cornel JH, Visser FC. Optimal viability criteria to predict functional recovery after revascularization [abstract]. Circulation 1997;96(Suppl I):I-194.
24. Martin WH, Delbeke D, Patton JA *et al.* FDG-SPECT: correlation with FDG-PET. J Nucl Med 1995;36:988-95.
25. Beller GA. Pharmacologic stress imaging. JAMA 1991;265:633-8.
26. Ragosta M, Beller GA, Watson DD, Kaul S, Gimple LW. Quantitative planar rest-redistribution 201-Tl imaging in detection of myocardial viability and prediction of improvement in left ventricular function after coronary artery bypass surgery in patients with severely depressed left ventricular function. Circulation 1993;87:1630-41.
27. Dilsizian V, Rocco TP, Freedman NM, Leon MB, Bonow RO. Enhanced detection of ischemic but viable myocardium by the reinjection of thallium after stress-redistribution imaging. N Engl J Med 1990;323:141-6.
28. Bax JJ, Cornel JH, Visser FC *et al.* Prediction of recovery of myocardial dysfunction after revascularization. Comparison of fluorine-18-fluorodeoxyglucose/thallium-201 SPECT, stress-reinjection SPECT and dobutamine echocardiography. J Am Coll Cardiol 1996;28:558-65.
29. Bax JJ, Cornel JH, Visser FC *et al.* Comparison of fluorine-18-FDG with rest-redistribution thallium-201 SPECT to delineate viable myocardium and predict functional recovery after revascularization. J Nucl Med 1998;39:1481-6.
30. Kitsiou AN, Srinivasan G, Quyyumi AA, Summers RM, Bacharach SL, Dilsizian V. Stress-induced reversible and mild-to-moderate irreversible defects: are they equally accurate for predicting recovery of regional left ventricular function after revascularization? Circulation 1998;98:501-8.
31. Cornel JH, Bax JJ, Fioretti PM *et al.* Prediction of improvement of ventricular function after revascularization. ^{18}F-fluorodeoxyglucose single photon emission computed tomography vs low-dose dobutamine echocardiography. Eur Heart J 1997;18:941-8.
32. Baer FM, Voth E, Deutsch HJ, Schneider CA, Schicha H, Sechtem U. Assessment of viable myocardium by dobutamine transesophageal echocardiography and comparison with fluorine-18 fluorodeoxyglucose positron emission tomography. J Am Coll Cardiol 1994;24:343-53.
33. Baer FM, Voth E, Deutsch HJ *et al.* Predictive value of low dose dobutamine transesophageal echocardiography and fluorine-18 fluorodeoxyglucose positron emission tomography for recovery of regional left ventricular function after successful revascularization. J Am Coll Cardiol 1996;28:60-9.

34. Sun KT, Czernin J, Krivokapich J *et al.* Effects of dobutamine stimulation on myocardial blood flow, glucose metabolism, and wall motion in normal and dysfunctional myocardium. Circulation 1996;94:3146-54.
35. Sawada S, Elsner G, Segar DS *et al.* Evaluation of patterns of perfusion and metabolism in dobutamine-responsive myocardium. J Am Coll Cardiol 1997;29:55-61.
36. Melon PG, De Landsheere CM, Degueldre C, Peters JL, Kulbertus HE, Pierard LA. Relation between contractile reserve and positron emission tomographic patterns of perfusion and glucose utilization in chronic ischemic left ventricular dysfunction: implications for identification of myocardial viability. J Am Coll Cardiol 1997;30:1651-9.
37. Cornel JH, Bax JJ, Elhendy A *et al.* Agreement and disagreement between "metabolic viability" and "contractile reserve" in akinetic myocardium. J Nucl Cardiol 1999;6:383-8.
38. Pagano D, Bonser RS, Townend JN, Parums D, Camici PG. Histopathological correlates of dobutamine echocardiography in hibernating myocardium [abstract]. Circulation 1996;94(8 Suppl):I543.
39. Bax JJ, Cornel JH, Visser FC *et al.* Prediction of improvement of contractile function in patients with ischemic ventricular dysfunction after revascularization by fluorine-18-fluorodeoxyglucose SPECT. J Am Coll Cardiol 1997;30:377-84.
40. Bax JJ, Cornel JH, Visser FC, Fioretti PM, Van Lingen A, Visser CA. Viability versus improvement of heart failure symptoms [abstract]. J Nucl Med 1998;39:18P.
41. Marwick TH, Nemec JJ, Lafont A, Salcedo EE, MacIntyre WJ. Prediction by postexercise fluoro-18 deoxyglucose positron emission tomography of improvement in exercise capacity after revascularization. Am J Cardiol 1992;69:854-9.
42. Eitzman D, Al-Aouar ZR, Kanter HL *et al.* Clinical outcome of patients with advanced coronary artery disease after viability studies with positron emission tomography. J Am Coll Cardiol 1992;20:559-65.
43. Lee KS, Marwick TH, Cook SA *et al.* Prognosis of patients with left ventricular dysfunction, with and without viable myocardium after myocardial infarction. Relative efficacy of medical therapy and revascularization. Circulation 1994;90:2687-94.
44. Di Carli M, Davidson M, Little R *et al.* Value of metabolic imaging with positron emission tomography for evaluating prognosis in patients with coronary artery disease and left ventricular dysfunction. Am J Cardiol 1994;73:527-33.
45. Vom Dahl J, Altehoefer C, Sheehan FH *et al.* Effect of myocardial viability assessed by technetium-99m-sestamibi SPECT and fluorine-18-FDG PET on clinical outcome in coronary artery disease. J Nucl Med 1997;38:742-8.
46. Ziegler SI, Enterrotacher A, Boning G *et al.* Performance characteristics of s dual head coincidence camera for the detection of small lesions [abstract]. J Nucl Med 1997;38(Suppl):206P.
47. Bax JJ, Veening MA, Visser FC *et al.* Optimal metabolic conditions during FDG imaging: a comparative study using different protocols. Eur J Nucl Med 1997;24:35-41.
48. Knuuti MJ, Yki-Järvinen H, Voipio-Pulkki LM *et al.* Enhancement of myocardial [fluorine-18] fluorodeoxyglucose uptake by a nicotinic acid derivative. J Nucl Med 1994;35:989-98.

8. Detection of myocardial viability by angiographic methods

WILLIAM WIJNS

Introduction

Historically, cardiac catheterization was instrumental in disclosing the fact that chronic contractile dysfunction in patients with coronary artery disease could be reversible following revascularization. Although the technique does not readily permit the study of regional myocardial blood flow or metabolism, prediction of potential recovery of function was shown to be possible prior to revascularization by studying the contraction response of dysfunctioning areas to inotropic stimulation. This approach can be considered as the forerunner of stress echocardiography. At present times, cardiac catheterization still plays a pivotal role in the clinical workup of patients with ventricular dysfunction in order to confirm the etiology, establish the prognosis,and explore the potential modes of treatment.

Historical importance of angiographic studies

As early as 1970, the group at the Montreal Heart Institute reported the observation that left ventricular dysfunction could be rapidly reversible following aorto-coronary bypass graft [1]. Out of 23 patients with abnormal preoperative ventriculograms and patent grafts between 12 and 20 days postoperatively, function had normalized in 30% and improved in 35%. Hypokinesia frequently returned to normal and akinesia improved in half of the cases. Similar observations were reported in 1971 by Rees et al. [2]. Improved left ventricular performance, i.e. increased ejection fraction and decreased end-systolic volume, 3 months after bypass surgery was associated with graft patency. The influence of revascularization on ventricular asynergy and function was carefully analyzed 2 weeks after surgery by Chatterjee et al. in 1973 [3]. Both in patients with and without prior infarction, functional improvement was apparent in many patients with depressed left ventricular function preoperatively. These "historical" observations, which were confirmed in the large randomized trials comparing bypass surgery with medical treatment [4], have convincingly shown that akinetic areas do not necessarily represent scar. Hence residual

A. E. Iskandrian and E. E. van der Wall (eds.), Myocardial Viability, 147-154.
© 2000 Kluwer Academic Publishers. Printed in the Netherlands.

"viability" must be retained in these areas since functional recovery eventually occurs. Subgroup analysis of the Coronary Artery Surgery Study (CASS) database already indicated that survival benefit from bypass surgery was most prominent in those patients with severe left ventricular dysfunction preoperatively [4]. Looking back at such data, it is worth considering that these observations were only made possible because cardiac surgeons disregarded the opinion of the cardiologists who would not recommend to bypass an "infarcted" area. Yet, placing a bypass on every graftable vessel led to the fortuitous observations mentioned earlier that even akinetic segments, previously thought to be irreversibly damaged, could regain contraction. This led Diamond et al. [5] to imply that "ischemic non-infarcted myocardium can exist in a state of function hibernation". As early as 1981, Flameng et al. [6] identified myocardial degeneration or dedifferentation as the main cause of reversible segmental asynergy by correlating pre- and post-operative angiographic findings with histopathological analysis of transmural biopsies obtained at the time of cardiac surgery. Finally, Rahimtoola used the term "hibernating myocardium" for the first time in 1984 [7] and he deserves the credit for conceptualizing the observations that were available since the late seventies as well as for emphasizing the clinical importance of this entity.

The intervention ventriculogram

The fact that "viable" dysfunctioning myocardium is able to respond to various inotropic stimuli by a transient improvement in contraction is known from angiographic studies since 1974. Intravenous infusion of epinephrine (1 to 4 µg/min) was used by Horn et al. [8] to challenge segments shown to be asynergic on the baseline angiography (Figure 1). Out of 44 dysfunctioning segments, 23 improved contraction during epinephrine ventriculography. The lack of improvement in 4 patients correlated with the presence of scar on pathological examination after aneurysmectomy. Nesto et al. [9] showed that the global left ventricular ejection fraction improved post-operatively in patients with a greater than 10 % increase in ejection fraction in response to inotropic stimulation.
Others have used the sublingual administration of nitroglycerin (0.4 mg) to unmask dysfunctioning areas with residual contractility. A positive response was shown to correlate with post-operative functional improvement in segmental function [10,11]. Bodenheimer et al. [12] demonstrated that nitroglycerin responsive asynergic areas generally comprised histologically intact myocardium while significant fibrosis was seen in unresponsive areas.
Limitations of the intervention ventriculography include the inconvenience and risks associated with additional contrast injections as well as the effects

of dye itself on the loading conditions and indexes of ventricular performance. These effects were particularly pronounced at the time when less toxic iso-osmolar contrast agents were not yet available. An appealing alternative is to take advantage of catheter-induced extrasystole which frequently occur during powered contrast injection. Following an early diastolic extrasystole, the post-extrasystolic beat is potentiated by the prolonged filling as well as by a direct inotropic effect such that viable asynergic areas were shown to improve contraction [13]. In another study, 6 of 7 patients with post-operative improvement in ejection fraction showed pre-operative post-extrasystolic potentiation. However, a positive response to extrasystole was observed in up to 40 % of patients without significant post-operative change in global function [14]. With the advent of percutaneous revascularization techniques, similar studies were performed in patients undergoing percutaneous transluminal coronary angioplasty (PTCA). For instance, Cohen *et al.* [15] identified 12 patients with post-extrasystolic potentiation of motion in the asynergic zone in whom resting function improved immediately after successful angioplasty. As a consequence, the global ejection fraction increased from 46±20 to 62±19% (p< 0.005).

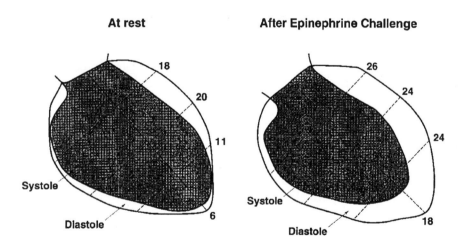

Figure 1. Left ventricular contours at enddiastole and endsystole under resting condition as well as after epinephrine infusion. Note the global improvement in function after epinephrine, particularly in the anterior, apical and inferior segments. Improved shortening results in an increase in ejection fraction from 32% at rest to 54% after inotropic stimulation. This response indicates to which extent functional recovery can be expected following successful revascularization (From Horn *et al.*, reference 8, with permission).

The relative accuracy of nitroglycerin administration, post-extrasystolic potentiation and their combination were compared by Banka et al. [16]. In responsive segments, percent shortening improved further following combined stimuli while no changes were observed in unresponsive segments, no matter which stimuli were applied. These observations imply that the combination of post-extrasystolic potentiation and nitroglycerin might unmask residual viability in asynergic areas that do not respond to either stimulus alone.

Again, the historical importance of these early studies cannot be overemphasized. The link between residual viability, contractile reserve, post-operative functional improvement and improved prognosis was already established in the late seventies. Yet, following the seminal report by Piérard et al. [17], the intervention ventriculogram has now been replaced by stress echocardiography. Standardized doses (5, 10, 20, up to 40 µg/kg/min) of dobutamine are given in steps of 3 minutes each and the response of regional and global function is analyzed throughout. Viable asynergic areas improve contraction at lower doses but may deteriorate again at high dose because of reduced flow reserve and ischemia. Although echocardiography has its own limitations, the advantages over contrast ventriculography are numerous. Being a tomographic technique, images of all segments of the ventricle can be obtained. Being noninvasive, data acquisition can be easily repeated and the dose-response is evaluated in each case. With ventriculography, at best biplane projections are obtained. As mentioned earlier, radiographic contrast agents cannot be injected repeatedly and only two datapoints (baseline and intervention) are available.

Clinical role of angiography

In patients with left ventricular dysfunction the results of cardiac catheterization play a pivotal role in the decision making process.

Coronary arteriography will contribute the following information:
- establish that ischemia causes the dysfunction,
- identify the presence of collateral flow to asynergic areas,
- determine which mode of revascularization is most appropriate,
- verify the adequacy of revascularization after PTCA or surgery.

First of all, in the presence of left ventricular dysfunction, coronary arteriography is essential in establishing the differential diagnosis (Figure 2). Chronic dysfunction can only be of ischemic origin when significant coronary stenoses are present. Whenever severe dysfunction is found in the absence of severe lesions, other potentially associated causes should be excluded, such as alcohol abuse [18], valvular disease or tachycardiomyopathy [19].

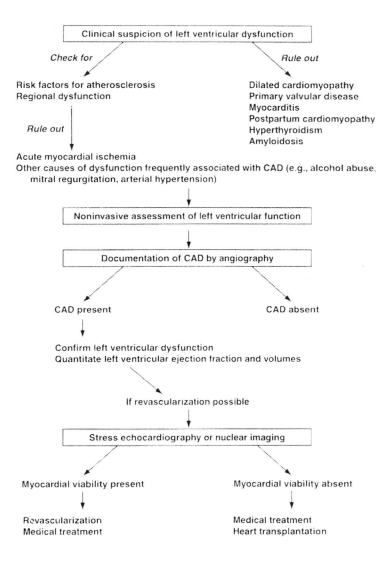

Figure 2. This decision tree indicates how patients presenting with left ventricular dysfunction should be investigated. Note that several causes of dysfunction are frequently associated in the same patient. In addition to the results of "viability" testing, the choice of therapy is also guided by age, the presence of diabetes, other comorbidity, coronary anatomy, availability of bypass conduits. In patients with severe ventricular arrhythmias the implantation of automatic defibrillators should also be considered.

The grade of collateral flow supply [20] to chronically dysfunctioning areas also provides some indication on the likelihood of residual viability and functional recovery following revascularization [21]. However, it should be remembered that angiographically visible collaterals only represent a small fraction of all potentially available channels. For instance, in the study by Vanoverschelde *et al.* [22], maximal coronary blood flow to collateral-dependent areas (measured with positron emission tomography after dipyridamole infusion) varied from no increase above baseline flow to normal flow reserve (up to fourfold increase) despite identical collateral grades at coronary angiography.

The results of coronary angiography have a powerful and independent prognostic value which is comparable to the prognostic value of the left ventricular volumes and function. It is frequently erroneously stated that the extent of coronary artery disease has no independent prognostic value. This is the case only when the results of the coronary angiogram are expressed in terms of 1, 2 or 3 vessel disease. As a matter of fact, several angiographic indices of disease severity and extent were shown to be predictive of long-term survival [23]. Although some of these scores are easily obtainable, it is unfortunate that they are not used in routine clinical practice.

The decision whether revascularization should be performed percutaneously or via bypass surgery likewise depends on the anatomy, the technicalities of PTCA or stenting, the suitability of the distal vessels for graft anastomosis and the availability of bypass conduits, all of which can only be defined by angiography. Most frequently, patients with severe left ventricular dysfunction have undergone several prior interventions which may preclude performing another revascularization procedure and stimulate newer approaches such as the intentional combination of PTCA and minimally invasive bypass surgery [24].

Lastly, coronary and graft angiography is extremely useful in evaluating the adequacy of revascularization. When PTCA has been performed, repeat angiography is frequently performed at 6 months in order to detect restenosis. Following surgery, repeat catheterization is usually only performed because of recurrent anginal symptoms. The majority of studies on the value of viability tests for the prediction of functional recovery following revascularization fail to verify graft patency and therefore likely underestimate the specificity of the tests [25].

Contrast ventriculography will permit to measure the baseline ejection fraction and most importantly, to calculate the ventricular volumes. While the ejection fraction can be accurately measured by various techniques including radionuclide angiography or magnetic resonance imaging, contrast angiography still remains the gold standard for the determination of left ventricular volumes. The endsystolic volume is a key determinant of prognosis in patients with coronary artery disease [26]. In patients with severe left ventricular dysfunction (ejection fraction below 35%), we have demonstrated that patients who improved left ventricular function postoperatively had smaller enddiastolic volumes prior to surgery [27]. By discriminant analysis, the two most powerful predictors of post-operative improvement were the responsiveness to dobutamine during stress echocardiography and the enddiastolic volume [27]. These data indicate that beyond a certain degree of ventricular remodeling (i.e. dilatation), function may no longer recover, even though asynergic areas may still be viable.

Conclusions

Despite all advances in medical therapy, the prognosis of patients with chronic ischemic left ventricular dysfunction remains poor. A wide array of accurate noninvasive tests is available for the identification and selection of those patients who might benefit from coronary revascularization because they have a sufficient amount of asynergic myocardium that remained viable. In clinical practice, the coronary angiogram and the baseline contrast ventriculogram still provide diagnostic and prognostic information that cannot be missed because it is essential for patient management.

References

1. Saltiel J, Lespérance J, Bourassa MG, Castonguay Y, Campeau L, Grondin P. Reversibility of left ventricular dysfunction following aorto-coronary by-pass grafts. Am J Roentgenol Radium Ther Nucl Med 1970;110:739-46.
2. Rees G, Bristow JD, Kremkau EL et al. Influence of aortocoronary bypass surgery on left ventricular performance. N Engl J Med 1971;284:1116-20.
3. Chatterjee K, Swan HJC, Parmley WW, Sustaita H, Marcus HS, Matloff J. Influence of direct myocardial revascularization on left ventricular asynergy and function in patients with coronary heart disease with and without previous myocardial infarction. Circulation 1973;47:276-86.
4. Alderman EL, Fisher LD, Litwin P et al. Results of coronary artery surgery in patients with poor left ventricular function (CASS). Circulation 1983;68:785-95.
5. Diamond GA, Forrester JS, deLuz PL, Wyatt HL, Swan HJC. Post-extrasystolic potentiation of ischemic myocardium by atrial stimulation. Am Heart J 1978;95:204-9.
6. Flameng W, Suy R, Schwarz F et al. Ultrastructural correlates of left ventricular contraction abnormalities in patients with chronic ischemic heart disease : determinants of reversible segmental asynergy postrevascularization surgery. Am Heart J 1981;102:846-57.
7. Rahimtoola SH. The hibernating myocardium. Am Heart J 1984;117:211-21.
8. Horn HR, Teichholz LE, Cohen PF, Herman MV, Gorlin R. Augmentation of left ventricular contraction pattern in coronary artery disease by an inotropic catecholamine. The epinephrine ventriculogram. Circulation 1974;49:1063-71.
9. Nesto RW, Cohn LH, Collins JJ Jr, Wynne J, Holman L, Cohn PF. Inotropic contractile reserve : a useful predictor of increased 5 year survival and improved postoperative left ventricular function in patients with coronary artery disease and reduced ejection fraction. Am J Cardiol 1982;50:39-44.

10. McAnulty JH, Hattenhauer MT, Rösch J, Kloster FE, Rahimtoola SH. Improvement in left ventricular wall motion following nitroglycerin. Circulation 1975;51:140-5.
11. Helfant RH, Pine R, Meister SG, Feldman MS, Trout RG, Banka VS. Nitroglycerin to unmask reversible asynergy. Correlation with post coronary bypass ventriculography. Circulation 1974;50:108-13.
12. Bodenheimer MM, Banka VS, Hermann GA, Trout RG, Pasdar H, Helfant RH. Reversible asynergy. Histopathologic and electrographic correlations in patients with coronary artery disease. Circulation 1976;53:792-6.
13. Dyke SH, Cohn PF, Gorlin R, Sonnenblick EH. Detection of residual myocardial function in coronary artery disease using post-extra systolic potentiation. Circulation 1974;50:694-9.
14. Popio KA, Gorlin R, Bechtel D, Levine JA. Postextrasystolic potentiation as a predictor of potential myocardial viability: preoperative analyses compared with studies after coronary bypass surgery. Am J Cardiol 1977;39:944-53.
15. Cohen M, Charney R, Hershman R, Fuster V, Gorlin R. Reversal of chronic ischemic myocardial dysfunction after transluminal coronary angioplasty. J Am Coll Cardiol 1988;12:1193-8.
16. Banka VS, Bodenheimer MM, Shah R, Helfant RH. Intervention ventriculography. Comparative value of nitroglycerin, post-extrasystolic potentiation and nitroglycerin plus post-extrasystolic potentiation. Circulation 1976;53:632-7.
17. Piérard LA, De Landsheere CM, Berthe C, Rigo P, Kulbertus HE. Identification of viable myocardium by echocardiography during dobutamine infusion in patients with myocardial infarction after thrombolytic therapy: comparison with positron emission tomography. J Am Coll Cardiol 1990;15:1021-31.
18. Demakis JG, Proskey A, Rahimtoola SH et al. The natural course of alcoholic cardiomyopathy. Ann Intern Med 1974;80:293-7.
19. Fenelon G, Wijns W, Andries E, Brugada P. Tachycardiomyopathy: mechanisms and clinical implications. Pacing Clin Electrophysiol 1996;19:95-106.
20. Cohen MV. Coronary collaterals: clinical and experimental observations. Mount Kisco, NY: Futura; 1985. pp. 93-185.
21. Melchior JP, Doriot PA, Chatelain P et al. Improvement of left ventricular contraction and relaxation synchronism after recanalization of chronic total coronary occlusion by angioplasty. J Am Coll Cardiol 1987;9:763-8.
22. Vanoverschelde JLJ, Wijns W, Depré C et al. Mechanisms of chronic regional postischemic dysfunction in humans. New insights from the study of noninfarcted collateral-dependent myocardium. Circulation 1993;87:1513-23.
23. Ringqvist I, Fisher LD, Mock M et al. Prognostic value of angiographic indices of coronary artery disease from the Coronary Artery Surgery Study (CASS). J Clin Invest 1983;71:1854-66.
24. Friedrich GJ, Bonatti J, Dapunt OE. Preliminary experience with minimally invasive coronary-artery bypass surgery combined with coronary angioplasty. N Engl J Med 1997; 336: 1454-5.
25. Bax JJ, Wijns W, Cornel JH, Visser FC, Boersma E, Fioretti PM. Accuracy of currently available techniques for prediction of functional recovery after revascularization in patients with left ventricular dysfunction due to chronic coronary artery disease : comparison of pooled data. J Am Coll Cardiol 1997;30:1451-60.
26. Hamer AW, Takayama M, Abraham KA et al. End-systolic volume and long-term survival after coronary artery bypass graft surgery in patients with impaired left ventricular function. Circulation 1994;90:2899-904.
27. Vanoverschelde JLJ, Gerber BL, D'Hondt AM et al. Preoperative selection of patients with severely impaired left ventricular function for coronary revascularization. Role of low-dose dobutamine echocardiography and exercise-redistribution-reinjection thallium SPECT. Circulation 1995;92(Suppl 2):II37-44.

9. Echocardiographic assessment of reversible left ventricular dysfunction

FAROOQ A. CHAUDHRY & KATHLEEN GALATRO

Introduction

Left ventricular function is one of the most important determinates of long term prognosis in patients with coronary artery disease [1]. In recent years it has become apparent that left ventricular dysfunction in patients with coronary artery disease is not always an irreversible process. Rahimtoola [2] and Bolli [3] have reported improvement in regional left ventricular function post-revascularization in patients with significant left ventricular dysfunction. In fact, restoration of blood flow to these severely dysfunctional regions, not only can improve regional and global left ventricular function post-revascularization, but may also impact on long term survival [4,5]. Therefore, identifying the degree and extent of viable myocardium in patients with significant left ventricular dysfunction is an essential part of risk stratification, including referral for revascularization for those patients in whom significant myocardial viability is determined. Low dose dobutamine echocardiography has gained significant attention in the identification of inotropic contractile reserve (myocardial viability) in patients with reversible left ventricular dysfunction and is the primary focus of this chapter.

Echocardiography assessment of reversible left ventricular dysfunction

Echocardiography

Myocardial thickening and endocardial excursion are both components of normal systolic wall motion seen by echocardiography. In patients with coronary artery disease, the presence of ischemia will result in the alteration of one or both of these components. A specific echocardiographic finding for ischemic muscle is an absence of, or decrease in systolic myocardial thickening and endocardial excursion. Normal segments adjacent to ischemic segments may appear hypokinetic as the motion of these normal segments is affected by the surrounding abnormal segments (tethering effect). This phenomenon would result in an

A. E. Iskandrian and E. E. van der Wall (eds.), Myocardial Viability, 155-175.
© 2000 *Kluwer Academic Publishers. Printed in the Netherlands.*

overestimation of ischemic myocardium. In addition, if the remaining normal segments demonstrate compensatory hyperkinesis, the amount of abnormal myocardium may be underestimated. In the setting of acute ischemia or infarction not only is myocardial wall motion abnormal, but systolic thinning may be present, whereby the thickness of the myocardial segment is greater in diastole than in systole. *Infarcted* myocardium may also appear thin in *both* systole and diastole with minimal to no thickening, and exhibit akinesis or dyskinesis. Acoustic changes occur within scarred myocardial tissue which result in enhanced echogenicity of these thinned walls [6]. Although baseline echocardiography provides information on resting left ventricular function, the assessment of reversibility requires pharmacological intervention.

Dobutamine echocardiography

Dobutamine, a synthetic catecholamine with positive inotropic effects mediated by β_1- adrenergic receptor stimulation, enhances regional systolic wall thickening and endocardial excursion at low dose, 4-8 μg/kg/min. In asynergic segments, contractile reserve is identified by improvement of wall thickening and endocardial excursion, and thus, represents areas of viable myocardium (Figure 1).

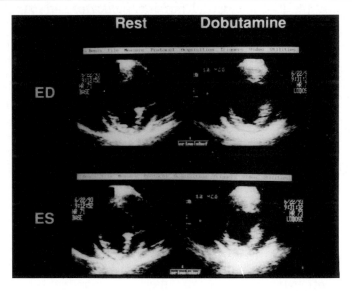

Figure 1. Short axis views representing end-diastolic frames (top left and top right panels) and end-systolic frames (bottom left and bottom right panels) at rest (left panel) and in response to dobutamine (right panel). With dobutamine infusion there is significant contractile reserve as evidenced by a decrease in both the enddiastolic and endsystolic dimensions and an increase in endocardial thickening and excursion (top right and bottom right panels).

Animal models of acute reversible left ventricular dysfunction have demonstrated the ability of low dose catecholamine stimulation to differentiate reversible from fixed dysfunction in regions of hypoperfusion [7]. Once higher doses are reached, and chronotropic effects predominate, myocardial demand increases, which is subsequently matched with an increase in regional myocardial blood flow. Areas of ischemia may be identified by resultant new reversible wall motion abnormalities in regions supplied by coronary arteries with flow limiting stenoses (Figure 2). Therefore, it is during low dose catecholamine stimulation, when inotropy predominates, that is effective in identifying regions of myocardial viability [8].

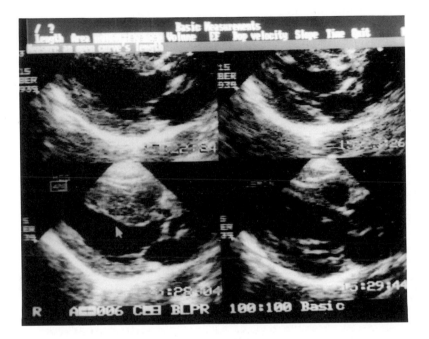

Figure 2. Parasternal long axis views demonstrating evidence of myocardial viability in the anteroseptal wall with concurrent evidence of ischemia in the posterior wall. Endsystolic frames at rest and during dobutamine stress echocardiography are shown. Echocardiographic images are displayed in a quad format representing baseline (upper left panel), low dose (upper right panel), peak dose (lower left panel) and recovery (lower right panel) phases. Severe anteroseptal hypokinesis is present at baseline (upper left panel). In response to low dose dobutamine infusion, there is a *decrease* in endsystolic dimension and an *increase* in endocardial thickening representing the presence of significant contractile reserve as evidence of myocardial viability (upper right panel). At peak dose dobutamine, there is an *increase* in end-systolic dimension and a *decrease* in endocardial thickening in the posterior segments representing evidence of ischemia (lower left panel).

Responses to dobutamine

During dobutamine infusion, there are four possible responses of asynergic myocardial segments (Figure 3):
1. continued improvement (monophasic)
2. initial improvement followed by subsequent deterioration (biphasic)
3. worsening (ischemic)
4. no change (nonphasic).

Both monophasic and biphasic responses to dobutamine identify regions of contractile reserve, and therefore, viable myocardium. The biphasic response (the presence of both contractile reserve and subsequent ischemia) is of particular importance in predicting improvement of regional left ventricular dysfunction post-revascularization [9,10].

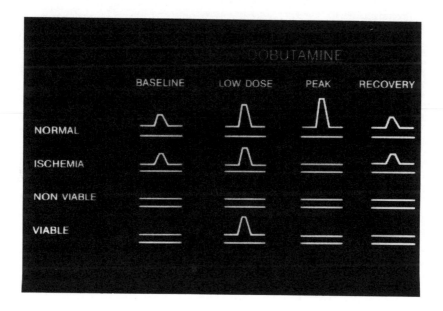

Figure 3. Diagrammatic representation of the possible responses of normal and abnormal myocardial segments to dobutamine infusion. Normal myocardial segments demonstrate increasing endocardial thickening and excursion with increasing doses of dobutamine. An ischemic response is represented by normal wall motion at baseline that demonstrates worsening of endocardial thickening and excursion during dobutamine infusion that reverts to normal in the recovery phase. Non-viable myocardium or non-phasic response is represented by abnormal endocardial thickening and excursion at baseline and the *absence* of improvement with dobutamine infusion. Viable myocardium, in this example, is represented by *abnormal* endocardial thickening and excursion at baseline, followed by improvement at low dose followed by subsequent deterioration at peak dose (biphasic response).

Safety of dobutamine echocardiography

The safety of dobutamine stress echocardiography has been reported in multiple studies. In a study by Mertes *et al.*, of 1,118 patients undergoing dobutamine stress echocardiography, no deaths, myocardial infarctions, or episodes of sustained ventricular tachycardia were reported. Arrhythmias, including premature ventricular contractions (15%) and frequent premature atrial contractions (8%), occurred in 35% of patients, but none were clinically or hemodynamically significant. Non-cardiac side effects including nausea, anxiety, headaches, tremor, and urgency did occur in 26% of patients. In only 3.2% of cases the test was terminated for any adverse side effect. The most common reasons for terminating the test were achieving target heart rate (52%), reaching maximal dose of dobutamine (21%), and anginal symptoms (13%) [11]. We have further extended these findings to patients with severe left ventricular dysfunction (mean left ventricular ejection fraction < 35%) [12]. In our laboratories, we have also demonstrated dobutamine stress echocardiography to be safe in the subset of patients with severe left ventricular dysfunction and laminated left ventricular apical thrombi [13]. More recently, Kumar *et al.* established the safety and efficacy of dobutamine echocardiography in the presence of multivessel coronary artery disease and acute myocardial infarction [14].

Dobutamine stress echocardiography protocol

Dobutamine infusion is started at 5 µg/kg/min and increased in a stepwise manner by 5 to 10 mcg/kg every 3 minutes. If the age-predicted heart rate is not attained, atropine may be administered in 0.25 mg increments up to a maximum dose of 2 mg. Dobutamine infusion is discontinued when one or more of the following criteria have been met:
1. A maximum infusion of 50 µg/kg/min was attained,
2. 85% of age predicted target heart rate was achieved, or
3. New wall motion abnormalities were identified in two or more segments in the same vascular distribution.

Echocardiographic images are obtained in the standard views: parasternal long axis, parasternal short axis, apical 4-chamber, and apical 2-chamber views, and, then, digitized online in a cine-loop format. Each standard echocardiographic view is displayed in a quad format representing baseline, low dose, peak dose, and recovery phases and are visually analyzed and assigned the appropriate response to dobutamine. Electrocardiogram, blood pressure, and rhythm strip are continuously monitored throughout the protocol.

Limitations to these methods include inability to visualize all myocardial segments, poor acoustic windows, and subjectivity of wall motion analysis.

In patients with poor acoustic windows, transesophageal echocardiography during dobutamine infusion, although not routinely performed for this purpose, is an useful alternative.

Dipyridamole echocardiography

Dipyridamole, through an adenosine A2-receptor mediated effect on arterioles, vasodilates, and therefore, increases blood flow. In regions of dysynergy, this increase in blood flow may result in an increase in myocardial contractility, thereby identifying regions of viability. Unlike dobutamine, the effect of dipyridamole is time-related rather than dose-related. After the administration of a predetermined dose of dipyridamole, an early inotropic phase followed by an ischemic phase, is identified [15,16]. Similar to dobutamine, the detection of myocardial viability is accomplished with a lower dose of pharmacologic agent than that used for inducing ischemia. Several studies have shown excellent concordance of dipyridamole echocardiography with low dose dobutamine for predicting functional recovery following successful revascularization. Varga *et al.* reported an overall concordance of 93% among 40 patients with coronary artery disease and left ventricular dysfunction who underwent both low dose dobutamine and dipyridamole echocardiography for the detection of myocardial viability. Follow-up resting echocardiography was obtained in 19 patients six weeks or more after successful revascularization. The sensitivity of dobutamine and dipyridamole for predicting recovery of regional left ventricular function was 76% and 78% (p = NS), respectively, and the specificity was 94% for both [17]. In a study by Picano *et al.*, the combined use of dipyridamole and low dose dobutamine to detect regions of myocardial viability improved the sensitivity for predicting recovery post revascularization in patients with baseline mild left ventricular dysfunction, as compared to either agent alone (sensitivities: 72% dobutamine, 67% dipyridamole, and 94% combined dipyridamole - dobutamine) [18]. The administration of dipyridamole prior to low dose dobutamine in patients with mild left ventricular dysfunction may help identify additional regions of selective myocardial viability which failed to demonstrate contractile reserve with either agent alone [18]. However, its usefulness in patients with severe left ventricular dysfunction has not yet been determined.

Nitroglycerine echocardiography

Evidence that regions of dysfunctional, but viable myocardium may respond to nitroglycerine was elucidated over two decades ago [19]. Rahimtoola *et al.* reported a sensitivity of 76% and a specificity of 65% with a predictive accuracy of 70% in the detection of viable myocardium with the use of nitroglycerin with left ventricular angiography [2]. Recently, there has been an increased interest in the administration of nitrates in echocardiographic imaging. In patients with critical stenoses, the administration of low dose dobutamine may induce ischemia prior to the detection of myocardial viability resulting in a false negative finding. Nitroglycerine, by increasing coronary blood flow, may allow the detection of viable myocardium prior to ischemia induced by low dose dobutamine. We have compared the use of nitroglycerin alone, low dose dobutamine and the combination of nitroglycerin and low dose dobutamine for the detection of myocardial viability. Of 272 abnormal segments at baseline, 144 (53%) segments were identified as viable by nitroglycerin alone, and 114 of these segments were concordant with those identified by low dose dobutamine alone. More importantly, 30 (11%) viable segments were identified with the use of nitroglycerin, but not with dobutamine. Similar results were obtained with the use of nitroglycerin and low dose dobutamine in combination, as compared to low dose dobutamine alone (108 segments concordant, 27 (10%) additional viable segments identified). Although, overall, the results are comparable with those of low dose dobutamine echocardiography, nitroglycerine echocardiography may identify additional viable segments not identified by low dose dobutamine alone, specifically regions with critical flow limiting stenoses [19].

Myocardial contrast echocardiography

Until recently, myocardial contrast echocardiography could only be utilized in the catheterization laboratory or in the operating room because the myocardial contrast agents required direct injection into the coronary arteries [20]. With newer second generation contrast agents and second harmonic imaging, although still experimental, myocardial perfusion assessment is now feasible with intravenous injections.

Myocardial contrast echocardiography utilizes the integrity of the microvasculature as a marker of myocardial viability. By using sonicated micro-bubbles similar in size to erythrocytes, blood flow through the microvasculature can be readily identified. Whereas coronary angiography can evaluate vessels as small as 100 microns, myocardial contrast echocardiography can detect flow in vessels as small as 10 microns. The degree of opacification is proportional to the amount of flow. DeFlippi *et al.* showed that, in patients with chronic ischemic heart disease, hypokinetic segments which demonstrated contractile reserve by dobutamine stress echocardiography and perfusion by myocardial contrast echocardiography were predictive of functional recovery post revascularization. Akinetic segments which did not improve post-revascularization, often demonstrated myocardial perfusion but no contractile reserve [20]. Therefore, the presence of contractile reserve during low dose dobutamine infusion is more specific, and has a better positive predictive value than perfusion by myocardial contrast echocardiography in predicting functional recovery post-revascularization in akinetic segments. With the use of intracoronary injection of myocardial contrast agent, Sabia *et al.* demonstrated that the presence of contrast in > 50% of the infarct zone predicts subsequent improvement in regional wall motion abnormality after successful reperfusion [21]. This study suggests that as long as microvasculature integrity is maintained, myocardial viability is preserved. Newer second generation contrast agents alone or in combination with technological advancements in ultrasound imaging are currently being investigated.

Acute reversible left ventricular dysfunction

In a pioneering study, Pierard *et al.*, evaluated the role of both low dose dobutamine echocardiography and positron emission tomography imaging in detecting acute reversible left ventricular dysfunction in patients who had acute anterior wall myocardial infarctions and received thrombolytic therapy [22]. Follow-up positron emission tomography and echocardiography were performed to assess the accuracy of these imaging studies to predict recovery of regional left ventricular function. Positron emission tomography and dobutamine echocardiography were concordant in detecting regions of viability and non-viability in 62 of 78 myocardial segments (79%). The regions that demonstrated viability by both positron emission tomography and dobutamine echocardiography improved in function post-revascularization. Regions with concordance regarding non-viability by the two techniques had persistent dysfunction. Interesting, all of the 9 discordant regions that were viable by positron emission tomography imaging, but did not demonstrate contractile reserve, did not improve in function post-revascularization. Six of these nine segments had metabolic evidence of necrosis on follow-up studies. Of the other seven regions that demonstrated contractile reserve (myocardial viability) by echocardiography, but necrosis by PET, five had improved function and normal metabolism on the follow-up study [22]. Several studies involving a total of 300 patients have further substantiated the role of low dose dobutamine echocardiography in the setting of acute myocardial infarction to predict the recovery of regional left ventricular function with sensitivity up to 86% and specificity up to 94% [23-27].

In 1991, Barilla *et al.*, reported on the positive utility of low dose dobutamine echocardiography in identifying "viable but non-contractile" myocardium in the setting of acute myocardial infarction. Marked improvement in response to low dose dobutamine was observed in the infarct-related segments, which was further reflected in a significant fall in wall motion score index. Furthermore, in those patients who demonstrated infarct zone contractile reserve and underwent revascularization, there was a greater improvement in regional left ventricular function compared to those who did not undergo revascularization [28].

Previtali *et al.* studied the role of dobutamine echocardiography for the early assessment of viability and ischemia in 59 patients with acute myocardial infarction who received thrombolytic therapy. In response to low dose dobutamine, a statistically significant drop in wall motion score index was observed in 73% of the patients, no significant change in 27% of the patients. The sensitivity, specificity and positive and negative predictive values of low dose dobutamine echocardiography in predicting recovery of regional left ventricular function were 79%, 68%, 89% and 50%, respectively [29]. Watada *et al.*, in a similar study reported a sensitivity and specificity of 83 and 86% [30].

Smart *et al.* studied the accuracy of segment response to low dose dobutamine in predicting recovery of regional left ventricular function in 115 patients, 2 to 7 days after acute myocardial infarction; 305 (44%) of 688 dysfunctional segments improved during the follow up period. A nonphasic response to dobutamine accurately predicted fixed dysfunction (318 (88%) of 360 segments), especially in akinetic or dyskinetic segments (276(91%) of 303 segments), independent of test interval and clinical or angiographic features. A biphasic or monophasic (continued improvement) response to dobutamine in baseline akinetic segments were highly predictive of reversible dysfunction (accuracy: 77% and 87%, respectively). However, among hypokinetic segments, accuracy was reduced primarily because of increased false positives (16%) [9].

Currently, there is overwhelming data to support the safety and usefulness of dobutamine echocardiography in the assessment of acute reversible left ventricular dysfunction.

Chronic reversible left ventricular dysfunction

The ability of low dose dobutamine echocardiography (LDDE) to predict the recovery of regional wall motion in patients with chronic left ventricular dysfunction secondary to coronary artery disease has been demonstrated in a number of studies with excellent results. These studies [31-36] have demonstrated that LDDE adequately predicts recovery of contractile function after revascularization with a mean sensitivity of 84% and a mean specificity of 81%. More importantly, the positive and negative predictive values of dobutamine echocardiography to predict improvement in regional left ventricular function after coronary artery bypass surgery have been excellent (87 and 84%, respectively). Meluzin *et al.* demonstrated a significant improvement of left ventricular ejection fraction after revascularization [LVEF, 38±5 to 42±5% (p<0.01)] in patients that demonstrated contractile reserve and no significant improvement in patients that did not demonstrate contractile reserve (LVEF, 38± 7% to 39± 8%, p=NS). Moreover, the magnitude of the change in left ventricular ejection fraction correlated linearly to the number of segments that demonstrated contractile reserve on low dose dobutamine echocardiography. Therefore, it is not only the presence, but the degree and extent of viable myocardium that determines the magnitude of improvement in regional left ventricular function [37]. Perrone-Filardi *et al.*, Bax *et al.*, and Vanoverschelde *et al.* have further confirmed these findings [31,38,39]. Perrone-Filardi *et al.*, LaConna *et al*, and Arnese *et al.*, have shown that low dose dobutamine echocardiography is a safe and accurate method for identifying reversible dysfunctional myocardium and predicts early reversibility of wall motion after surgical revascularization [31,32,36]. We have demonstrated that low dose dobutamine stress echocardiography in patients with severe left ventricular dysfunction, can predict left ventricular ejection fraction post surgical revascularization. Left ventricular ejection fraction determined during low dose dobutamine echocardiography correlated well with post-coronary artery bypass left ventricular ejection fractions (r =0.87) [40].

Afridi *et al.* determined the optimal dosing of dobutamine and compared the echocardiographic segment responses to the revascularization results. The biphasic response had the highest positive predictive value (72%) for subsequent recovery of left ventricular regional function [10]. Cornel *et al.* has shown that the diagnostic accuracy of dobutamine echocardiography in predicting recovery is dependent on three factors: the combining of low and high dose of dobutamine dosages, the severity of regional dyssynergy, and the timing of evaluation [42]. Senior *et al.* has shown that the detection of myocardial ischemia may be significantly enhanced by utilizing the biphasic response during serial stress dobutamine echocardiography in patients with baseline wall motion abnormalities [43]. Because dysfunctional, yet viable myocardium, can exhibit both inotropic reserve as well as inducible ischemia, it is not surprising the a biphasic response had the highest positive predictive value for predicting improvement after revascularization. Demonstrating contractile reserve and inducible ischemia in the same segments is fairly definitive proof that these segments will improve after revascularization. Dobutamine echocardiography should be considered the imaging technique of choice for accurate prediction of regional and global left ventricular function after surgical revascularization.

Risk stratification and prognosis

Low dose dobutamine has been shown to be an accurate method for identifying viable myocardium and predicting improvement of regional left ventricular dyssynergy post surgical revascularization. Table 1 summarizes the sensitivity and specificity for low dose dobutamine echocardiography for detection of improved regional contractile function after revascularization among the current published data. The presence of inotropic contractile reserve with low dose dobutamine echocardiography predicts a better initial survival compared to the absence of inotropic contractile reserve, independent of symptoms, baseline left ventricular function or coronary anatomy. By performing dobutamine echocardiography in patients with severe left ventricular dysfunction secondary to coronary artery disease, patients can be further risk stratified based on the extent and degree of contractile reserve. Meluzin *et al* have shown that the presence of a large amount of dysfunctional but viable myocardium detected by low dose dobutamine echocardiography identifies patients with the best prognosis [44]. Thus, in patients with similar ejection fractions, demonstrating contractile reserve stratifies them to a lower risk group than patients without contractile reserve. These findings were most recently confirmed by Afridi *et al* in a study of 318 patients with coronary artery disease and ejection fraction less than or equal to 35% who underwent dobutamine echocardiography and were followed up for 18 months. In those patients that demonstrated myocardial viability during low dose dobutamine echocardiography, revascularization improved survival as compared to medical therapy alone (mortality; 6 % vs. 20%, respectively. P = 0.001) [45].

Carlos *et al.* demonstrated that dobutamine stress echocardiography provided incremental value over clinical and resting echocardiographic data in predicting future cardiac events in patients after myocardial infarction. Identification of *nonviability* in the infarct zone and echocardiographic evidence of multivessel disease in patients with significant left ventricular dysfunction was highly predictive of cardiac events. Conversely, the presence of *viability* in the infarct zone, regardless of the extent of coronary artery disease, predicted a good outcome. Furthermore, the detection of multivessel disease by dobutamine stress echocardiography was more predictive of adverse outcome than the extent of coronary artery disease detected by angiography [46].

In a study by Picano *et al.*, 314 medically treated patients underwent dobutamine stress echocardiography to detect myocardial viability and myocardial ischemia. During the follow-up period of 9 ± 7 months, those patients that demonstrated more contractile reserve (Δ WMSI > 0.25), therefore more myocardial viability, had a better survival than those who demonstrated less contractile reserve (Δ WMSI < 0.25), therefore less

Table 1. Sensitivity and specificity for low dose dobutamine echocardiography for detection of improved regional contractile function after revascularization. Adapted from Bax *et al.* JACC 1997;30:1451-60 (with permission).

Study	No. of pts	Male (%)	Mean age (yr)	Mean LVEF (SD) (%)	Pts with MVD (%)	Pts with Prev MI (%)	Segs. with recovery (%)	Technique after revasc.	Sens (%)	Spec (%)
Charney et al.	17	59	63	46(±9)	76	65	53	Echo	71	93
Arnese et al.	38	68	59	31(NA)	92	100	22	Echo	74	96
Perrone-Filardi et al.	34	NA	NA	39(±14)	NA	NA	28	Echo	74	89
Afridi et al.	20	85	60	NA	40	55	33	Echo	76	74
Vanoverschelde et al.	73	85	59	36(±12)	79	68	38	Echo/RNV	79	80
Qureshi et al.	18	NA	61	NA	76	56	69	Echo	79	83
Marzullo et al.	14	79	54	39(±7)	93	100	65	Echo	82	94
Bax et al.	17	82	57	36(±11)	100	100	29	Echo	85	63
Senior et al.	22	95	61	26(±8)	86	NA	70	Echo	87	82
Perrone-Filardi et al.	18	94	59	43(±12)	50	89	61	Echo	88	87
La Canna et al.	33	97	56	33(±8)	94	70	65	Echo	92	75
Haque et al.	26	81	55	43(±14)	56	88	77	Echo	94	80
Baer et al.	42	90	59	40(±13)	74	100	62	Echo	96	69
DeFilippi et al.	23	100	NA	38(±10)	NA	NA	61	Echo	97	75
Average	28	86	58	36	78	78	52		84	
Weighted mean										81

LEVF = left ventricular ejection fraction; MI = myocardial infarction; MVD = multivessel disease; segs = segments; sens = sensitivity; spec = specificity myocardial viability or no contractile reserve (no myocardial viability) (100%, 94.1%, 95.6%, respectively, p<0.04) [47]. Therefore, it is not only the presence, but also the extent of myocardial viability that is predictive of survival. Similarly, in our laboratory, we have demonstrated that the presence of significant contractile reserve ($\geq$ 5 segments) in patients with severe left ventricular dysfunction secondary to coronary artery disease predicts a better initial survival than those without significant contractile reserve, independent of symptoms, baseline left ventricular function or coronary anatomy. Furthermore, those patients with significant contractile reserve who undergo early surgical revascularization have an improved survival as compared to medical management alone, or as compared to those patients with little or no contractile reserve regardless of revascularization. Those patients with little or no contractile reserve who undergo revascularization had the worst prognosis (Figure 4) [48].

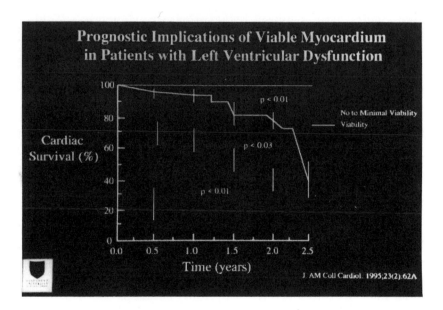

Figure 4. Survival curves demonstrating that those patients with significant viability as detected by dobutamine stress echocardiography, who underwent revascularization had the best survival over a 2.5 year follow-up(top solid line) as compared to those patients that demonstrated significant viability and were treated with medical therapy alone(second solid line) or with those patients with little to no viability regardless of revascularization(dashed lines). In addition, those patients who demonstrated little to no viability and underwent revascularization had the worst prognosis(bottom-most dashed line). J Am Coll Cardiol 1998 (in press).

Similarly, in a recent study by Senior *et al.*, 87 patients with congestive heart failure and chronic left ventricular dysfunction due to coronary artery disease were evaluated for the presence of myocardial viability by dobutamine stress echocardiography and followed for a period of 40 ± 17 months. Those patients with significant myocardial viability by dobutamine stress echocardiography (improvement in at least 5 of 12 myocardial segments) showed improvement in New York Heart Association class, global left ventricular systolic function and survival after revascularization as compared to those with significant myocardial viability who did not undergo revascularization or those without significant myocardial viability who did undergo revascularization (p< 0.01) [49].

Comparative studies

Several studies have compared dobutamine echocardiography with other imaging modalities to assess myocardial viability including 18 FDG PET [50-54], thallium-201 [55-62]. Technetium-99m MIBI SPECT [63,64], magnetic resonance imaging (MRI) [65,66] and myocardial contrast echocardiography [67]. As compared to thallium imaging techniques or PET, dobutamine echocardiography consistently had a much better specificity and positive predictive value in identifying and predicting improvement in regional left ventricular function after revascularization. Le Feuvre *et al.* studied 50 patients post acute myocardial infarction who underwent dobutamine echocardiography and rest redistribution thallium-201 SPECT imaging. The detection of myocardial viability by these two techniques were concordant in 163 of the 235 (69%) dyssynergic segments. The positive and negative predictive values for the prediction of recovery of acute reversible left ventricular dysfunction post revascularization by thallium-201 SPECT were 80% and 69%, respectively, and by dobutamine echocardiography were 91% and 70%, respectively [57]. Smart *et al.* compared dobutamine echocardiography and resting Thallium-201 SPECT imaging for detection of reversible dysfunction during the first week after acute myocardial infarction. The presence of a biphasic or monophasic (continued improvement) during dobutamine echocardiography were more accurate than thallium-201 uptake by SPECT scintigraphy for predicting regions of reversible dysfunction. Low dose dobutamine echocardiography had both higher sensitivity (81% versus 73%) and specificity (75% versus 35%) compared to thallium imaging [58]. Claeys *et al.* compared technetium 99m–sestamibi with dobutamine echocardiography in detecting myocardial viability in patients early after myocardial infarction. They concluded that technetium 99m–sestamibi may underestimate residual viability within the infarct region as compared to dobutamine echocardiography, especially in regions of abnormal flow states due to severe infarct related stenosis or late reperfusion therapy [66].

In the setting of chronic left ventricular dysfunction, Arnese *et al.* reported that thallium imaging had a higher sensitivity (74% for low dose dobutamine echocardiography versus 89% for thallium) for improvement of segmental function following revascularization, although low dose dobutamine echocardiography had a higher specificity (95% versus 48%, respectively) and positive predictive value (85% versus 33%, respectively) for predicting improvement of left ventricular function [36]. A study by Charney supports the conclusion that thallium SPECT imaging has better sensitivity (95% versus 71%), but lower specificity (85% versus 93%) than low dose dobutamine echocardiography. More importantly, low dose dobutamine echocardiography has a better positive predictive value (92% versus 90%) compared to thallium SPECT imaging for subsequent improvement in regional left ventricular function following successful revascularization [61].

Most recently, Bax *et al.* [70] in a meta-analysis, examined the most frequently used techniques for predicting improvement in regional contractile function after coronary revascularization in patients with left ventricular dysfunction secondary to coronary artery disease. Their meta-analysis revealed that the sensitivities for predicting improvement in regional contractile function after revascularization were high for all techniques analyzed (weighted means, range 83 – 90%); and the specificities for all techniques were low (weighted means, range 47 – 81%). Specificity is highest for low dose dobutamine echocardiography and lowest for thallium-201 stress redistribution–reinjection and thallium-201 rest–redistribution, favoring the use of low dose dobutamine echocardiography as the preferred technique for the prediction of regional functional recovery of left ventricular dysfunction post revascularization.

The data of Pierard *et al.* suggests that, while PET imaging overestimates viable myocardium, low dose dobutamine echocardiography has a better positive predictive value than PET imaging for predicting improvement of regional left ventricular function [23]. Since Pierard, several studies using 18-FDG PET to predict functional recovery in patients with coronary artery disease and chronic left ventricular dysfunction undergoing revascularization have been published [50-56]. Over 332 patients have been evaluated with nearly 400 segments analyzed. The reported mean sensitivity and specificity of PET techniques is 88% and 73% respectively. Thus, although PET and dobutamine echocardiography concur in the majority of the regions, data from several studies indicated that PET consistently overestimates the presence and extent of viability. More myocardial segments appear viable with thallium and PET imaging, therefore overestimating myocardial viability as compared to dobutamine echocardiography. However, many of the "viable" segments as determined by thallium imaging or PET, do not improve after revascularization leading to lower specificity for these two imaging modalities. This indicates that some regions although still metabolically viable, lack inotropic reserve. Blood flow and flow reserve may be so low that contractile reserve is lost despite preservation of trans-membrane pump activity. Alternatively, thallium and PET imaging may detect small regions of viability that are below a threshhold of critical "mass" to detect any regional improvement in left ventricular function. These regions of viability detected by thallium and PET imaging and not low dose dobutamine echocardiography, may involve primarily the *epicardial* and outer zones of the myocardium, and, therefore, unable to demonstrate inotropic contractile reserve which depends upon improvement of *endocardial* thickening.

Contrast MRI also shows excellent promise with concordant results with thallium-201 SPECT and dobutamine echocardiography. Rogers *et al.* recently demonstrated three abnormal patterns on contrast-enhanced MRI after reperfused myocardial infarction. Regions of initial normal signal followed by delayed hyperenhancement may represents predominantly viable myocardium [67]. Ramani *et al.* recently demonstrated that delayed hyperenhancement with gadolinium diethylenetriamine pentaacetic acid (Gd-DTPA) occurs frequently in areas of regional left ventricular dysfunction and correlates with thallium-201 scintigraphy and dobutamine echocardiography, particularly in regions demonstrating akinesis or dyskinesis at baseline [68].

Marwick *et al.* evaluated the accuracy of myocardial contrast echocardiography for the detection of segments and patients who had myocardial infarction with moderate and severe perfusion defects by SPECT. The segmental sensitivity for the detection of moderate to severe perfusion defects by myocardial contrast echocardiography ranged from 14% to 65 % and the specificity from 78% to 95%. Although accuracy was enhanced with the use of harmonic imaging in the triggered mode, myocardial contrast echocardiography underestimated the extent of SPECT defects [71]. More reliable methods of image acquisition and interpretation are currently under investigation.

Conclusions

The degree and extent of left ventricular function has important implications for risk stratification and prognosis [72,73]. Thus, it is imperative to identify reversible left ventricular dysfunction in patients with coronary artery disease because of the significant implications regarding risk stratification, prognosis, and the need for revascularization. Low dose dobutamine echocardiography is safe and has excellent sensitivity, specificity, and more importantly positive predictive accuracy in identifying both acute and chronic reversible left ventricular dysfunction.

References

1. Hammermeister KE, DeRouen TA, Dodge HT. Variables predictive of survival in patients with coronary disease. Selection by univariate and multivariate analysis from the clinical, electrocardiographic, exercise, arteriographic, and quantitative angiographic evaluation. Circulation 1979;59:421-30.
2. Rahimtoola SH. The hibernating myocardium. Am Heart J 1989;117:211-21.
3. Bolli R. Myocardial stunning in man. Circulation 1992;86:1671-91.
4. Alderman EL, Fisher LD, Litwin P *et al.* Results of coronary artery surgery in patients with poor left ventricular function (CASS). Circulation 1983;68:785-95.
5. Pigott JD, Kouchoukos NT, Oberman A, Cutter GR. Late results of surgical and medical therapy for patients with coronary artery disease and depressed left ventricular function. J Am Coll Cardiol 1985;5:1036-45
6. Feigenbaum H. Echocardiography. 4th ed. Philadelphia: Lea & Febiger; 1986.
7. Schulz R, Myazaki S, Miller M *et al.* Consequences of regional inotropic stimulation of ischemic myocardium on regional myocardial blood flow and functon in anesthetized swine. Circ Res 1989;64:1116-26.
8. Willerson JT, Hutton I, Watson JT, Platt MR, Templeton GH. Influence of dobutamine on regional myocardial blood flow and ventricular performance during acute and chronic myocardial ischemia in dogs. Circulation 1976;53:828-33.
9. Sehgal R, Lambert KL, Saham GM, Bonow RO, Chaudhry FA. Prediction of viable myocardium by dobutamine echocardiography in patients with chronic left-ventricular dysfunction [abstract]. Clin Res 1993;41:A683.
10. Afridi I, Kleiman NS, Raizner AE, Zoghbi WA. Dobutamine echocardiography in myocardial hibernation. Optimal dose and accuracy in predicting recovery of ventricular function after coronary angioplasty. Circulation 1995;91:663-70.
11. Mertes H, Sawada SG, Ryan T *et al.* Symptoms, adverse effects, and complications associated with dobutamine stress echocardiography. Experience in 1118 patients. Circulation 1993;88:15-9.
12. Singh K, Tauke JT, Bonow RO. Chaudry FA. Safety of dobutamine stress echocardiography in patients with severe left-ventricular dysfunction [abstract]. Clin Res 1994;42:358A.
13. Cusick DA, Aliwadi G, Tauke JT, Parker MA, Bonow RO, Chaudhry FA. Presence of left ventricular apical thrombus predicts lack of myocardial viability: a dobutamine stress echocardiographic study [abstract]. J Am Coll Cardiol 1996;27(2 Suppl A):369A.
14. Kumar R, Dwivedi SK, Puri VK, Saran RK, Narain VS, Hasan M. Predischarge dobutamine induced distant wall motion abnormalities after acute myocardial infarction predict multi-vessel disease. Indian Heart J 1995;47:349-52.
15. Picano E, Lattanzi F. Dipyridamole echocardiography. A new diagnostic window on coronary artery disease. Circulation 1991; 83:III19-26.
16. Picano E, Bento de Sousa MJ, de Moura Duarte LF, Pingitore A, Sicari R. Detection of viable myocardium by dobutamine and dipyridamole stress echocardiography. Herz 1994;19:204-9.
17. Varga A, Ostojic M, Djordjevic-Dikic A *et al.* Infra-low dose dipyridamole test. A novel dose regimen for selective assessment of myocardial viability by vasodilator stress echocardiography. Eur Heart J 1996;17:629-34.

18. Picano E, Ostojic M, Varga A *et al.* Combined low dose dipyridamole-dobutamine stress echocardiography to identify myocardial viability. J Am Coll Cardiol 1996;27:1422-8.
19. Helfant R, Pine R, Meister SG, Feldman MS, Trout RG, Banka VS. Nitroglycerine to unmask reversible asynergy. Correlation with post coronary bypass ventriculography. Circulation 1974;50:108-13.
20. Valentini W, Pappas EP, Parker MA, Bonow RO, Chaudhry FA. Does nitroglycerin enhance the identification of viable myocardium by dobutamine echocardiography? [abstract] J Investig Med 1995;43:390A.
21. DeFilippi C, Willett DL, Irani WN, Eichhorn EJ, Velasco CE, Grayburn PA. Comparison of myocardial contract echocardiography and low-dose dobutamine stress echocardiography in predicting recovery of left ventricular function after coronary revascularization in chronic ischemic heart disease. Circulation 1995;92:2863-8.
22. Sabia PJ, Powers ER, Ragosta M, Sarebock IJ, Burwell LR, Kaul S. An association between collateral blood flow and myocardial viability with recent myocardial infarction. N Engl J Med 1992;327:1825-31.
23. Pierard L, De Landsheere CM, Berthe C, Rigo P, Kulbertus HE. Identification of viable myocardium by echocardiography during dobutamine infusion in patients with myocardial infarction after thrombolytic therapy: comparison with positron emission tomography. J Am Coll Cardiol 1990;15:1021-31.
24. Barilla F, Gheorghiade M, Alam M, Khaja F, Goldstein S. Low dose dobutamine in patients with acute myocardial infarction identifies viable but not contractile myocardium and predicts the magnitude of improvement in wall motion abnormalities in response to coronary revascularization. Am Heart J 1991;122:1522-31.
25. Smart S, Sawada S, Ryan T. *et al.* Low dose dobutamine echocardiography detects reversible dysfunction after thrombolytic therapy of acute myocardial infarction. Circulation 1993;88:405-15.
26. Previtali M, Poli A, Lanzarini L, Fetiveau R, Mussini A, Ferrario M. Dobutamine stress echocardiography for assessment of myocardial viability and ischemia in acute myocardial infarction treated with thrombolysis. Am J. Cardiol 1993;72:124G-130G.
27. Watada H, Ito H, Oh H *et al.* Dobutamine stress echocardiography predicts reversible dysfunction and quantitates the extent of irreversibly damaged myocardium after reperfusion of anterior myocardial infarction. J Am Coll Cardiol 1994;24:624-30.
28. Salustri A, Elhendy A, Garyfallydis P *et al.* Prediction of improvement of ventricular function after first acute myocardial infarction using low-dose dobutamine stress echocardiography. Am J Cardiol 1994;74:853-6.
29. Barilla F, Gheorghiade M, Alam M, Khaja F, Goldstein S. Low-dose dobutamine in patients with acute myocardial infarction identifies viable but not contractile myocardium and predicts the magnitude of improvement in wall motion abnormalities in response to coronary revascularization. Am Heart J 1991;122:1522-31.
30. Previtali M, Poli A, Lanzarini L, Fetiveau R, Mussini A, Ferrario M. Dobutamine stress echocardiography for assessment of myocardial viability and ischemia in acute myocardial infarction treated with thrombolysis. Am J Cardiol 1993;73(19):124G-130G.
31. Watada H, Ito H, Oh H, Masuyama T, Aburaya M, Hori M, Iwakura M, Higashino Y, Fujii K, Minamino T. Dobutamine stress echocardiography predicts reversible dysfunction and quantitates the extent of irreversibly damaged myocardium after reperfusion of anterior myocardial infarction. J Am Coll Cardiol 1994;24:624-30.
32. Smart S, Wynsen J, Sagar K. Dobutamine-atropine stress echocardiography for reversible dysfunction during the first week after acute myocardial infarction: limitations and determinants of accuracy. J Am Coll Cardiol 1997;30:1669-78.
33. Perrone-Filardi P, Pace L, Prastaro M *et al.* Dobutamine echocardiography predicts improvement of hypoperfused dysfunctional myocardium after revascularization in patients with coronary artery disease. Circulation 1995;91:2556-65.

34. La Canna G, Alfieri O, Giubbini R, Gargano M, Ferrari R, Visioli O. Echocardiography during infusion of dobutamine for identification of reversible dysfunction in patients with chronic coronary artery disease. J Am Coll Cardiol 1994,23:617-26.

35. Charney R, Swinger ME, Cohen MV, Menegus M, Spindola-Franco H, Greenberg MA. Dobutamine echocardiography predicts recovery of hibernating myocardium following coronary revascularization [abstract]. J Am Coll Cardiol 1992;19(3 Suppl A):176A.

36. Cigarroa CG, DeFilippi CR, Brickner ME, Alvarez LG, Wait MA, Grayburn PA. Dobutamine stress echocardiography identifies hibernating myocardium and predicts recovery of left ventricular function after coronary revascularization. Circulation 1993;88:430-6.

37. Arnese M, Cornel JH, Salustri A *et al.* Prediction of improvement of regional left ventricular function after surgical revascularization: a comparison of low-dose dobutamine echocardiography with 201-Tl SPECT. Circulation 1995;91:2748-52.

38. Meluzin J, Cigarroa CG, Brickner ME *et al.* Dobutamine echocardiography in predicting improvement in global left ventricular systolic function after coronary bypass or angioplasty in patients with healed myocardial infarcts. Am J Cardiol 1995;76:877-80.

39. Bax JJ, Cornel JH, Visser FC *et al.* Prediction of recovery of myocardial dysfunction following revascularization: comparison of F18-flurorodeoxyglucose/thallium-201 single photon emission computed tomography, thallium-201 stress-reinjection single photon emission computed tomography and dobutamine echocardiography. J Am Coll Cardiol 1996;28:558-64.

40. Vanoverschelde JL, D'Hondt AM, Marwich T *et al.* Head-to-head comparison of exercise-redistribution-reinjection thallium single-photon emission computed tomography and low dose dobutamine echocardiography for prediction of reversibility of chronic left ventricular ischemic dysfunction. J Am Coll Cardiol 1996;28:432-42.

41. Singh B, Singh V, Ghandi S *et al.* Detection of myocardial viability and prediction of post revascularization ejection fraction in the presence of severe left ventricular dysfunction. [abstract] J Am Coll Cardiol 1999;33(Suppl A):175A

42. Cornel JH, Bax JJ, Elhendy A, Maat APWM *et al.* Biphasic response to dobutamine predicts improvement of global left ventricular function after surgical revascularization in patients with stable coronary artery disease. J Am Coll Cardiol 1998;31:1002-10.

43. Senior R, Lahiri A. Enhanced detection of myocardial ischemia by stress dobutamine echocardiography utilizing the "biphasic" response of wall thickening during low and high dose dobutamine infusion. J Am Coll Cardiol 1995;26:26-32.

44. Meluzin J, Cerny J, Frelich M *et al.* Prognostic value of the amount of dysfunctional but viable myocardium in revascularized patients with coronary artery disease and left ventricular dysfunction. J Am Coll Cardiol 1998;32:912-20.

45. Afridi I, Grayburn PA, Panza JA, Oh JK, Zoghbi WA, Marwich TH. Myocardial viability during dobutamine echocardiography predicts survival in patients with coronary artery disease and severe left ventricular systolic dysfunction. J Am Coll Cardiol 1998;32:921-6.

46. Carlos ME, Smart SC, Wynsen JC, Sagar KB. Dobutamine stress echocardiography for risk stratification after myocardial infarction. Circulation 1997;95:1402-10.

47. Picano E, Sicari R, Landi P *et al.* Prognostic value of myocardial viability in medically treated patients with global left ventricular dysfunction early after an acute uncomplicated myocardial infarction: a dobutamine stress echocardiographic study. Circulation 1998;98:1078-84.

48. Chaudhry FA, Tauke JT, Alessandrini RS, Vardi G, Parker MA, Bonow RO. Prognostic implications of myocardial contractile reserve in patients with coronary artery disease and left ventricular dysfunction. J Am Coll Cardiol. In press 1999.

49. Senior R, Kaul S, Lahiri A. Myocardial viability on echocardiography predicts long-term survival after revascularization in patients with ischemic congestive heart failure. J Am Coll Cardiol 1999;33:1848-54.
50. Baer FM, Voth E, Deutsch HJ, Schneider CA, Schicha H, Sechtem U. Assessment of viable myocardium by dobutamine transesophageal echocardiography and comparison with fluorine-18 fluorodeoxyglucose positron emission tomography. J Am Coll Cardiol 1994;24:343-53.
51. Tamaki N, Kawamot M, Tadamura E et al. Prediction of reversible ischemia after revascariztion. Perfusion and metabolic studies with positron emission tomography. Circulation 1995;91:1697-705.
52. Tillisch J, Brunken R, Marshall R et al. Reversibility of cardiac wall-motion abnormalities predicted by positron tomography. N Engl J Med 1986;314: 884-8.
53. Lucignani G, Paolini G, Landoni C et al. Presurgical identification of hibernating myocardium by combined use of technetium-99m hexakis 2-ethoxyisobutylisonitrile single photon emission computed tomography and fluorine-18 fluoro-2-deoxy-D-glucose positron emission tomography in patients with coronary artery disease. Eur J Nucl Med 1992;19:874-81.
54. Carrel T, Jenni R, Haubold-Reuter S, Von Schulthess G, Pasic M, Turina M. Improvement of severely reduced left ventricular function after surgical revascularization in patients with preoperative myocardial infarction. Eur J Cardiothorac Surg 1992;6:479-84.
55. Gropler RJ, Geltman EM, Sampathkumaran K et al. Comparison of carbon-11 acetate with fluorine-18 fluorodeoxyglucose for delineating viable myocardium by positron emisson tomography. J Am Coll Cardiol 1993;22:1587-97.
56. Vom Dahl J, Altehoefer C, Sheehan FH et al. Recovery of myocardial function following coronary revascularization: impact of viability and long-term vessel patency as assessed by preoperative F-18 FDG PET and serial angiography [abstract]. J Nucl Med 1993;34(5 Suppl):23P.
57. Le Feuvre C, Baubion N, Aubry N, Metzger JP, de Vernejoul P, Vacheron A. Assessment of reversible dyssynergic segments after acute myocardial infarction: Dobutamine echocardiography versus thallium-201 single photon emission computed tomography. Am Heart J 1996;131:668-75.
58. Smart S, Stoiber T, Hellman R et al. Low dose dobutamine echocardiography is more predictive of reversible dysfunction after acute myocardial infarction than resting single photon emission computed tomographic thallium-201 scintigraphy. Am Heart J 1997;134:822-34.
59. Haque T, Furukawa T, Takahashi M, Kinoshita M. Identification of hibernating myocardium by dobutamine stress echocardiography: comparison with thallium-201m reinjection imaging. Am Heart J 1995;130:553-63.
60. Panza JA, Dilsizian V, Laurienzo JM, Curiel RV, Katsiyiannis PT. Relation between thallium uptake and contractile response to dobutamine. Implications regarding myocardial viability in patients with chronic coronary artery disease and left ventricular dysfunction. Circulation 1995;91:990-8.
61. Charney R, Schwinger ME, Chun J et al. Dobutamine echocardiography and resting-redistribution thallium-201 scintigraphy predicts recovery of hibernating myocardium after coronary revascularization. Am Heart J 1994;128:864-9.
62. Perrone-Filardi P, Pace L, Prastaro M et al. Assessment of myocardial viability in patients with chronic coronary artery disease. Rest-4-hour-24-hour 201Tl tomography versus dobutamine echocardiography. Circulation 1996;94:2712-9.
63. Qureshi U, Nagueh SF, Afridi I et al. Dobutamine echocardiography and quantitative rest-redistribtuion 201Tl tompgraphy in myocardial hypernation. Relation of contractile reserve to 201Tl uptake and comparative prediction of recovery of function. Circulation 1997;95:626-35.

64. Senior R, Glenville B, Basu S *et al.* Dobutamine echocardiography and thallium-201 imaging predict functional improvement after revascularization in severe ischaemic left ventricular dysfunction. Br Heart J 1995;74:358-64.

65. Marzullo P, Parodi O, Reisenhofer B *et al.* Value of rest thallium-201/technetium-99m sestamibi and dobutamine echocardiography for detecting myocardial viability. Am J Cardiol 1993;71:166-72.

66. Claeys MJ, Rademakers FE, Vrints CJ *et al.* Comparative study of rest technetium-99m sestamibi SPECT and low-dose dobutamine stress echocardiography for the early assessment of myocardial viability after acute myocardial infarction: importance of the severity of the infarct related stenosis. Eur J Nucl Med 1996;23:748-55.

67. Rogers WJ Jr, Kramer CM, Geskin G *et al.* Early contrast-enhanced MRI predicts late functional recovery after reperfused myocardial infarction. Circulation 1999;99:744-50.

68. Ramani K, Judd RM, Holly TA *et al.* Contrast magnetic resonance imaging in the assessment of myocardial viability in patients with stable coronary disease and left ventricular dysfunction. Circulation 1998;98:2687-94.

69. Bolognese L, Antoniucci D, Rovai D *et al.* Myocardial contrast echocardiography versus dobutamine echocardiography for predicting functional recovery after acute myocardial infarction treated with primary coronary angioplasty. J Am Coll Cardiol 1996;28:1677-83.

70. Bax JJ, Wijns W, Cornel JH, Visser FC, Boersma E, Fioretti PM. Accuracy of currently available techniques for prediction of functional recovery after revascularization in patients with left ventricular dysfunction due to chronic coronary artery disease: comparisons of pooled data. J Am Coll Cardiol 1997;30:1451-60.

71. Marwick TH, Brunken R, Meland N *et al.* Accuracy and feasibility of contrast echocardiography for detection of perfusion defects in routine practice: comparison with wall motion and technetium-99m sestamibi single-photon emission computed tomography. The Nycomed NC100100 Investigators. J Am Coll Cardiol 1998;32:1260-9.

72. Iskandrian AS, Van der Wall EE, editors. Myocardial viability: detection and clinical relevance. Dordrecht: Kluwer Academic Publishers; 1994.

73. Hendel RC, Chaudhry FA, Bonow RO. Myocardial viability. Curr Probl Cardiol 1996;21:145-221.

10. Role of magnetic resonance techniques in viability assessment

ERNST E. VAN DER WALL, JEROEN J. BAX, HUBERT W. VLIEGEN, ALBERT V.G. BRUSCHKE & ALBERT DE ROOS

Introduction

With the application of magnetic resonance (MR) techniques in clinical cardiology, important tools have been added to the currently available diagnostic arsenal for the evaluation of patients with coronary artery disease. In patients with coronary artery disease it is of paramount importance to distinguish between viable myocardium and areas of myocardial fibrosis. Viable myocardial areas are most likely to benefit from revascularization, whereas revascularization of fibrotic myocardium will not lead to improvement of left ventricular function. For the prospective identification of jeopardized but viable myocardium for purposes of guiding therapeutic interventions in individual patients the following three standards for myocardial viability can be used;
1.   preserved myocardial perfusion and perfusion reserve
2.   preserved systolic wall motion and thickening
3.   preserved myocardial metabolism
The current MR techniques provide a great potential to measure all *three* standards of viability. Systolic wall motion, thickness and thickening can be assessed by *cine MR imaging*, adequate perfusion and perfusion reserve by *spin-echo MR imaging* or *ultrafast MR imaging*, and the presence of metabolic integrity by *MR spectroscopy*.
These noninvasive and versatile techniques have led towards and increasing interest and research in the past years. Particular strengths of the MR techniques are: 1) the inherent three-dimensional data acquisition without radiation exposure, 2) the intrinsic soft tissue contrast which allows tissue characterization, 3) the excellent spatial resolution (in the 1-2 mm range) which permits the evaluation of regional abnormalities, 4) multitomographic imaging capabilities which allow acquisition of cardiac images in any plane, 5) the inherent sensitivity to blood and wall motion, and 6) the potential of in vivo measurement of myocardial metabolism using MR spectroscopy.
Recently, the clinical role of MR techniques in cardiovascular disease has been defined in a Task Force Report instituted by a Task Force of the

A. E. Iskandrian and E. E. van der Wall (eds.), Myocardial Viability, 177-197.
© 2000 *Kluwer Academic Publishers. Printed in the Netherlands.*

European Society of Cardiology, in Collaboration with the Association of European Paediatric Cardiologists composed by Sechtem *et al.* [1]. Table 1 lists the most important indications for MR imaging in clinical cardiology. Although the use of MR techniques in the detection of coronary artery disease is still being considered as investigational, assessment of myocardial viability may become one of the first-line issues in clinical cardiac MR imaging (Table 2). Before dwelling into the value of MR imaging in assessing myocardial viability, the currently used MR techniques are shortly described.

Table 1. Current indications for cardiac MR imaging

Primary indications
Congenital heart disease
Great vessel disease
(Para)cardiac masses
Pericardial processes

Secondary indications
Congestive heart failure
Myocardial tissue abnormalities
Valvular heart disease

Investigational
Aortocoronary bypass angiography
Coronary angiography
Ischemic heart disease

Spin-echo MR imaging

Multislice spin-echo MR imaging, with triggering of the image acquisition to the R-wave of the electrocardiogram, is the most commonly used strategy for defining the morphology of the heart and great vessels [2]. The flowing blood provides natural contrast, thereby allowing anatomical evaluation of cardiovascular pathology. Slice thickness, image orientation and image contrast can be selected by the operator, depending on the anatomical structures under investigation. The MR imaging approach provides unlimited access to the chest without the problems of obtaining adequate imaging windows inherent to echocardiography. Spin-echo MR images, however, provide only static information, require relatively long acquisition times, and may be degraded by motion or flow artefacts.

Table 2. Indications for magnetic resonance imaging in patients with coronary artery disease

Indication	Class
Assessment of myocardial function	III
Detection of coronary artery disease	
Analysis of regional left ventricular function during stress	III
Assessment of myocardial perfusion	Inv
Coronary angiography	Inv
Bypass graft angiography	III
Assessment of coronary flow	Inv
Detection and quantification of acute myocardial infarcts	IV
Sequelae of myocardial infarction	
Myocardial Viability	**II**
Ventricular septal defect	III
Mitral regurgitation	III
Intraventricular thrombus	II

Class I - provides clinically relevant information and is usually appropriate ; may be used as a first line imaging technique
Class II - provides clinically relevant information and is frequently useful, but similar information may be provided by other imaging techniques
Class III - may provide clinically relevant information but is infrequently used because information from other imaging techniques is usually adequate
Class IV - does not provide clinically useful information
Inv - potentially useful, but still under investigation
(Reproduced from Sechtem *et al.*, reference 1 with permission)

Gradient-echo MR imaging

In contrast to spin-echo sequences, gradient-echo MR imaging provides dynamic information on blood flow and cardiac function [3]. Gradient-echo images display blood flow as a bright signal, whereas spin-echo images show blood flow generally as a dark signal or no signal. Flow disturbances, like those associated with valvular stenoses and insufficiencies, are visualized because of low-signal turbulent jet effects contrasting with the bright signal of normal flowing blood. The images are acquired with high temporal resolution with 20 or more phases per cardiac cycle. They can be displayed in a pseudo-real-time movie loop format to provide a dynamic impression of flow and function. However, gradient-echo acquisitions require ECG gating and are not real time.

High-speed MR imaging

Ultrafast MR imaging techniques and real-time echo-planar techniques have recently become available. High-speed MR imaging will reduce image degradation from physiological motion effects such as respiration. Echo-planar imaging operates in a single-shot or multi-shot format, allowing the reduction of acquisition times to 50 ms or less per image [4]. It may become clinically useful in imaging the entire heart with multiple imaging sections within a single breathhold. These fast techniques may be particularly useful in assessing function, flow and myocardial perfusion. However, echo-planar technology places heavy demands on the MR gradient system and the radiofrequency receiver of the MR imaging machine.

MR angiography

MR angiography is based on gradient-echo sequences that allow visualization and quantification of blood flow non-invasively without the use of contrast agents [5]. Such techniques are categorized as time-of-flight or phase-contrast methods. In the resulting angiographic image the vessels are depicted as a bright signal against a dark background because of the phenomenon of 'flow-related enhancement'. The phase-contrast method is based on velocity-induced phase shifts of spins in blood flow in the presence of a magnetic field gradient. The measured phase shift is proportional to flow velocity, which allows the extraction of quantitative data on flow velocity and volume. MR flow mapping is widely used to measure blood flow in the aorta, pulmonary circulation, intracardiac flow, native coronary vessels and coronary artery bypass grafts, as well as a number of other vascular areas throughout the body.

MR spectroscopy

MR spectroscopy is an exciting tool for evaluation of cardiac metabolism by direct measurement of changes in high-energy phosphates using surface coils directly applied to the surface of the chest wall. These changes can be observed by generating spectra from the myocardial wall. As the signal intensities of the high-energy phosphates are dependent on metabolic conditions, such as ischemia or hypoxia, MR spectroscopy should be very well suited to study myocardial viability based on differences in spectra [6].

Myocardial perfusion

Ultrafast MR imaging

MR perfusion imaging, with the aid of contrast agents for MR imaging such as the paramagnetic contrast agent gadolinium-diethylene-triaminepenta-acetic acid (Gd-DTPA), may be used to assess the functional significance of coronary artery stenoses by demonstrating perfusion abnormalities in the myocardial bed distal to the stenoses. Ultrafast gradient-echo sequences only require a fraction of a second for data acquisition and is therefore also known as subsecond MR imaging or high-speed MR imaging [7]. Coupled with the bolus administration of contrast media and the acquisition of first-pass images of the right and left ventricular cavity, ultrafast MR imaging has great potential in the assessment of regional myocardial perfusion. The technique has advantages over the conventional techniques as a result of higher spatial resolution, and less attenuation related to patient motion during the imaging procedure as a result of the short duration of the procedure. In addition, ultrafast imaging enables the study of fast physiological processes, such as cardiac first-pass effects.

Atkinson *et al.* [8] demonstrated that a T1 weighted ultrafast imaging technique can provide adequate temporal and spatial resolution to permit first-pass perfusion studies of the heart. In studies of human subjects, it was possible to show dynamically the first-pass transit of a Gd-DTPA bolus, administered in a peripheral vein, through the four cardiac chambers and into the left ventricular myocardium. Wilke *et al.* [9] showed in a dog model that MR first pass technique using Gd-DTPA as an indicator is well suited to obtain myocardial perfusion images and has the potential to assess relative myocardial perfusion quantitatively. Manning *et al.* [10] used ultrafast MR imaging for the assessment of coronary artery stenosis in patients with chest pain. Regional myocardium perfused by a diseased vessel demonstrated a lower peak signal intensity and lower rate of signal increase than did myocardium perfused by coronary arteries without stenosis. Repeat MR imaging study after revascularization showed an increase in peak signal intensity. Van Rugge *et al.* [11,12] evaluated the value of ultrafast MR imaging for the assessment of dynamic contrast enhancement and myocardial perfusion abnormalities in 7 healthy volunteers and in 20 patients after myocardial infarction. After Gd-DTPA administration, infarcted myocardium demonstrated a signal intensity enhancement of 50% whereas in normal myocardium an enhancement of 134% was obtained. The infarct site on MR imaging corresponded with the location of wall motion asynergy determined by echocardiography. It was concluded that Gd-DTPA-enhanced ultrafast MRI provides noninvasive assessment of myocardial viability in patients with suspected and proven coronary artery disease. Matheijssen *et al.* [13] compared dipyridamole MR imaging with technetium-99m sestamibi single photon emission computed tomography (SPECT) in 10 patients with single-vessel disease. Both SPECT and MR imaging had a 100% sensitivity for detection of coronary artery disease. Agreement in localization of stenosis was 90% between MR imaging and SPECT and 70% between MR imaging and contrast angiography. It should be realized that in most ensuing studies differences in regional perfusion were based on differences in signal intensity rather than on visually judged differences. Wilke *et al.* [14] showed that first-pass

MR imaging can be used to quantitatively assess myocardial perfusion reserve. First pass images were obtained at rest and during adenosine infusion and it was shown that accurate estimates of the perfusion index, corresponding to the ratio of resting and hyperemic myocardial blood flow, can be obtained in patients with decreased myocardial perfusion reserve due to microvascular dysfunction. Lauerma et al. [15] used multislice MR imaging (3 sections) in the detection of myocardial ischemia and the assessment of revascularization on tissue perfusion in 11 patients with single-vessel coronary artery disease. Revascularization normalized enhancement patterns of formerly underperfused myocardium and decreased infarct size in the MR imaging sections. A linear correlation in defect size between MR imaging and thallium-201 scintigraphy was observed, implying the potential of multislice MR imaging in assessing myocardial viability. Recently, Dendale et al. [16] used ultrafast contrast-enhanced MR imaging in 20 patients with a first myocardial infarction to distinguish open and closed infarct-related arteries. An open artery was characterized by both a faster rise and fall in signal intensity than an occluded artery .

Apart from ultrafast first-pass MR imaging, paramagnetic contrast agents may be used to vizualize the myocardium over a longer period of time based on a high specific affinity to irreversibly injured myocardium, which can be visualized by spin-echo imaging. The paramagnetic contrast agent Gd-DTPA positively stains the infarcted area 30-60 minutes after intravenous administration, which can be visualized by spin-echo MR imaging. A considerable advantage of this approach is the ability to image the myocardium with high spatial resolution, as the contrast agent has to reach an equilibrium state. Myocardial patterns with hyperenhancement may be indicative of compromised myocardial viability or infarction. This approach might therefore be effective in discriminating hibernating but viable myocardium from nonviable myocardial tissue [17]. Several studies from our institution in patients with (sub) acute myocardial infarcts [18,19] showed differences in signal intensity and morphological appearance of contrast enhancement between reperfused and nonreperfused myocardial areas. In reperfused areas increased signal intensities and a homogeneous enhancement pattern was observed, whereas the nonreperfused areas showed diminished signal intensity and a heterogeneous aspect [20,21]. In addition, Gd-DTPA determined infarct size was significantly smaller in patients with documented reperfusion compared to patients in whom no reperfusion was established.

Until now, only one MR imaging viability study showed prognostic significance. Wu et al. [22] recently demonstrated that patients with microvascular obstruction after acute myocardial infarction, as assessed by MR imaging, was associated with a poor prognosis. In 44 patients, who were studied 2 weeks after acute myocardial infarction, microvascular obstruction was defined as hypoenhancement 5-10 minutes following contrast injection. Patients were followed for approximately 1.5 years and patients with microvascular obstruction had significantly more cardiac events than patients without microvascular obstruction (45% versus 9%). It was concluded that the microvascular status following myocardial infarction, as determined by contrast-enhanced MR imaging, is a strong prognostic marker for future cardiac events.

Cardiac wall motion

Cine MR imaging

By assessing wall motion dynamics cine MR imaging can be considered as the next standard of viability. The temporal resolution attained by cine MR imaging has extended the application of MR imaging to the assessment of cardiac function. Cine MR imaging can be performed sequentially, so that the severity of cardiac disease states can be monitored and the response to interventions determined. Since both the endocardial and epicardial borders are well defined by MR imaging, it is possible to assess wall thickness and thickening during the cardiac cycle and to detect regional myocardial dysfunction. The capability of MR imaging to provide sequential information about the state of pathologically altered myocardium in combination with assessment of diastolic wall thickness and systolic wall thickening makes it suitable for identification of viable myocardium in areas previously affected by myocardial infarction. In the following sections we describe the value of MR imaging in delineating myocardial ischemia and viability.

Myocardial ischemia

Similar to stress echocardiography, the hallmark of myocardial ischemia is the presence of resting wall motion abnormalities or stress-induced abnormalities. Since physical exercise during MR imaging is difficult because of motion artifacts and space restriction, pharmacological stress has been used in these studies. Pennell *et al.* [23] were the first to report on the use of MR imaging in combination with dipyridamole. The authors performed a direct comparison between thallium-201 scintigraphy and MR imaging in 40 patients with coronary artery disease. The sensitivity of dipyridamole MR imaging for the detection of coronary artery disease was 62% and the agreement between reversible thallium-201 defects and wall motion abnormalities was 67%. Hence, dipyridamole did not induce wall motion abnormalities in 33% of the regions exhibiting a perfusion defect on thallium-201 imaging. Baer *et al.* [24] using dipyridamole MR imaging showed a sensitivity of 78% in the detection of wall motion abnormalities. In a subsequent study, Pennell *et al.* [25] compared dobutamine MR imaging with thallium-201 SPECT in 22 patients with coronary artery disease. Twenty-one of the patients showed ischemia on thallium-201 SPECT imaging, with 20 (95%) exhibiting new wall motion abnormalities during dobutamine MR imaging, indicating a high sensitivity for the detection of coronary artery disease. In a subsequent study, Baer *et al.* [26] compared technetium-99m sestamibi SPECT with dobutamine MR imaging and reported almost similar sensitivities for MR imaging and technetium-99m sestamibi SPECT: 84% and 87%, respectively.

In our institution, Van Rugge *et al.* [27] gained extensive experience with dobutamine MR based on quantitative evaluation of regional and global heart function using our home-made MR Analytical Software System (MASS 3.0), which is a dedicated software package for automatic delineation of the subepicardial and subendocardial borders [28]. Wall motion abnormalities, either induced by pharmacological stress or following myocardial infarction [29] can be accurately and reliably assessed using the MASS-derived centerline method. Using this technique, a sensitivity of 91% and a specificity of 80% were obtained [27]. An overview of the results of the available MR imaging studies in detecting coronary artery disease is presented in Table 3.

Table 3. Accuracy of MR imaging in the detection of coronary artery disease

Author	Year	No. of pts	Stressor	MPI agent	MPI sens	MR sens
Pennell *et al.*[23]	1990	40	dipy	Tl-201	92%	62%
Baer *et al.*[24]	1992	23	dipy	-	-	78%
Pennell *et al.*[25]	1992	22	dobu	Tl-201	95%	91%
Baer *et al.*[26]	1994	35	dobu	MIBI	87%	84%
Van Rugge *et al.*[27]	1994	39	dobu	-	-	91%

dipy: dipyridamole; dobu: dobutamine; MIBI: technetium-99m sestamibi; MPI: myocardial perfusion imaging; sens: sensitivity; spec: specificity; Tl-201: thallium-201 chloride.

Myocardial viability

Based on the Task Force Report of the European Society of Cardiology [1], the clinically most useful approach of MR imaging in coronary artery disease is the assessment of myocardial viability (Class II indication, Table 2). Various studies with MR imaging have focused on the assessment of myocardial viability [30-42]. Four markers of viability have been used in these studies: 1) increased signal intensity, 2) enddiastolic wall thickness, 3) systolic wall thickening at rest, and 4) contractile reserve during dobutamine stimulation. The available studies concerning the assessment of myocardial viability with MR imaging are summarized in Table 4.

Table 4. Experience of MR imaging in the assessment of myocardial viability

Author	Year	No. pts	Viability marker	Outcome
Johnston et al.[30]	1993	24	ISI, SWT	MR imaging is superior over Tl-201 stress-redistribution for assessment of viability
Lawson et al.[31]	1997	24	EDWT, SWT	EDWT and SWT correlate well with Tl-201 uptake
Baer et al.[32]	1992	20	EDWT, SWT	good agreement between absent SWT or reduced EDWT and scar on MIBI SPECT
Baer et al.[33]	1994	55	EDWT, SWT	good agreement between absent SWT or reduced EDWT and scar on MIBI SPECT
Baer et al.[34]	1995	35	EDWT, CR	comparison with FDG PET; optimal detection of viability by combining EDWT and CR
Perrone-Filardi et al.[35]	1992	25	EDWT, SWT	viable segments on Tl-201 reinjection or FDG PET have preserved EDWT and SWT
Perrone-Filardi et al.[36]	1992	25	EDWT, SWT	EDWT and SWT underestimate viability as compared to PET
Morguet et al.[37]	1996	30	EDWT,SWT	SWT absent in severe persistent Tl-201 defects
Baer et al.[38]	1998	43	EDWT, CR	CR is superior over EDWT in the prediction of functional outcome after revascularization
Baer et al.[39]	1996	43	CR	CR on MR imaging or low-dose dobutamine echocardiography correlates well with viability on FDG PET
Dendale et al.[40]	1995	37	CR	CR on MR imaging predicts recovery of function after acute myocardial infarction
Dendale et al.[41]	1998	26	CR	dobutamine MR imaging has an 80% accuracy to predict outcome after myocardial infarction
Gunning et al.[42]	1998	30	CR	CR is very specific, whereas myocardial scintigraphy is very sensitive for identification of reversible myocardial dysfunction

CR: contractile reserve during dobutamine stimulation; EDWT: enddiastolic wall thickness; FDG: F18-fluorodeoxyglucose; ISI: increased signal intensity; PET: positron emission tomography; SWT: systolic wall thickening at rest; Tl-201: thallium-201 chloride.

Comparative studies with radionuclide markers have shown excellent correlations between MR imaging techniques and scintigraphic modalities. Johnston *et al.* [30] evaluated 24 patients with MR imaging and stress-rest thallium-201 scintigraphy. Viability criteria on MR imaging were increased signal intensity and preserved systolic wall thickening. The authors demonstrated that 91% of the patients with redistribution on thallium-201 scintigraphy had preserved increased signal intensity and systolic wall thickening on MR imaging, while 46% of the patients with a fixed defect were also classified viable by MR imaging. It was concluded that MR imaging is capable of detecting myocardial viability and that conventional thallium-201 stress-redistribution imaging underestimates the presence of viable tissue.

Lawson *et al.* [31] showed a good correlation between end-diastolic/systolic wall thickness and thallium-201 uptake in 24 patients with acute and healed infarcts. Baer *et al.* [32,33] performed two studies evaluating the value of end-diastolic wall thickness and systolic wall thickening at rest for the presence or absence of viability and compared the results to resting technetium-99m sestamibi SPECT. Both studies indicated segments with end-diastolic wall thickness >2.5SD below the mean value and absent systolic wall thickening at rest demonstrated scar on technetium-99m sestamibi SPECT (tracer uptake<50%). In a more recent study, Baer *et al.* [34] compared MR imaging with fluoro-deoxyglucose positron emission tomography (FDG PET) in akinetic myocardial segments of 35 patients with sustained (>4 months old) myocardial infarction. Segments were considered viable on FDG PET when the uptake was 50% or more; on MR imaging segments were considered viable when end-diastolic wall thickness was ≥5.5 mm (Figure 1). FDG uptake correlated with end-diastolic wall thickness; considering FDG PET as the gold standard, end-diastolic wall thickness had a sensitivity of 72%, a specificity of 89%, and a positive predictive accuracy of 91%.

Two studies by Perrone-Filardi *et al.* [35,36] compared FDG PET and thallium-201 reinjection scintigraphy with MR imaging. In one study the authors showed that the majority of segments with viability on FDG PET and thallium-201 reinjection imaging exhibited preserved end-diastolic wall thickness and systolic wall thickening at rest [35]. In the other study the authors showed that many regions with reduced end-diastolic wall thickness and absent systolic wall thickening at rest were viable on FDG PET, indicating underestimation of viability by the parameters derived from MR imaging [36]. Morguet *et al.* [37] compared thallium-201 SPECT findings with cine MR imaging in 30 patients with coronary artery disease. All patients had persistent defects at thallium-201 reinjection imaging. The authors showed that the mild and moderate persistent defects still contained viable tissue, whereas the severely persistent defects predominantly represented nonviable myocardium without having any regional contractile function. Recently, Baer *et al.* [38] tested the predictive value of end-diastolic wall thickness against outcome after revascularization. In a study comprising 40 patients, enddiastolic wall thickness had a high sensitivity (93%) with a low specificity (60%) to predict functional outcome after revascularization (Table 5). Hence, segments with <5.5 mm enddiastolic wall thickness are likely to represent transmural scars and will not recover function after revascularization. On the other hand, segments with preserved enddiastolic wall thickness do not always recover function after revascularization. The most likely explanation for this finding is the presence of subendocardial scars: these segments frequently have a pre-served end-diastolic wall thickness but will not improve in function after revascularization. The number of segments with contractile reserve correlated significantly with the magnitude of improvement of left ventricular ejection fraction after revascularization.

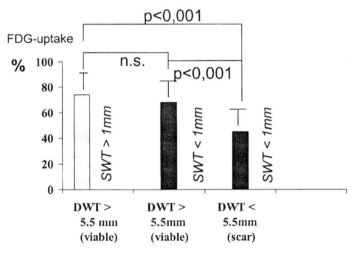

Figure 1. Segmental [^{18}F] fluorodeoxyglucose uptake related to enddiastolic wall thickness (DWT) and systolic wall thickening (SWT) at rest as assessed by MR imaging. (Adapted from Baer et al. Circulation 1995:91;1006-15, with permission).

Table 5. Accuracy of MR viability testing in predicting recovery of function after revascularization. 40 Patients, turbo field GRE-MRI control 4-6 months after successful revascularization (From Baer *et al.,* reference 38).

MR viability criterium	(Detection of viability)	Specificity (Detection of scar)	Positive predictive accuracy (%)
Dobutamine contractile reserve	88 (22/25)	93 (15/15)	96
Preserved enddiastolic wall thickness	92 (23/25)	60 (8/15)	79

The last criterium indicating viability that can be derived from MR imaging is the presence of contractile reserve during stimulation with low-dose dobutamine (10 μg/kg/min). Baer *et al.* [34]   showed that ≥1mm dobutamine-induced systolic wall thickening (Figure 2) is a better predictor of residual metabolic activity than ≥5.5mm wall thickness (sensitivity 81%, specificity 95%, positive predictive accuracy 96%).

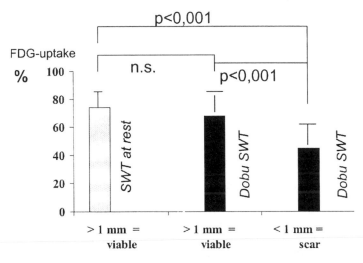

Figure 2. Segmental [¹⁸F]-fluorodeoxyglucose uptake related to dobutamine-induced systolic wall thickening as assessed by MR imaging. Dobu-SWT indicates dobutamine-induced systolic wall thickening in akinetic segments at rest; SWT at rest, systolic wall thickening at rest (Adapted from Baer et al. Circulation 1995:91;1006-15, with permission).

More recently, Baer *et al.* [39] compared the presence of contractile reserve of MR imaging and dobutamine transesophageal echocardiography in 43 patients with chronic ischemic left ventricular dysfunction following myocardial infarction (Figure 3). Using FDG PET as gold standard, it was shown that MR imaging had a slightly higher sensitivity and specificity than transesophageal echocardiography for detection of myocardial viability (sensitivity 81% vs 77%, specificity 100% vs 94%, respectively). Dendale *et al.* [40] studied 37 patients with a recent myocardial infarction and showed that patients with dobutamine-induced (5 μg/kg/min) contractile reserve on MR imaging did recover function 3 to 6 months after infarction (Figures 4,5). MR data were compared with two-dimensional echocardiographic data, and concordancy between the two techniques was observed in 81% of patients (Figure 6). In a more recent study [41], these authors reported an accuracy of 80% of dobutamine MR imaging in predicting functional outcome after myocardial infarction. Very recently, Gunning *et al.* [42] examined hibernating myocardium in 30 patients with

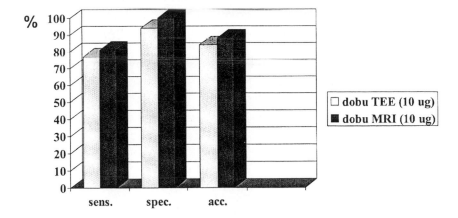

Figure 3. Assessment of myocardial viability by dobutamine (dobu) transesophageal echocardiography (TEE) and dobutamine MR imaging comparison with [^{18}F]-fluorodeoxyglucose uptake (FDG-PET). Sens.=sensitivity, spec.= specificity, acc.=accuracy (Adapted from Baer et al. Am J Cardiol 1996:78;415-9, with permission).

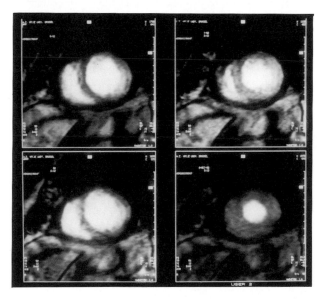

Figure 4. Enddiastolic (left) and endsystolic (right) short-axis myocardial cine MR images (upper panels) of a patient after myocardial infarction. Comparable images (lower panels) after administration of dobutamine. The images demonstrate a hypokinetic segment of the anterior wall of the left ventricle. Recovery of wall motion in this segment after dobutamine administration demonstrates viability (Courtesy P. Dendale, VUB Brussels).

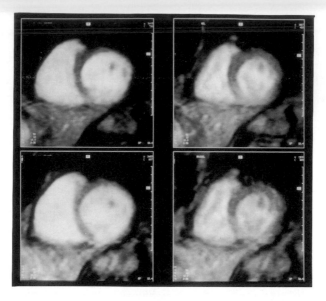

Figure 5. Enddiastolic (left) and endsystolic (right) short-axis cine MR images (upper panels) of the heart of a patient after myocardial infarction. Comparable images (lower panels) after administration of dobutamine. The images demonstrate a hypokinetic nonviable segment of the inferior wall of the left ventricle (Courtesy P. Dendale, VUB Brussels).

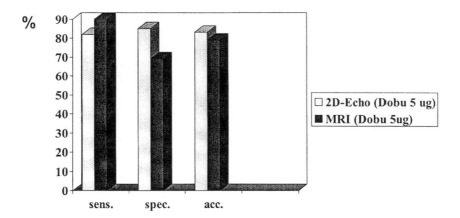

Figure 6. Comparison between MR imaging and 2D-echocardiography for prediction of recovery of function at follow-up. No significant differences were found in sensitivity, specificity, or accuracy. Sens.=sensitivity, spec.= specificity, acc.=accuracy (Adapted from Dendale et al. Am Heart J 1995:130;134-40, with permission).

three-vessel disease and impaired left ventricular function who underwent coronary artery bypass surgery. They compared thallium-201 and technetium-99m tetrofosmin tomographic imaging with dobutamine MR imaging (5-10 μg/kg/min) for the identification of reversible myocardial dysfunction following surgery. It was shown that the tracer techniques were very sensitive but moderately specific, whereas dobutamine MR imaging was very specific (81%) but only moderately sensitive (50%). Using a combined approach, it was claimed that the relative merits of myocardial scintigraphy and dobutamine MR imaging may be applied to full advantage. In conclusion, different markers for viability can be derived from MR imaging and it appears that assessment of contractile reserve during dobutamine MR imaging may provide the most accurate information on the presence or absence of residual myocardial viability.

Myocardial tagging

Myocardial tagging permits determination of the absolute motion and thickening of specific myocardial segments [43]. This can be used to evaluate myocardial rotational deformation and differences in subendocardial and epicardial wall motion. MR imaging with tissue tagging allows accurate noninvasive assessment of systolic wall thickening. Power *et al.* [44] using MR tagging in 13 healthy volunteers, showed that mean circumferential shortening was the preferred measure contractile function during dobutamine stimulation. Kramer *et al.* [45] studied 23 patients one week after acute onset of myocardial infarction with MR tagging and showed significantly reduced intramyocardial circumferential shortening in the infarct zones compared to normally perfused regions. In a subsequent study, Kramer *et al.* [46] examined the relation between regional changes in intramyocardial function and global left ventricular remodeling in the first 8 weeks after reperfused first anterior wall myocardial infarction in 26 patients. An increase in left ventricular end-diastolic volume was seen, which was not related to changes in global and regional function. Marcus *et al.* [47] studied 10 patients with a first myocardial infarction at an average of 8 days after the acute onset. MR tagging clearly distinguished regions with normal function and dysfunctional regions and, in addition, delineated hyperfunction in regions remote from the infarcted area. It is presaged that MR tagging will very likely become one of the reference standards for assessment of wall motion and wall thickening, and hence viability, in the setting of acute and chronic myocardial infarction.

Cardiac metabolism

MR spectroscopy

Preserved metabolism can be considered as the third MR standard of myocardial viability. Using phosphorus-31 (31-P) MR spectroscopy, changes in high-energy phosphate metabolism of myocardial cells resulting from ischemia or infarction can be studied [48,49]. Concentrations and kinetics of metabolically important compounds can be determined, intracellular pH be measured, and the fate of exogenously administered tracers be followed. Three-dimensionally localized 31-P spectra are obtained from the myocardium using a surface coil placed on the chest over the cardiac apex. The spectrum provides quantitative information on the concentration of multiple high-energy phosphate compounds, including inorganic phosphate (Pi), phosphodiesters, phosphocreatine (PCr), and the three peaks from adenosine triphosphate (ATP) .

Several human studies performed with MR spectroscopy have focused on the changes during ischemia [50,51]. The diagnosis of myocardial ischemia with 31-P MR spectroscopy in man has been limited by the inability to measure accurately myocardial Pi due to the overlapping signal from the 2,3-diphosphoglycerate of chamber blood. Thus, calculation of the Pi/PCr ratio, shown previously to be a sensitive marker of ischemia in experimental models, might be difficult in humans. In normal individuals, Bottomley *et al.* [52] first demonstrated the capability of measuring cardiac PCr and ATP. The authors calculated a PCr/ATP ratio of 1.3, which was in agreement with earlier values obtained from animal hearts. In human hearts, 5 to 9 days post myocardial infarction, a low PCr/ATP ratio (approximately 1.1) and elevated Pi levels were observed in regions that corresponded with the infarcted region. Blackledge *et al.* [52] found a myocardial PCr/ATP ratio of 1.55 in 6 normal subjects. Schaefer *et al.* [53] used image-selected in-vivo spectroscopy (ISIS), a technique that allows three-dimensional localization of the volume of interest, and reported a myocardial PCr/ATP ratio of 1.33 in 12 young healthy volunteers. It is now more or less accepted that the limits of normal for the PCr/ATP ratio should be between 1.6 and 2.0 [54,55]. Lamb *et al.* [56] studied 22 healthy volunteers during atropine-dobutamine stress and showed a decrease in PCr/ATP ratio from 1.42 ± 0.18 at rest to 1.22 ± 0.18 during stress, suggesting inadequate adaptation of oxidative phosphorylation of the normal heart to high work states. Weiss *et al.* [57] studied regional myocardial metabolism of high-energy phosphates during isometric exercise in patients with coronary artery disease. At rest, the PCr/ATP ratio of left ventricular myocardium was 1.72 ± 0.15 in 11 normal subjects as compared to 1.45 ± 0.31 in 16 patients with coronary artery disease. During exercise, the PCr/ATP ratio did not change in the normal group, but changed significantly to 0.91±0.18 (p<0.001) in the group with coronary artery disease and recovered to 1.27±0.38 two minutes after exercise. Repeat exercise testing in 5 patients after revascularization yielded values of 1.60±0.20 at rest and 1.62±0.18 during exercise (NS), as compared to 1.51±0.19 at rest and 1.02±0.26 during exercise before revascularization (p<0.02). Yabe *et al.* [58] showed that the PCr/ATP ratio was significantly altered by handgrip exercise in patients with reversible thallium defects. They studied 27 patients with severe stenosis of the left anterior descending artery, using both 31-P MR spectroscopy and thallium-201 scintigraphy. The patients with reversible defects showed a change of PCr/ATP ratio from 1.60±0.19 to 0.96±0.28 (p<0.001) compared to 1.24±0.30 to 1.19±0.28 (p=NS) in the patients with fixed defects. It was concluded that the decrease in PCr/ATP ratio reflects a transient imbalance between oxygen supply and demand in myocardium with compromised blood flow. Similarly, Yabe *et al.* [59] showed in a subsequent study that PCr content was significantly decreased in patients with both reversibele and fixed thallium defects, but that the ATP content was also reduced in the patients with fixed defect, resulting in a decreased PCr/ATP ratio in reversibly injured viable myocardium versus a normal ratio in irreversibly damaged nonviable myocardium. Stress testing with 31-P MR spectroscopy seems therefore to be a useful method of assessing the effect of ischemia on myocardial metabolism of high-energy phosphates and of monitoring the response to treatment. Neubauer *et al.* [60] showed very nicely that the PCr/ATP ratio might be used as a predictor of mortality in patients with dilated cardiomyopathy. The mortality rate was 40% in patients with a PCr/ATP ratio of < 1.60 and only 11% with a PCr/ATP ratio of ≥1.60. Recently, Bottomley and Weiss [61] investigated creatine content in the myocardium using water-suppressed hydrogen (1-H) MR spectroscopy. They studied 10 patients with sustained myocardial infarction and showed creatine depletion in nonviable myocardium. The detection of regional creatine depletion by 1-H MR spectroscopy may provide a metabolic means to distinguish viable from nonviable myocardium.

Conclusions

The unique features of MR techniques like good anatomical and temporal resolution, three-dimensional representation, easy reproducibility, an unlimited field of view and lack of radiation, and the possibility of in vivo measurement of myocardial biochemistry render the MR techniques a modality especially suited for determination of myocardial viability in patients with coronary artery disease [62]. Sofar, MR techniques are valuable in the detection of a wide range of pathophysiological entities such as myocardial perfusion and perfusion reserve, wall motion, wall thickness and thickening, and myocardial metabolism. As acquisition times improve and real time imaging becomes a reality, MR imaging and spectroscopy will likely become very accurate tools for assessing functional reserve and metabolic myocardial activity. This will give the MR techniques an expanding role in the assessment of myocardial viability in patients with coronary artery disease, keeping pace with echocardiographic techniques and nuclear cardiology approaches [63].

References

1.   The clinical role of magnetic resonance in cardiovascular disease. Task Force of the European Society of Cardiology, in collaboration with the Association of European Paediatric Cardiologists. Eur Heart J 1998;19:19-39.
2.   Longmore DB, Klipstein RH, Underwood SR et al. Dimensional accuracy of magnetic resonance studies of the heart. Lancet 1985;1:1360-2.
3.   Sechtem U, Pflugfelder PW, White RD et al. Cine MR imaging: potential for the evaluation of cardiovascular function. AJR Am J Roentgenol 1987;148:239-46.
4.   Wetter DR, McKinnon GC, Debatin JF, Von Schulthess GK. Cardiac echo-planar MR imaging: comparison of single- and multiple shot techniques. Radiology 1995;194:765-70.
5.   Rebergen SA, Van der Wall EE, Doornbos J, De Roos A. Magnetic resonance measurement of velocity and flow: technique, validation, and cardiovascular applications. Am Heart J 1993;126:1439-56.
6.   Beyerbacht HP, Vliegen HW, Lamb HJ et al. Magnetic resonance spectroscopy of the human heart: current status and clinical implications. Eur Heart J 1996;17:1158-66.
7.   Frahm J, Merboldt KD, Bruhn H, Gyngell ML, Hanicke W, Chien D. 0.3-second FLASH MRI of the human heart. Magn Reson Med 1990;13:150-7.
8.   Atkinson DJ, Burstein D, Edelman RR. First-pass cardiac perfusion: evaluation with ultrafast MR imaging. Radiology 1990;174:757-62.
9.   Wilke N, Simm C, Zhang J et al. Contrast-enhanced first pass myocardial perfusion imaging: correlation between myocardial blood flow in dogs at rest and during hyperemia. Magn Reson Med 1993;29:485-97.
10.   Manning WJ, Atkinson DJ, Grossman W, Paulin S, Edelman RR. First-pass nuclear magnetic resonance imaging studies using gadolinium-DTPA in patients with coronary artery disease. J Am Coll Cardiol 1991;18:959-65.
11.   Van Rugge FP, Boreel JJ, van der Wall EE et al. Cardiac first-pass and myocardial perfusion in normal subjects assessed by sub-second Gd-DTPA enhanced MR imaging. J Comput Assist Tomogr 1991;15:959-65.
12.   Van Rugge FP, van der Wall EE, van Dijkman PRM, Louwerenburg HW, de Roos A, Bruschke AVG. Usefulness of ultrafast magnetic resonance imaging in healed myocardial infarction. Am J Cardiol 1992;70:1233-7.
13.   Matheijssen NAA, Louwerenburg HW, Van Rugge FP et al. Comparison of ultrafast dipyridamole magnetic resonance imaging with dipyridamole SestaMIBI SPECT for detection of perfusion abnormalities in patients with one-vessel cornary artery disease: assessment by quantitative model fitting. Magn Reson Med 1996;35:221-8.
14.   Wilke N, Jerosch-Herold M, Wang Y et al. Myocardial perfusion reserve: assessment with multisection, quantitative, first-pass MR imaging. Radiology 1997;204:373-84.
15.   Lauerma K, Virtanen KS, Sipilä LM, Hekali P, Aronen HJ. Multislice MRI in assessment of myocardial perfusion in patients with single-vessel proximal left anterior descending coronary artery disease before and after revascularization. Circulation 1997;96:2859-67.

16. Dendale P, Franken PR, Meusel M, Van der Geest R, De Roos A. Distinction between open and occluded infarct-related arteries using contrast-enhanced magnetic resonance imaging. Am J Cardiol 1997;80:334-6.
17. Van der Wall EE, Van Dijkman PRM, De Roos A *et al.* Diagnostic significance of gadolinium-DTPA (diethylenetriamine penta-acetic acid) enhanced magnetic resonance imaging in thrombolytic treatment for acute myocardial infarction: its potential in assessing reperfusion. Br Heart J 1990;63:12-7.
18. De Roos A, Van Rossum AC, Van der Wall EE *et al.* Reperfused and nonreperfused myocardial infarction: diagnostic potential of Gd-DTPA-enhanced MR imaging. Radiology 1989;172:717-20.
19. De Roos A, Matheijssen NAA, Doornbos J, Van Dijkman PRM, Van Voorthuisen AE, Van der Wall EE. Myocardial infarct size after reperfusion therapy: assessment with Gd-DTPA-enhanced MR imaging. Radiology 1990;176:517-21.
20. Yokota C, Nonogi H, Miyazaki S *et al.* Gadolinium-enhanced magnetic resonance imaging in acute myocardiol infarction. Am J Cardiol 1995;75:577-581
21. Dendale P, Franken PR, Block P, Pratikakis Y, de Roos A. Contrast enhanced and functional magnetic resonance imaging for the detection of viable myocardium after infarction. Am Heart J 1998;135:875-80.
22. Wu KC, Zerhouni EA, Judd RM *et al.* Prognostic significance of microvascular obstruction by magnetic resonance imaging in patients with acute myocardial infarction. Circulation 1998;97:765-72.
23. Pennell DJ, Underwood SR, Ell PJ, Swanton RH, Walker JM, Longmore DB. Dipyridamole magnetic resonance imaging dipyridamole: a comparison with thallium-201 emission tomography. Br Heart J 1990;64:362-9.
24. Baer FM, Smolarz K, Jungehülsing M *et al.* Feasibility of high-dose dipyridamole-magnetic resonance imaging for detection of coronary artery disease and comparison with coronary angiography. Am J Cardiol 1992;69:51-6.
25. Pennell DJ, Underwood SR, Manzara CC *et al.* Magnetic resonance imaging during dobutamine stress in coronary artery disease. Am J Cardiol 1992;70:34-40.
26. Baer FM, Voth E, Theissen P, Schicha H, Sechtem U. Coronary artery disease: findings with GRE MR imaging and Tc-99m methoxyisobutyl-isonitrile SPECT during simultaneous dobutamine stress. Radiology 1994;193:203-9.
27. Van Rugge FP, Van der Wall EE, Spanjersberg SJ *et al.* Magnetic resonance imaging during dobutamine stress for detection and localization of coronary artery disease. Quantitative wall motion analysis using a modification of the centerline method. Circulation 1994;90:127-38.
28. Buller VGM, Van der Geest RJ, Kool MD, Van der Wall EE, De Roos A, Reiber JHC. Assessment of regional left ventricular wall parameters from short-axis magnetic resonance imaging using a three-dimensional-extension to the improved centerline method. Invest Radiol 1997;32:529-39.
29. Holman ER, Buller VGM, De Roos A *et al.* Detection and quantification of dysfunctional myocardium by magnetic resonance imaging. A new three-dimensional method for quantitative wall thickening analysis. Circulation 1997;95:924-31.
30. Johnston DL, Gupta VK, Wendt RE, Mahmarian JJ, Verani MS. Detection of viable myocardium in segments with fixed defects on thallium-201 scintigraphy: usefulness of magnetic resonance imaging early after acute myocardial infarction. Magn Reson Imaging 1993;11:949-56.
31. Lawson MA, Johnson LL, Coghlan L *et al.* Correlation of thallium uptake with left ventricular wall thickness by cine magnetic resonance imaging in patients with acute and healed myocardial infarcts. Am J Cardiol 1997;80:434-41.
32. Baer FM, Smolarz K, Jungehülsing FM *et al.* Chronic myocardial infarction: assessment of morphology, function, and perfusion by gradient echo magnetic resonance imaging and ^{99m}Tc-methoxyisobutyl-isonitrile SPECT. Am Heart J 1992;123:636-45.

33. Baer FM, Smolarz K, Theissen P, Voth E, Schicha H, Sechtem U. Regional ^{99m}Tc-methoxyisobutyl-isonitrile-uptake at rest in patients with myocardial infarcts: comparison with morphological and functional parameters obtained from gradient-echo magnetic resonance imaging. Eur Heart J 1994;15:97-107.

34. Baer FM, Voth E, Schneider CA, Theissen P, Schicha H, Sechtem U. Comparison of low-dose dobutamine-gradient-echo magnetic resonance imaging and positron emission tomography with [18F]fluorodeoxyglucose in patients with chronic coronary artery disease. A functional and morphological approach to the detection of residual myocardial viability. Circulation 1995;91:1006-15.

35. Perrone-Filardi P, Bacharach SL, Dilsizian V, Maurea S, Frank JA, Bonow RO. Regional left ventricular wall thickening. Relation to regional uptake of 18Fluorodeoxyglucose and 201Tl in patients with chronic coronary artery disease and left ventricular dysfunction. Circulation 1992;86:1125-37.

36. Perrone-Filardi P, Bacharach SL, Dilsizian V et al. Metabolic evidence of viable myocardium in regions with reduced wall thickness and absent wall thickening in patients with chronic ischemic left ventricular dysfunction. J Am Coll Cardiol 1992;20:161-8.

37. Morguet AJ, Kögler A, Schmitt HA, Emrich D, Kreuzer H, Munz DL. Assessment of myocardial viability in persistent defects on thallium-201 SPECT after reinjection using gradient-echo MRI. Nuklearmedizin 1996;35:146-52.

38. Baer FM, Theissen P, Schneider CA et al. Dobutamine magnetic resonance imaging predicts contractile recovery of chronically dysfunctional myocardium after successful revascularization. J Am Coll Cardiol 1998;31:1040-8.

39. Baer FM, Voth E, LaRosee K et al. Comparison of dobutamine transesophageal echocardiography and dobutamine magnetic resonance imaging for detection of residual myocardial viability. Am J Cardiol 1996;78:415-9.

40. Dendale PA, Franken PR, Waldman GJ et al. Low-dosage dobutamine magnetic resonance imaging as an alternative to echocardiography in the detection of viable myocardium after acute infarction. Am Heart J 1995;130:134-40.

41. Dendale P, Franken PR, Holman E, Avenarius J, Van der Wall EE, De Roos A. Validation of low-dose dobutamine magnetic resonance imaging for assessment of myocardial viability after infarction by serial imaging. Am J Cardiol 1998;82:375-7.

42. Gunning MG, Anagnostopoulos C, Knight CJ et al. Comparison of ^{201}Tl, ^{99m}Tc-tetrofosmin, and dobutamine magnetic resonance imaging for identifying hibernating myocardium. Circulation 1998;98:1869-74.

43. Zerhouni EA, Parish DM, Rogers WJ, Yang A, Shapiro EP. Human heart: tagging with MR imaging - a method for noninvasive assessment of myocardial motion. Radiology 1988;169:59-63.

44. Power TP, Kramer CM, Shaffer AL et al. Breath-hold dobutamine magnetic resonance myocardial tagging: normal left ventricular response. Am J Cardiol 1997;80:1203-7.

45. Kramer CM, Rogers WJ, Geskin G et al. Usefulness of magnetic resonance imaging early after acute myocardial infarction. Am J Cardiol 1997;80:690-5.

46. Kramer CM, Rogers WJ, Theobald TM, Power TP, Geskin G, Reichek N. Dissociation between changes in intramyocardial function and left ventricular volumes in the eight weeks after first anterior myocardial infarction. J Am Coll Cardiol 1997;30:1625-32.

47. Marcus JT, Götte MJW, Van Rossum AC et al. Myocardial function in infarcted and remote regions early after infarction in man: assessment by magnetic resonance tagging and strain analysis. Magn Reson Med 1997;38:803-10.

48. De Roos A, van der Wall EE. Magnetic resonance imaging and spectroscopy of the heart. Curr Opin Cardiol 1991;6:946-52

49. Bottomley PA. MR spectroscopy of the heart: the status and the challenges. Radiology 1994;191:593-612.

50. De Roos A, Doornbos J, Luyten PR, Oosterwaal LJMP, Van der Wall EE, Den Hollander JA. Cardiac metabolism in patients with dilated and hypertrophic

cardiomyopathy: assessment with proton decoupled P-31 MR spectroscopy. J Magn Reson Imaging 1992;2:711-9.

51. Bottomley PA. Noninvasive study of high-energy phosphate metabolism in human heart by depth-resolved 31P NMR spectroscopy. Science 1985;229:769-72.

52. Blackledge MJ, Rajagopalan B, Oberhaensli RD, Bolas NM, Styles P, Radda G. Quantitative studies of human cardiac metabolism by 31P rotation-frame NMR. Proc Natl Acad Sci USA 1987;84:4283-7.

53. Schaefer S, Gober J, Valenza M et al. Nuclear magnetic resonance imaging-guided phosphorus-31 spectroscopy of the human heart. J Am Coll Cardiol 1988;12:1449-55.

54. Lamb HJ, Doornbos J, Den Hollander JA *et al.* Reproducibility of human cardiac 31P-NMR spectroscopy. NMR Biomed 1997;9:217-27.

55. Bottomley PA. The trouble with spectroscopy papers. Radiology 1991;181:344-50.

56. Lamb HJ, Beyerbacht HP, Ouwerkerk R *et al.* Metabolic response of normal human myocardium to high-dose atropine-dobutamine stress studied by P31-MRS. Circulation 1997;96:2969-77.

57. Weiss RG, Bottomley PA, Hardy CJ, Gerstenblith G. Regional myocardial metabolism of high-energy phosphates during isometric exercise in patients with coronary artery disease. N Engl J Med 1990;323:1593-600.

58. Yabe T, Mitsunama K, Okada M, Morikawa S, Inubushi T, Kinoshita M. Detection of myocardial ischemia by 31P magnetic resonance spectroscopy during handgrip exercise. Circulation 1994;89:1709-16.

59. Yabe T, Mitsunami K, Inubishi T, Kinoshita M. Quantitative measurements of cardiac phosphorous metabolites in coronary artery disease by 31P magnetic resonance spectroscopy. Circulation 1995;92:15-23.

60. Neubauer S, Horn M, Cramer M *et al.* Myocardial phosphocreatine-to-ATP ratio is a predictor of mortality in patients with dilated cardiomyopathy. Circulation 1997;96:2190-6.

61. Bottomley PA, Weiss RG. Non-invasive magnetic-resonance detection of creatine depletion in non-viable infarcted myocardium. Lancet 1998;351:714-8.

62. Van der Wall EE, Vliegen HW, De Roos A, Bruschke AVG. Magnetic resonance imaging in coronary artery disease. Circulation 1995;92:2723-9.

63. Van der Wall EE, Bax JJ. Current clinical relevance of cardiovascular magnetic resonance and its relationship to nuclear cardiology. J Nucl Cardiol 1999;6:462-9.

11. Viability assessment: clinical applications

AMI E. ISKANDRIAN

Introduction

Myocardial viability assessment is indicated in patients with severe coronary artery disease (CAD) and severe left ventricular (LV) dysfunction (Table 1) [1-10]. In many other patients, viability assessment is not indicated (Table 2). There are different endpoints for viability assessment (Table 3). These endpoints need to be assessed quantitatively, and be tailored to the individual patient, for example, in an asymptomatic patient improvement in survival is desirable, while in an elderly patient with heart failure improvement in the quality of life may be more important. In some patients, all endpoints may be achievable because they are interdependent ie., improvement in wall motion, ejection fraction (EF), quality of life and survival. Improvement in survival may occur without improvement in wall motion or EF, possibly because coronary revascularization in patients with viable myocardium may prevent further deterioration of LV dysfunction or death (Table 4). It is also conceivable that the timing after coronary revascularization is crucial for the detection of improvement of LV function. Histological changes of de-differentiation in severe cases of hibernation may be slow to recover; improvement may occur at 6 to 12 months rather than 3 to 6 weeks, which is the conventional time period for follow-up studies [4-6]. In other patients, improvement may not occur because of subendocardial scarring. It is presumed that the inner most layer of the myocardium is responsible for the resting wall motion. Therefore, though there is sufficient viable myocardium in the outer layer to result in improvement in quality of life and survival after coronary revascularization, there is no improvement in regional function. More recently using magnetic resonance imaging with a tagging technique, a significant role of the subepicardium to regional LV function has been demonstrated. After coronary revascularization, the subepicardial viable myocardium has been shown to result in improvement in regional function and if such improvement involves a sufficient zone of the myocardium, there is also increase in EF [11]. Thus, while improvement in wall motion (or EF) are appropriate endpoints for viability assessment, it is possible that improvement in quality of life and survival could be achieved with modest or no change in regional function. It should also be noted that improvement

A. E. Iskandrian and E. E. van der Wall (eds.), Myocardial Viability, 199-227.
© 2000 *Kluwer Academic Publishers. Printed in the Netherlands.*

in wall motion is often assessed subjectively and precise registration on segmental basis is difficult when different methods are used to assess perfusion and function (see below). There are other potential reasons for discordance between viability assessment and endpoints (Table 5) [1-3]. It is possible that LV volume affects significantly the ability of revascularization to improve regional and global LV function and survival even if there is reversible myocardial ischemia [12].

Table 1. Appropriate candidates for viability studies

1.	Patients with chronic ischemic cardiomyopathy (EF<35% and severe MVD)
	a. Asymptomatic
	b. Mild angina
	c. Heart failure
	d. Survivors of sudden cardiac death/life threatening ventricular arrhythmias
2.	Patients after acute myocardial infarction with a large area of severe wall motion abnormality in the presence of a significant stenosis in the culprit artery

EF: ejection fraction; MVD: multivessel disease

Table 2. Inappropriate candidates for viability studies

1.	Mild CAD and LV dysfunction
2.	Severe CAD but normal or near normal LV function.
3.	Primary cardiomyopathy
4.	Valvular heart disease with the exception of mitral regurgitation if deemed secondary to ischemic cardiomyopathy
5.	Congenital heart disease
6.	One-vessel disease and severe LV dysfunction out of proportion to degree of LV dysfunction
7.	Unstable angina requiring urgent revascularization
8.	Co-morbid conditions that limit good outcome after coronary revascularization
9.	Inoperable CAD (poor run off) unless alternative therapy is available*
10.	Severe LV dilation - alternative therapy is available*

*Alternative therapy: transmyocardial and endomyocardial laser revascularization and neo-angiogenesis using growth factors

Table 3. Endpoints after coronary revascularization of viability assessment

1.	Improvement of regional function
2.	Improvement of ejection fraction
3.	Improvement of quality of life
4.	Improvement of survival
5.	Cost-effectiveness

Table 4. Potential benefit of coronary revascularization unrelated to recovery of regional left ventricular (LV) function

---

1. Prevent further worsening of LV function due to:
    a. prevent future acute myocardial infarction
    b. prevent repetitive stunning
    c. prevent apoptosis
    d. prevent further LV dilation
2. Prevent sudden arrhythmic death

Table 5. Reasons for discordant results between viability assessment and endpoints such as wall motion improvement or outcome after coronary revascularization

---

1. Incomplete revascularization
2. Diffuse distal disease
3. Graft occlusion or restenosis
4. Perioperative infarction
5. Inappropriate timing of post-revascularization study

For these reasons, it may be appropriate to distinguish reversible LV dysfunction from "viable myocardium". While reversible LV dysfunction represents "viable myocardium", the reverse is not necessarily true i.e., "viable myocardium" does not have to be reversible. The distinction between these two terms is important for study design and endpoints. For example, using perfusion imaging the tracer uptake at rest of technetium-99m (Tc-99m) sestamibi, Tc-99m tetrofosmin or thallium is a good marker of viable myocardium and patient outcome (survival and quality of life). On the other hand, the presence of stress-induced reversible defects is a stronger predictor of recovery of regional LV function than mild to moderate fixed defects.[13] Therefore, whether a rest study or a stress study is needed may depend on the endpoint of the study. The advantage of thallium over Tc-labeled tracers may be related to its ability to detect "rest hypoperfusion" in subgroup of patients with classic hibernating myocardium (reduced resting flow).

Despite large numbers of patients who may benefit from viability studies, there are only few multicenter studies and no prospective randomized studies. Most of the available data are obtained from single center studies in fairly small number of patients who are scheduled for revascularization i.e., the study itself was not used in the decision-making process. It is conceivable however that there is a hidden bias and that the decision for or against coronary revascularization was based at least in part on the viability assessment.

Patient selection

Most candidates for viability assessment require both a viability study and coronary angiography. Exceptions occur when coronary angiography is performed first and the anatomy is deemed not suitable for revascularization; in such patients viability assessment is not necessary. Conversely, if viability assessment is performed initially and shows the lack of substantial viable myocardium, then subsequent coronary angiography in such patients may not be necessary. In the vast majority of patients, however the two studies need to be performed and the results integrated. It is conceivable that in the future, transmyocardial lasar, endomyocardial lasar, Fibroblast Growth Factor, Vascular Endothelial Growth Factor and other neo-angiogenesis growth factors may provide alternative options of revascularizations in patients with inoperable CAD and may broaden the need of viability studies to these patients as well [14]. As shown in Table 1, patient selection depends on clinical presentation. In addition to patients who present with angina pectoris, It is estimated that in the United States, there are 4.7 million patients with heart failure, 460,000 new cases each year and 40,000 deaths per year. Most patients who die are over the age of 65 years. Although some of the patients with heart failure have diastolic dysfunction or other causes of heart failure, roughly, 70-75% have CAD [1-3]. The mortality remains high especially in patients with NYHA Class III/IV, despite improvement in therapeutic options. Medical therapy includes diuretics, digoxin, angiotension converting enzyme inhibitors, hydrallazine, and beta-blockers including carvidolol which has a vasodilator property as well. Most deaths in heart failure especially in patients in NYHA Class I/II are sudden presumably due to ventricular arrhythmias. Most antiarrhythmic medications have either a neutral or negative effect on survival and automatic implantable cardiovertors defibrillators (ICD) are gaining momentum as first-line therapy in patients with serious ventricular arrhythmias [15]. There are other medical options that need to be considered such as aggressive cholesterol lowering therapy, cessation of smoking, antiplatelet and anticoagulation[8]. The SOLVD, the CARE and the 4S trials have shown reduction in heart failure, acute myocardial infarction and improvement of endothelial function [16-19]. Progression of heart failure, due to discrete episodes of ischemia or infarction or to ongoing apoptosis, maybe prevented or retarded by such therapy [20].

The alternative treatment in heart failure includes cardiac transplantation, but the major problem is the shortage of heart donors. Louie *et al.* examined their experience in 270 patients with ischemic cardiomyopathy awaiting heart transplantation [21]. Eighty-three received transplants and 22 patients underwent coronary revascularization. The 3-year mortality was 72% in the revascularized patients and 73% in the transplanted patients. The functional class (NYHA) improved from 3.9 to 1.2 in the revascularized patients, and the EF increased from 25% to 36%. The patients who did not receive transplantation had a 50% one-year mortality. Twelve of the revascularized patients had positron emission tomography (PET) viability studies which showed viable myocardium in 10 patients and nonviable in 2 patients. The 10 patients with viable myocardium had successful revascularization and the 2 patients with nonviable myocardium had unsuccessful revascularization. This study therefore suggested that coronary revascularization is an acceptable option in some patients awaiting cardiac transplantation.

In addition to patients with CAD and LV dysfunction who are either asymptomatic or present with angina or heart failure (or both), there are approximately 300,000 patients who are survivors of sudden cardiac death per year [15]. Although sudden cardiac death in some patients may be due to life threatening ventricular arrhythmias induced by ischemia, in the vast majority, it is however due to severe LV dysfunction. In our experience in 210 such patients, the degree of perfusion abnormality assessed by SPECT thallium imaging was the single most important market by multivariate analysis that predicted patient outcome; patients with large abnormality had worse outcome (Figure 1) [22,23].

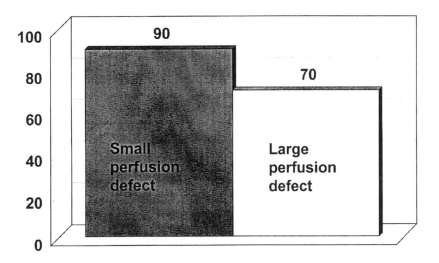

Figure 1. Kaplan-Meier Survival in patients with life threatening ventricular arrhythmias treated medically with ICD. Patients with large perfusion abnormality had lower survival.

Such patients with viable myocardium therefore may benefit from coronary revascularization. In fact, the CABG-PATCH trial showed that in patients with CAD, decreased EF, ventricular premature beats and a positive signal averaged electrocardiograms, coronary artery bypass surgery alone was as effective as surgery and ICD implantation [23,24]. It should however be recognized that the 2-year mortality in the trial was 18%, the patient included in the trial did not have life threatening ventricular arrhythmias, and there were no viability studies. Margonato *et al.* found a higher prevalence of ischemia (by SPECT) and viable myocardium (by PET) in the infarct zone in patients with than without exercise induced ventricular arrhythmias [25].

Finally, there are 1.5 million patients a year who suffer from acute myocardial infarction, 300,000 of whom die before reaching the hospital. In the remaining patients, the mortality is 5-30% during the first year. An unknown but probably a substantial number of these patients may have severe wall motion abnormality and significant stenosis in the culprit artery whom may benefit from viability assessments. Clearly, survival after acute myocardial infarction has improved and some have suggested that the increasing prevalence of heart failure is partly because of better survival during initial hospitalization for acute myocardial infarction.

These entities: acute myocardial infarction, sudden cardiac death/life-threatening ventricular arrhythmias, angina pectoris and heart failure are not necessarily mutually exclusive as patients with myocardial infarction may present with heart failure and patient with heart failure may experience sudden cardiac death. Since heart failure increases with aging, one can argue that in the elderly patients improvement in quality of life may be an important endpoint for viability assessment, and may be even more important than improvement in survival.

Outcome studies

Acute myocardial infarction

Studies in patients after acute myocardial infarction are complicated by at least four reasons. First, there is a natural tendency for improvement in LV function with time even without coronary interventions probably because of resolution of stunning; second, it is important to know whether or not there is a severe residual stenosis in the culprit artery. It is only when such a stenosis is present that viability assessment is useful to determine the need for coronary intervention and third, the presence and extent of ischemia in the remote zones may affect outcome independent of viability in infarct territory and lastly, there are obviously other important risk factors such as age, gender, race, diabetes, renal failure, stroke, and other co-morbid conditions that affect outcome.

Huitink *et al.* used thallium/FDG (F-18 fluorodeoxyglucose) imaging in 53 patients and found higher even rate (death, recurrent myocardial infarction, late revascularization and unstable angina) in patients with a mismatch pattern (19 of 39[49%]) than patients with a match pattern (1 of 14 [7%]) during a mean follow-up of 47 months.[26] Sicari *et al.* from the multicenter International study using dobutamine echocardiography found that the event-free survival at 10 months was 77% in patients with viable myocardium and 89% in patients with non-viable myocardium [27]. The events in this study were defined as death, recurrent myocardial infarction and unstable angina pectoris. Myocardial viability was defined as improvement in wall motion at low dose dobutamine. Carlos *et al.* found that ischemia or infarction at distance and the presence of non-viability in the infarct zone to be the strongest predictor of future events [28]. One of the differences between this study and that of Sicari *et al.* is that many patients in the Carlos study had prior coronary interventions following acute infarction. Basu *et al.* studied 100 patients after acute myocardial infarction and found that patients with reversible ischemia detected by stress-nitroglycerin rest thallium imaging had higher event-rate during a 21 month follow-up than patients with no ischemia [29]. Events were defined as death, recurrent infarction, unstable angina and heart failure. The event rate was 49% in patients with reversible ischemia and 13% in those without (33 of 68 vs 4 of 32). Petretta *et al.* showed that the hard event-free survival (free of death or re-infarction) was 60% in patients with viable myocardium (>25% of myocardium with reversible or mild fixed thallium defects) and 84% in patients with less viable myocardium [30].

Patients with chronic ischemic cardiomyopathy

These results are summarized in Table 6 and Figure 2 [2,31-42]. In 947 patients reported in 11 studies, 84% were men with a mean age of 63 years. The mean EF was 32% and 83% of patients had multivessel CAD. During a follow-up of 22 months, the annual cardiac event rate was 27% in patients with viable myocardium treated medically and 7% in patients with viable myocardium treated with coronary revascularization. The events were death in 7 studies and death plus re-infarction, unstable angina, revascularization or transplantation in 4 studies. In patients with nonviable myocardium, the event rate was not different in those treated medically or with coronary revascularization.

Table 6. Event rate in Viability Studies in patients with ischemic cardiomyopathy

Author	Imaging	Viability	#pts	% men	Age	EF (%)	% MVD	F/U (months)	Events	Annual event rate (%) Viable		Annual event rate (%) Nonviable	
										Medical	Rev	Medical	Rev
Haas et al[31]	PET NH₃/FDG	Mismatch	34	91	63	28	100	12	D	NA	3	NA	NA
Pageley et al[32]	Rest/redist Tl	Median score	70	77	66	28	100	39	D/Tx	NA	6	NA	14
Vom Dahl et al[33]	MIBI/FDG	Mismatch	135	89	56	45	69	29	D	9	0	5	3
Gioia et al[34]	Rest/redist Tl	RD	81	73	68	26	86	31	D	23	NA	10	NA
Gioia et al[35]	Rest/redist Tl	RD	85	75	65	30	92	31	D	17	6	10	NA
DiCarli et al[36]	NH₃/FDG	Mismatch	93	84	65	25	78	14	D	50	12	8	6
Dreyfus et al[37]	H₂0²/FDG	Mismatch	46	98	58	23	91	18	D	NA	6	NA	NA
Lee et al[38]	Rb/FDG	Mismatch	129	79	62	38	74	17	D	10	6	9	4
Tamaki et al[39]	NH₃/FDG	Mismatch	84	93	59	48	66	23	D/MI//Rev	17	NA	2	NA
Eitzman et al[40]	NH₃/FDG	Mismatch	82	88	59	34	70	12	D/MI	50	8	8	0
Williams et al[41]	dob ECHO	Ischemia/CR	108	80	67	30	NA	16	D/MI/UA	43	NA	8	NA
Petretta et al[42]	Rest/redist	N,RD,FD	82	82	54	40	90	25	D/MI	14	NA	2	NA
Total/mean	NA	NA	1029	84	62	33	83	22	NA	27	6	7	5

Abbreviation: PET: Positron emission tomography, TL: thallium-201, RI: reinjection, MIBI: Tc-99m sestamibi, redist: redistribution, RD: reversible defect, MFD: Mild fixed defect, pt: patient, EF: ejection fraction, MVD: multivessel disease, F/U: follow-up, D: death, Tx: transplant, MI: myocardial infarction, UP: unstable angina, Rev: revascularization, FDG: F-18 fluorodeoxyglucose, NH_3:N-13 Ammonia, UA:unstable angina, dob:dobutamine, CR:contractile response, NA:not available or applicable, N:normal, MFD:mild fixed defect. Reproduced with permission [2].

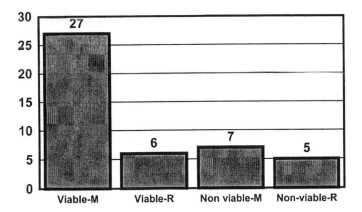

Figure 2. Annual death rate in patients with chronic ischemic cardiomyopathy treated with coronary revascularization (R) or medically (M) according to the status of myocardial viability (Reproduced with permission) [2].

Because of the variability between the various studies, a few comments may be useful regarding each study. Haas *et al.* studied two groups of patients both had angiographically severe CAD and LV dysfunction with suitable anatomy for coronary artery bypass grafting [31]. In group 1, the decision for surgery was based on angiographic finding alone but in group 2 the patients were required to have viable myocardium (at least 40% in at least two vascular territories) by positron emission tomography (these results are shown in table 1). The perioperative mortality was 11% in group 1 and 0% in group 2; the length of stay in the intensive care unit was shorter in group 2 than in group 1; there was less need of inotropic support in group 2 than group 1 and finally at one year 14% in group 1 and only 3% in group 2 died. In group 2 there was also improvement in EF (28% to 35%) and functional class after revascularization (74% vs 6% in NYHA class III/IV). This by far is the most convincing study showing that assessment of myocardial viability added incremental value to angiography in predicting outcome. It is important however to remember that all group 2 patients had viable myocardium and there was no medical arm. The results of this study are different than the study by Elefteriades *et al.*, which showed that the perioperative event is low and long-term survival is good in unselected patients with severe LV dysfunction after CABG [42]. The later results suggests that viability assessment is not indicated in such patients. The last study is however also at variance from our experience [44] and those of others [31,32] but the precise reasons are not clear.

In the study by Pagley *et al.* rest-redistribution thallium, imaging was used and the tracer uptake was quantified in multiple segments. All patients underwent CABG [32]. The patients were divided into 2 groups; group 1 with substantial viability (n:34) and group 2 with lesser viability (n:37) based on the median thallium score in the entire group. This study is in agreement with a previous work done by the same group, which showed that the number of segments with viable myocardium (defined in a similar fashion) predicted improvement in EF after CABG [45]. In the current study, patients with substantial viability had significantly less late events (death or transplantation) and less morbidity in the perioperative period than patients with lesser amount of viable myocardium.

In the study by vom Dahl et al. there were four groups of patients, viable myocardium with revascularization, (n:36), viable myocardium with medical therapy, (n:9), nonviable myocardium with revascularization (n:27) and nonviable myocardium with medical therapy (n:63) [33]. Viability was defined as a mismatch pattern using FDG with positron emission tomography and sestamibi with SPECT. The best outcome was in patients with viable myocardium treated with revascularization. In the viable group who underwent coronary revascularization, functional class (NYHA) improved in 31% of the patients and the EF increased from 46% to 54%.

Gioia et al. in the first of two studies used rest-redistribution thallium imaging and defined viable myocardium as the presence of reversible rest hypoperfusion [34,35]. All patients were treated medically. The death rate was significantly higher in patients with viable myocardium (n:38) compared to nonviable myocardium (n:43). In the second study, again using rest-redistribution thallium imaging and using hypoperfusion as evidence of hibernation, the event rate was significantly lower in patients with thallium redistribution treated with coronary revascularization (n:38) than patients with thallium redistribution treated medically (n:20) or patients with no thallium redistribution treated medically (n:27).

In the study of DiCarli et al., a mismatch pattern using N-13 ammonia and FDG by PET was used to define viable myocardium [36]. The death rate was significantly lower in the group of patients with viable myocardium treated with revascularization (n:26) than those treated medically (n:17). The death rate was not significantly different in the groups of patients with nonviable myocardium treated with revascularization (n:17) or with medical therapy (n:33). In patients with viable myocardium who underwent coronary revascularization, there was symptomatic improvement; 81% before and only 23% after coronary revascularization were in NYHA Class III/IV.

In the study by Dreyfus et al., only patients with viable myocardium showing mismatch pattern by PET undergoing coronary revascularization were included [37]. There were no other groups for comparison. The EF increased from 23% before to 39% after coronary revascularization and all patients had improvement in symptoms by at least one functional class (NYHA).

In the study by Lee *et al.*, the death rate was lower in the group of patients with viable myocardium treated with revascularization (n:49) than those treated medically (n:21) [38].
Viability was defined as mismatch between perfusion assessed by rubidium 82 and metabolism assessed by FDG.
In the study by Tamaki *et al.*, events (defined as death, myocardial infarction, unstable angina and coronary revascularization) were significantly higher in medically treated patients with viable myocardium (n:48) than in patients with nonviable myocardium (n:36). Viability was assessed as a mismatch pattern using N-13 ammonia and FDG [39].
In the study by Eitzman *et al.*, the hard event rate (defined as death or myocardial infarction) was lower in the group of patients with viable myocardium treated with revascularization (n:26) than those treated medically (n:18) [40]. Improvement in symptoms was noted in 31% of patients (at least one functional class according to NYHA) after coronary revascularization. In the study of Williams *et al.* events were more frequent in patients with ischemia or viable myocardium (presence of contractile response) during dobutamine echocardiography than patients with scar [41].
Finally, in the study by Petretta *et al.* [42] multivariate analysis of clinical, echocardiographic, coronary angiographic and thallium results showed that the extent of viable myocardium (normal uptake, reversible defect or mild moderate fixed defect) and age were independent predictors or events. The patients with viable myocardium in ≥ 6 of 13 segments had worse outcome than patients with lesser degree of viability.
There are only preliminary data from two multicenter studies in chronic ischemic cardiomyopathy; these studies are not randomized and one of them is a registry. In one multicenter study that assessed myocardial viability by SPECT I-123 IPPA (IodoPhenylPentadecanoicAcid), the preliminary data showed that patients with viable myocardium treated with revascularization had less events (deaths) than patients with nonviable myocardium [46]. This study however was not powered to look for survival differences. The second multicenter study is a registry and again showed results favoring coronary revascularization in patients with severe LV dysfunction who have viable myocardium [47].

Methodology of a novel myocardial viability protocol

There are two main problems with existing imaging protocols. First, it is difficult to assure precise registration between perfusion and functional data when these two measurements are obtained by different techniques such as SPECT perfusion imaging and 2-dimensional echocardiography and

second, the inability to define the pathophysiologic mechanisms (hibernation vs repetitive stunning) responsible for LV dysfunction [48].
We hypothesized that a dual isotope gated SPECT imaging can be used to determine the presence of hibernation, stress-induced reversible deficit and regional LV function. Dobutamine unlike exercise, adenosine or dipyridamole can be infused at a low dose during SPECT imaging to assess contractile response.
With this background, we describe a new viability protocol. This protocol is feasible and safe and has been used in our laboratory for more than 2 years. The protocol is as follows (Figure 3) [49].

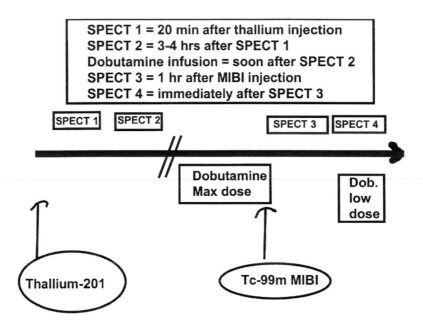

Figure 3. Design of a novel viability protocol (Reproduced with permission) [44].

1. After an overnight fast, 3 mCi thallium-201 is injected intravenously at rest, and SPECT images are obtained 20 minutes and 3 to 4 hours later as rest-redistribution) (SPECT 1 and SPECT 2).
2. Dobutamine is infused to a maximum tolerated dose and technetium 99m sestamibi (20 to 30 mCi) is injected intravenously at peak infusion. The dobutamine infusion is discontinued. Gated SPECT sestamibi is performed 1 hour later. Earlier imaging is discouraged because it is conceivable that in some patients, post-stress stunning may occur (SPECT-3).

3. Dobutamine is then infused at a low dose (5 μg/kg/min), and gated SPECT scstamibi images are acquired <u>during</u> the infusion (SPECT 4).

4. Data analysis with a 20-segment model is used to assess regional perfusion (thallium and MIBI) and regional function (wall motion and wall thickening) either by a scoring system (0 absent, 4 normal) or quantitatively using an automated method as percent uptake (perfusion), % thickening and absolute wall motion (mm). The LVEF and volumes are also measured from SPECT 3 and 4 (Figures 4-6).

Image analysis

On the basis of SPECT 1 and 2, the perfusion is defined as normal, reversible, mild-to-moderate fixed and severe fixed defect. On the basis of SPECT 3 and 1, stress-induced ischemia (reversible defect) is noted as well as regional wall motion, wall thickening, EF, end-diastolic volume. end-systolic volume. On the basis of SPECT 4 and 3, the following information is obtained: improvement in segmental wall motion and wall thickening (contractile response positive) or lack of improvement (contractile response negative) and changes in EF and volume.

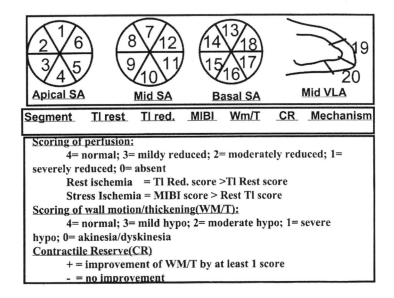

Figure 4. Assessment of regional perfusion and function using segmental semi-quantitative method. Shown are selected slices, polar maps, 3D perfusion images and quantitative estimated of defect size and sites.

Novel viability protocol

Rest- redistribution thallium

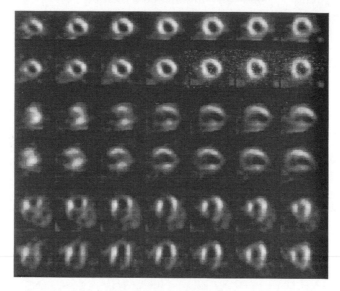

Dobutamine MIBI/rest thallium

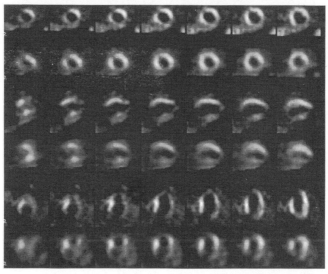

Figure 5. Assessment of regional perfusion and function using automated quantitative method.

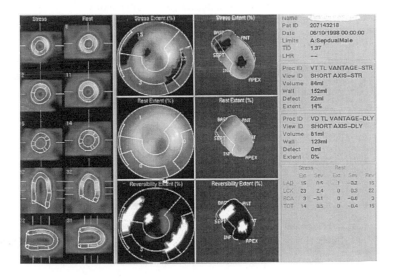

Figure 6. SPECT images of a patients with chronic ischemic cardiomyopathy rest/redistribution thallium (left) and dobutamine sestamibi/rest thallium (right). There are multiple stress-induced defects.

Synthesis of data

On the basis of segmental perfusion and function, the following definitions are used in dysfunctional segments (Table 7)

1. Myocardial hibernation: segments with regional dysfunction and reversible thallium defects (SPECT 1 vs 2)
2. Myocardial stunning: segments with regional dysfunction and reversible sestamibi defects (SPECT 3 vs 1)
3. Myocardial remodeling: segments with regional dysfunction and normal thallium and normal sestamibi uptake (no ischemia) (SPECT 3 vs 1)
4. Myocardial scarring: segments with regional dysfunction with severe fixed defects and no evidence of ischemia on either thallium or sestamibi (SPECT 3,2 and 1).

The segment is considered normal if it had normal function and normal perfusion.

This protocol allows incorporation of echocardiographic assessment for research purposes (see below).

Results: In our initial experience in 54 patients with chronic ischemic cardiomyopathy using this protocol, all patients also had 2-dimensional echocardiography simultaneously with SPECT (Table 8) [49,50].

Table 7. Characterization of pathophysiological state of myocardium

Myocardial state	Perfusion	Wall motion/thickness
Normal	Normal	Normal
Stunned	Stress-ischemia	Abnormal
Remodeled	Normal	Abnormal
Hibernation	Rest-ischemia	Abnormal
Scar	Abnormal	Abnormal

Table 8. The Demographics in Study Group

Age	65 ($\pm$9.2)

Gender	
Male	45 (83%)
Female	9 (17%)
Old MI	44 (82%)
PTCA	10 (19%)
Bypass Surgery	13 (24%)
Risk Factors	
Diabetes	23 (43%)
Hypertension	31 (57%)
Hyperlipidemia	25 (26%)
Tobacco	15 (28%)
Family History	22 (40%)
Medications	
Beta-blocker	29 (54%)
Ca^{++}-blocker	13 (24%)
ACE inhibitor	40 (74%)
Digoxin	27 (50%)
Nitroglycerin	25 (26%)
Electrocardiogram-baseline	
Q-wave	34 (63%)
Left BBB	6 (11%)
LVH	3 (6%)
ST abnormality	39 (72%)
Pacemaker	3 (6%)
Angiographic Disease	
Single vessel	7 (13%)
Two vessel	13 (24%)
Triple vessel	34 (63%)

Using gated SPECT, perfusion and wall motion/thickening were assessed in a total of 1080 myocardial segments (20 segments per patients). Of 1080 segments, 584 (54%) demonstrated severe wall motion/thickening abnormality. Of these 584 segments, the thallium perfusion showed a normal pattern in 239 segments (41%), reversible defects in 140 segments (24%), mild-to-moderate fixed defects in 74 segments (13%) and severe fixed defects in 131 segments (22%). The dobutamine sestamibi images showed inducible ischemia in 88 of the 239 (37%) normal thallium segments, 91 of 140(65%) reversible thallium defects, 51 of 74 (69%) mild-to-moderate fixed thallium defects and 26 of 131 (20%) severe fixed thallium defects. Based on combination of function and perfusion in these 584 segments, 24% (n=140) of dysfunctional segments were labeled as hibernating, 28% (n=165) as stunned, 20%(n=174) as remodeled and 18% (n=105) as scar. Contractile response by gated SPECT was observed in 83% of stunned, 59% of hibernating, 35% of remodeled and 13% of scarred myocardial segments. (Figure 7-12).

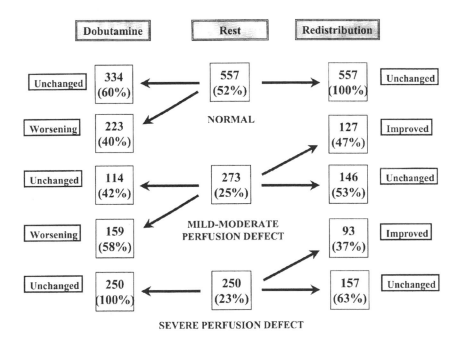

Figure 7. Results of SPECT thallium and sestamibi assessment in 54 patients with ischemic cardiomyopathy. (Reproduced with permission) [45].

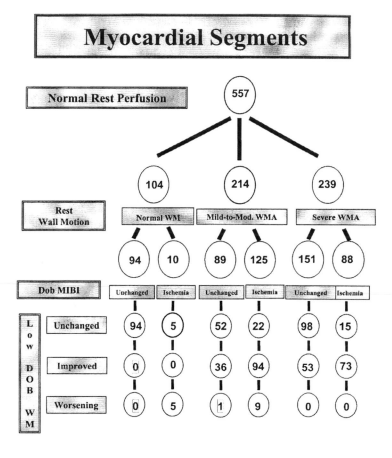

Figure 8. Results of SPECT sestamibi and function in segments with normal thallium. WMA = wall motion abnormalities.

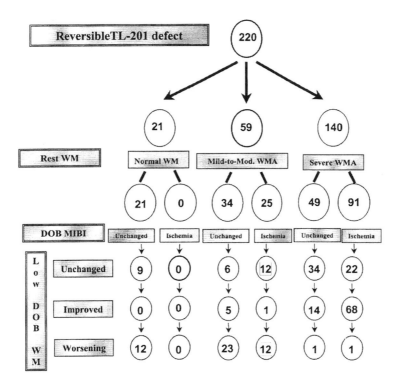

Figure 9. Results of SPECT sestamibi and function in segments with reversible thallium (Tl-201) defects.

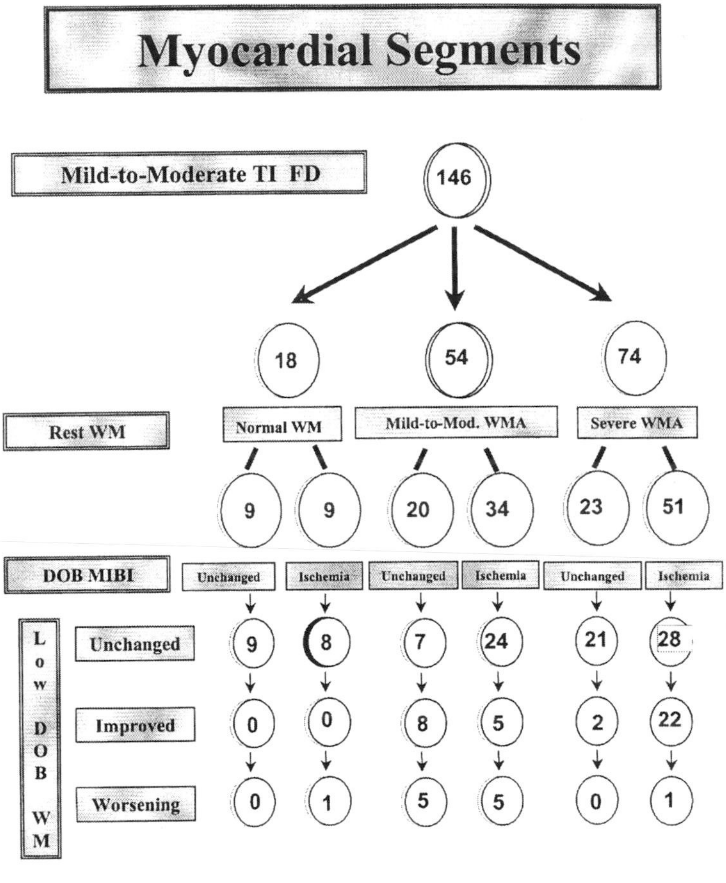

Figure 10. Results of SPECT sestamibi and function in segments with mild-to-moderate fixed thallium defects (Tl TD). WMA = wall motion abnormalities.

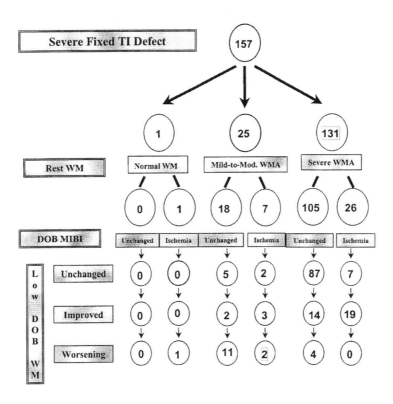

Figure 11. Results of SPECT sestamibi and function in segments with severe fixed thallium defects. WMA = wall motion abnormalities

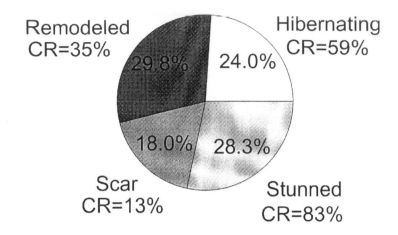

Figure 12. Contractile response in relation to dysfunctional myocardium by gated SPECT

These results of SPECT were compared to dobutamine stress echocardiography (DSE) in the same patients using a 16-segment model (864 segments). Wall motion abnormality was present in 796 segments (92%), contractile reserve during dobutamine infusion was seen in 400 of these segments (50%). Contractile reserve by echocardiography was seen in 331 of 509 (65%) hypokinetic segments and 69 of 287 (24%) akinetic/dyskinetic segments (p<0.001). Contractile reserve was more frequent in segments with normal thallium uptake (64%), reversible thallium defects (42%) or mild to moderate fixed thallium defects (48%) than severely fixed defects (22%) (p<0.05 each). Concordant information about viability by thallium imaging and DSE was obtained in 62% of segments. Dobutamine sestamibi ischemia was seen in 518 of 796 segments (65%) compared to 265 segments (33%) by DSE (p<0.001) (Figure 13). Scintigraphic ischemia was noted in 126 of 195 segments (65%) demonstrating biphasic response, 129 of 205 (63%) segments showing sustained improvement, 42 of 70 (60%) segments deteriorating during dobutamine infusion and 221 of 326 (68%) segments demonstrating no significant change (Figure 14).

In summary, in patients with ischemic cardiomyopathy contractile reserve is more frequent in hypokinetic segments than akinetic/dyskinetic segments. There is a relationship between contractile response and tracer uptake. The number of segments with normal or near normal thallium uptake or with scintigraphic ischemia is significantly greater than the number of those capable of increasing contractile function or demonstrating ischemic response during dobutamine echocardiography.

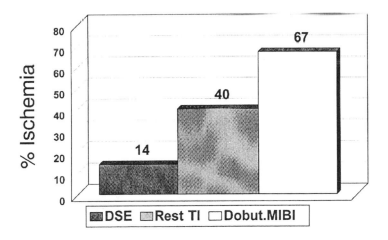

Figure 13. Prevalence of reversible defects by rest thallium, dobutamine echocardiography and dobutamine sestamibi

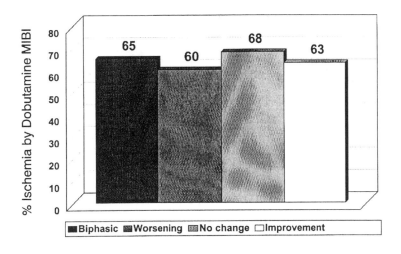

Figure 14. Reversible defects in relation to wall motion response by dobutamine echocardiography

Thus, rest-redistribution thallium perfusion scintigraphy with low-dose and high-dose dobutamine stress gated SPECT allow precise registration of myocardial perfusion and function and assessment of contractile reserve in the same segments. This technique allows characterization of dysfunctional myocardial segments into stunned, hibernating, remodeled and non-viable myocardial substrates. Both stunning and hibernation may contribute to reversible LV dysfunction. In some segments both co-existed i.e., stunning on the top of hibernation (Figure 15). We also identified another important mechanism for dysfunction, referred to as remodeling probably related to LV remodeling and increased wall stress. Remodeling was recognized by others as regional dysfunction with normal myocardial blood flow by nitrogen-13 ammonia and normal FDG uptake [51].

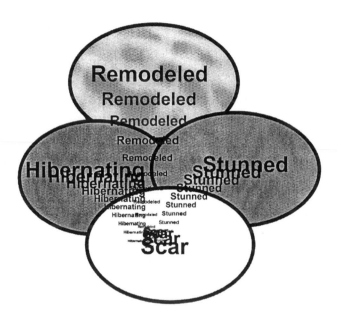

Figure 15. Co-existence of hibernation, stunning, remodeling and scar: an ischemic presentation.

Designs for prospective studies

Design of prospective studies in myocardial viability raises moral and ethical issues. For example, it is probably unethical to randomize patients with angina (and severe LV dysfunction) who clearly have evidence of viable myocardium to medical therapy because there is sufficient evidence that these patients do better with coronary revascularization. On the other hand, it is probably also unethical to randomize patients with heart failure and nonviable myocardium to coronary revascularization. Therefore, the design of study depends on the initial presentation i.e., angina or heart failure and the presence or absence of viability (Figure 16). In the future when neo-angiogenesis therapy proves beneficial using Fibroblast Growth Factor, Vascular Endothelial Growth Factor or other newer factors or by laser therapy especially using endomyocardial approach, the randomization process may change and may include subgroups of patients previously excluded (Figure 17).

The need for randomized prospective studies is clearly indicated because of the magnitude of the problem and the tremendous health costs (estimated that heart failure patients alone consume 20 billion dollars a year in the United States). These studies should use novel protocols such as the one described here and should address clinical and pathophysiological concepts, summarized in Table 9. Until further data became available, the presence of at least 40% viable myocardium in at least two of the three vascular beds is needed to achieve a good clinical outcome after coronary revascularization [31].

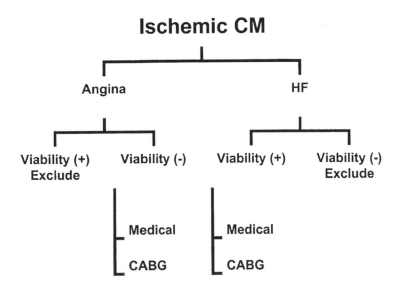

Figure 16. Scheme for prospective randomized studies. CABG = coronary artery bypass surgery; CM = cardiomyopathy; HF = heart failure.

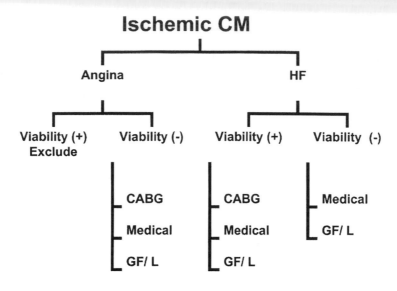

Figure 17. Scheme for prospective randomized studies that include alternative therapies. GF = growth factor; L = laser

Table 9. Direction in future viability studies

Hibernation vs repetitive stunning
Natural history
Prevalence in heart failure
Most cost-effective diagnostic method
Benefit of revascularization independent of functional improvement
Extent of hibernation that impact benefit on survival quality of life and EF

References

1. Iskandrian AS, Heo J, Schelbert HR. Myocardial viability: methods of assessment and clinical relevance. Am Heart J 1996;132:1226-35.
2. Iskander S, Iskandrian AE. Prognostic utility of myocardial viability assessment. Am J Cardiol 1999;83:696-702.
3. Iskandrian AE, Verani MS: Myocardial viability. In: Iskandrian AE, Nuclear cardiac imaging: principles and applications. 2nd edition. Philadelphia: FA Davis; 1996. p. 305-21.
4. Kloner RA, Bolli R, Marban E, Reinlib L, Braunwald E. Medical and cellular implications of stunning, hibernation, and preconditioning: an NHLBI workshop. Circulation 1998;97:1848-67.
5. Camici PG, Wijns W, Borgers M *et al.* Pathophysiological mechanisms of chronic reversible left ventricular dysfunction due to coronary artery disease (hibernating myocardium). Circulation 1997;96:3205-14.
6. Vanoverschelde JL, Wijns W, Borgers M *et al.* Chronic myocardial hibernation in humans. From bedside to bench. Circulation 1997;95:1961-71.
7. Bax JJ, Cornel JH, Visser FC *et al.* Prediction of recovery of myocardial dysfunction after revascularization. Comparison of fluorine-18 fluorodeoxyglucose/thallium-201 SPECT, thallium-201 stress-reinjection SPECT and dobutamine echocardiography. J Am Coll Cardiol 1996;28:558-64.
8. Gheorghiade M, Bonow RO. Chronic heart failure in the United States: a manifestation of coronary artery disease. Circulation 1998;97:282-9.
9. Udelson JE. Steps forward in the assessment of myocardial viability in left ventricular dysfunctions. Circulation 1998;97:833-8.
10. Dilsizian V. Myocardial viability: contractile reserve or cell membrane integrity? J Am Coll Cardiol 1996;28:443-6.
11. Bogaert J, Maes A, Van de Werf F *et al.* Functional recovery of subepicardial myocardial tissue in transmural myocardial infarction after successful reperfusion: an important contribution to the improvement of regional and global left ventricular function. Circulation 1999;99:36-43
12. Yamaguchi A, Ino T, Adachi H *et al.* Left ventricular volume predicts postoperative course in patients with ischemic cardiomyopathy. Ann Thorac Surg 1998,65:434-8.
13. Kitsiou AN, Srinivasan G, Quyumi AA, Summers RM, Bacharach SL, Dilsizian V. Stress-induced reversible and mild-to-moderate irreversible thallium defects: are they equally accurate for predicting recovery of regional left ventricular function after revascularization? Circulation 1998;98:501-8.
14. Schumacher B, Pecher P, von Specht BU, Stegmann T. Induction of neoangiogenosis in ischemic myocardium by human growth factors: first clinical results of a new treatment of coronary heart disease. Circulation 1998;97:645-50.
15. Myerburg RJ, Mitrani R, Inerian A Jr, Castellanos A. Interpretation of outcomes of antiarrhythmic clinical trials: design features and population impact. Circulation 1998;97:1514-21.
16. The SOLVD Investigators. Effect of enalapril on survival in patients with reduced left ventricular ejection fractions and congestive heart failure. N Engl J Med 1991;325:293-302.
17. Sacks FM, Pfeffer MA, Moye LA *et al.* The effect of pravastatin or coronary events after myocardial infarction in patients with average cholesterol levels. Cholesterol and Recurrent Events Trial investigators. N Engl J Med 1996;335:1001-9.
18. Pedersen TR, Kjekshus J, Berg K *et al.* Cholesterol lowering and the use of healthcare resources. Results of the Scandinavian Simvastatin Survival Study. Circulation 1996;93:1796-802.
19. Mancini GBJ, Henry GC, Macaya C *et al.* Angiotensin-converting enzyme inhibition with quinapril improves endothelial vasomotor dysfunction in patients with coronary

artery disease: The TREND (Trial on Reversing Endothelial Dysfunction) Study. Circulation. 1996;94:258-65.

20. Chen C, Ma L, Linfert DR *et al*. Myocardial cell death and apoptosis in hibernating myocardium. J Am Coll Cardiol 1997;30:1407-12.

21. Louie HW, Laks H, Milgalter E *et al*. Ischemic cardiomyopathy. Criteria for coronary revascularization and cardiac transplantation. Circulation 1991;84(5 Suppl):III290-5.

22. Gioia G, Bagheri B, Gottlieb CD *et al*. Prediction of outcome of patients with life-threatening ventricular arrhythmias treated with automatic implantable cardioverter-defibrillators using SPECT perfusion imaging. Circulation 1997;95:390-4.

23. Kothari M, Bagheri B, Hessen S *et al*. Outcome of patients with life-threatening ventricular arrhythmias [abstract]. J Am Coll Cardiol 1998;31(2 Suppl A):181A.

24. Bigger JT Jr. Prophylactic use of implanted cardiac defibrillators in patients at high risk for ventricular arrhythmias after coronary artery bypass graft surgery. Coronary Artery Bypass Graft (CABG) Patch Trial Investigators. N Engl J Med 1997;337:1569-75.

25. Margonato A, Mailhac A, Bonetti F *et al*. Exercise-induced ischemic arrhythmias in patients with previous myocardial infarction: role of perfusion and tissue viability. J Am Coll Cardiol 1996;27:593-8.

26. Huitink JM, Visser FC, Bax JJ *et al*. Predictive value of planar 18F-fluorodeoxyglucose imaging for cardiac events in patients after acute myocardial infarction. Am J Cardiol 1998;81:1072-7.

27. Sicari R, Picano E, Landi P *et al*. Prognostic value of dobutamine-atropine stress echocardiography early after acute myocardial infarction. Echo Dobutamine International Cooperative (EDIC) Study. J Am Coll Cardiol 1997;29:254-60.

28. Carlos ME, Smart SC, Wynsen JC, Sagar KB. Dobutamine stress echocardiography for risk stratification after myocardial infarction. Circulation 1997;95:1402-10.

29. Basu S, Senior R, Raval U, Lahiri R. Superiority of nitrate-enhanced ^{201}Tl over conventional redistribution ^{201}Tl imaging for prognostic evaluation after myocardial infarction and thrombolysis. Circulation 1997;96:2932-7.

30. Petretta M, Cuocolo A, Bonaduce D *et al*. Incremental prognostic value of thallium reinjection after stress-redistribution imaging in patients with previous myocardial infarction and left ventricular dysfunction. J Nucl Med 1997;38:195-200.

31. Haas F, Haehnel CJ, Picker W *et al*. Preoperative positron emission tomographic viability assessment and perioperative and postoperative risk in patients with advanced ischemic heart disease. J Am Coll Cardiol 1997;30:1693-700.

32. Pagley PR, Beller GA, Watson DD, Gimple LW, Ragosta M. Improved outcome after coronary bypass surgery in patients with ischemic cardiomyopathy and residual myocardial viability. Circulation 1997;96:793-800.

33. Vom Dahl J, Altehoefer C, Sheehan FH *et al*. Effect of myocardial viability assessed by technetium-99m-sestamibi SPECT and fluorine-18-FDG PET on clinical outcome in coronary artery disease. J Nucl Med 1997;38:742-8.

34. Gioia G, Milan E, Guibbini R, De Pace N, Heo J, Iskandrian AS. Prognostic value of tomographic rest-redistribution thallium-201 imaging in medically treated patients with coronary artery disease and left ventricular dysfunction. J Nucl Cardiol 1996;3:150-6.

35. Gioia G, Powers J, Heo J, Iskandrian AS. Prognostic value of rest-redistribution tomographic thallium-201 imaging in ischemic cardiomyopathy. Am J Cardiol 1995;75:759-62.

36. Di Carli MF, Davidson M, Little R *et al*. Value of metabolic imaging with positron emission tomography for evaluating prognosis in patients with coronary artery disease and left ventricular dysfunction. Am J Cardiol 1994;73:527-33.

37. Dreyfus GD, Duboc D, Blasco A *et al*. Myocardial viability assessment in ischemic cardiomyopathy: benefits of coronary revascularization. Ann Thorac Surg 1994;57:1402-8.

38. Lee KS, Marwick TH, Cook SA *et al*. Prognosis of patients with left ventricular dysfunction, with and without viable myocardium after myocardial infarction. Relative efficacy of medical therapy and revascularization. Circulation 1994;90:2687-94.
39. Tamaki N, Kawamoto M, Takahashi N, *et al*. Prognostic value of an increase in fluorine-18 deoxyglucose uptake in patients with myocardial infarction: Comparison with stress thallium imaging. J Am Coll Cardiol 1993;22:1621-7.
40. Eitzman D, Al-Aouar Z, Kanter HL *et al*. Clinical outcome of patients with advanced coronary artery disease after viability studies with positron emission tomography. J Am Coll Cardiol 1992;20:559-65.
41. Williams MJ, Odabashian J, Lauer MS, Thomas JD, Marwick TH. Prognostic value of dobutamine echocardiography in patients with left ventricular dysfunction. J Am Coll Cardiol 1996;27:132-9.
42. Petretta M, Cuocolo A, Nicolai E, Acampa W, Salvatore M, Bonaduce D. Combined assessment of left ventricular function and rest-redistribution regional myocardial thallium-201 activity for prognostic evaluation of patients with chronic coronary artery disease and left ventricular dysfunction. J Nucl Cardiol 1998;5:378-86.
43. Elefteriades JA, Morales DL, Gradel C, Tolis G Jr, Levi E, Zaret BL. Results of coronary artery bypass grafting by a single surgeon in patients with left ventricular ejection fractions < or = 30%. Am J Cardiol 1997;79:1573-8.
44. Iskandrian S, Gioia G, Pancholy S, Dileva K, Heo J, Iskandrian AS. Prognosis of patients with severe left ventricular dysfunction after coronary artery bypass grafting. Am J Cardiol 1996;77:199-200.
45. Ragosta M, Beller GA, Watson DD, Kaul S, Giumple LW. Quantitative planar rest-redistribution ^{201}Tl imaging in detection of myocardial viability and prediction of improvement in left ventricular function after coronary bypass surgery in patients with severely depressed left ventricular function. Circulation 1993;87:1630-41.
46. Orlandi C, Quin JB, Iskandrian AE *et al*. Prediction of outcome after coronary revascularization in patients with left ventricular dysfunction: the I-123-IPPA viability multicenter study [abstract]. J Am Coll Cardiol 1998;31(2 Suppl A):260A.
47. Marzullo P. Revascularization of viable myocardium favourably influences long-term outcome of patients with severe but not moderate ischemic left ventricular dysfunction [abstract]. J Am Coll Cardiol 1998;31(2 Suppl A):375A.
48. Iskandrian AE, Acio E. Methodology of a novel myocardial viability protocol. J Nucl Cardiol 1998;5:206-9.
49. Narula J, Dawson MS, Mishra J *et al*. Noninvasive characterization of stunned, hibernating, remodeled and nonviable myocardium in ischemic cardiomyopathy. In press 1999.
50. Amanullah AM, Chaudhry FA, Narula J *et al*. Contractile reserve and myocardial ischemia in patient with ischemic cardiomyopathy. Comparison of dobutamine echocardiography, dobutamine SPECT sestamibi and rest-redistribution thallium-201 SPECT. Iin press 1999.
51. Sun KT, Czernin J, Krivokapich J *et al*. Effects of dobutamine stimulation on myocardial blood flow, glucose metabolism, and wall motion in normal and dysfunctional myocardium. Circulation 1996;94:3146-54.

12. Summary

AMI S. ISKANDRIAN & ERNST E. VAN DER WALL

The previous chapters discussed in details the various methods for assessment of myocardial viability (Tables 1 and 2). Newer methods are being introduced such as measurement of intracavitary voltage by electromechanical mapping. The endocardial voltage in myocardial segments with reversible defects is reported to be higher than that in segments with fixed defects [1] (Figure 1). The ultimate utility of this method, however, remains to be determined.

The terms viable myocardium and reversible left ventricular (LV) dysfunction are not identical; viability may produce improvement in survival or quality of life (or both) yet recovery of function may not be realized after coronary revascularization. The various reasons have been addressed elsewhere in this book. The continued use of these two terms as if though they are identical is an important reason for the confusion in this subject. The threshold of viable myocardium that is necessary to produce improvement in function vs survival benefit vs enhancement of quality of life measures is not yet defined. Neither do we know precisely of why some patients have improvement in LV function, survival and quality of life while others have only one or two of these (after revascularization). These issues need to be addressed in future studies.

There is an urgent need to explore the role of viability assessment in patients who present with heart failure rather than angina. The number of patients with heart failure continues to grow, and the prognosis of such patients remains dismal despite multiple new therapeutic options; cardiac transplantation is feasible in minority of these patients because of shortage in donor hearts. Rough estimates will suggest that at least 10% of the total group and 20% of those with ischemic cardiomyopathy will benefit from coronary revascularization (Table 3). The zealous, technology oriented researchers sometimes forget the clinical problem. The magnitude of this clinical problem is likely to keep all technologies viable!

A. E. Iskandrian and E. E. van der Wall (eds.), Myocardial Viability, 229-231.
© 2000 *Kluwer Academic Publishers. Printed in the Netherlands.*

Table 1. Assessment of myocardial viability

1 – Nuclear
2 - 2DE
3 – MRI
4 – EPS
5 – Contrast angiography

2DE = two-dimensional echocardiography; MRI = magnetic resonance imaging; EPS = electrophysiologic study

Table 2. Myocardial viability: nuclear imaging methods

PET	SPECT
○ 1 – MBF	○ 1 – Thallium-201
♦ O-15 Water	
♦ N-13 Ammonia	○ 2 – Technetium-Tracers
○ 2 – MBF/FDG	○ 3 – Dual isotope
○ 3 – Metabolism	○ 4 – Nitroglycerine
♦ F-18 FDG	
♦ C-11 Palmitate	○ 5 – I-123 IPPA/BMIPP
♦ C-11 Acetate	
♦ C-11 Citrate	○ 6 – F-18 FDG
♦ N-13 Glutamate	
	○ 7 – Technetium-Tracer/FDG
○ 4 – Rb-82	

Table 3. Coronary revascularization in heart failure

No. of pts with HF	~5,000,000
Systolic dysfunction (%HF)	~70% (~3,500,000)
CAD (% systolic dysfunction)	~70% (~2,500,00)
Viable myocardium (% CAD)	~20% (~500,000)

CAD = coronary artery disease; HF = heart failure

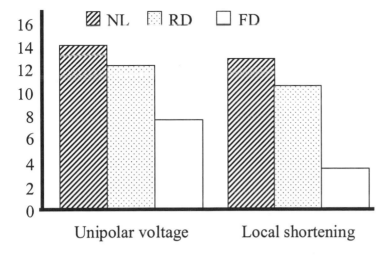

NL = normal myocardium; RD = reversible defects; FD = fixed defects

Figure 1. Based on Kornowski *et al.* [1] (Circulation 1998;98:1837-41).

References

1. Kornowski R, Hong MK, Leon MB. Comparison between left ventricular electromechanical mapping and radionuclide perfusion imaging for detection of myocardial viability. Circulation 1998;98:1837-41

INDEX

233

Developments in Cardiovascular Medicine

Developments in Cardiovascular Medicine

138. A.-M. Salmasi and A.S. Iskandrian (eds.): *Cardiac Output and Regional Flow in Health and Disease.* 1993
ISBN 0-7923-1911-7
139. J.H. Kingma, N.M. van Hemel and K.I. Lie (eds.): *Atrial Fibrillation, a Treatable Disease?* 1992
ISBN 0-7923-2008-5
140. B. Ostadel and N.S. Dhalla (eds.): *Heart Function in Health and Disease.* Proceedings of the Cardiovascular Program (Prague, Czechoslovakia, 1991). 1992
ISBN 0-7923-2052-2
141. D. Noble and Y.E. Earm (eds.): *Ionic Channels and Effect of Taurine on the Heart.* Proceedings of an International Symposium (Seoul, Korea, 1992). 1993
ISBN 0-7923-2199-5
142. H.M. Piper and C.J. Preusse (eds.): *Ischemia-reperfusion in Cardiac Surgery.* 1993 ISBN 0-7923-2241-X
143. J. Roelandt, E.J. Gussenhoven and N. Bom (eds.): *Intravascular Ultrasound.* 1993 ISBN 0-7923-2301-7
144. M.E. Safar and M.F. O'Rourke (eds.): *The Arterial System in Hypertension.* 1993 ISBN 0-7923-2343-2
145. P.W. Serruys, D.P. Foley and P.J. de Feyter (eds.): *Quantitative Coronary Angio- graphy in Clinical Practice.* With a Foreword by Spencer B. King III. 1994
ISBN 0-7923-2368-8
146. J. Candell-Riera and D. Ortega-Alcalde (eds.): *Nuclear Cardiology in Everyday Practice.* 1994
ISBN 0-7923-2374-2
147. P. Cummins (ed.): *Growth Factors and the Cardiovascular System.* 1993
ISBN 0-7923-2401-3
148. K. Przyklenk, R.A. Kloner and D.M. Yellon (eds.): *Ischemic Preconditioning: The Concept of Endogenous Cardioprotection.* 1993
ISBN 0-7923-2410-2
149. T.H. Marwick: *Stress Echocardiography.* Its Role in the Diagnosis and Evaluation of Coronary Artery Disease. 1994
ISBN 0-7923-2579-6
150. W.H. van Gilst and K.I. Lie (eds.): *Neurohumoral Regulation of Coronary Flow.* Role of the Endothelium. 1993
ISBN 0-7923-2588-5
151. N. Sperelakis (ed.): *Physiology and Pathophysiology of the Heart.* 3rd rev. ed. 1994 ISBN 0-7923-2612-1
152. J.C. Kaski (ed.): *Angina Pectoris with Normal Coronary Arteries: Syndrome X.* 1994
ISBN 0-7923-2651-2
153. D.R. Gross: *Animal Models in Cardiovascular Research.* 2nd rev. ed. 1994
ISBN 0-7923-2712-8
154. A.S. Iskandrian and E.E. van der Wall (eds.): *Myocardial Viability.* Detection and Clinical Relevance. 1994
ISBN 0-7923-2813-2
155. J.H.C. Reiber and P.W. Serruys (eds.): *Progress in Quantitative Coronary Arteriography.* 1994
ISBN 0-7923-2814-0
156. U. Goldbourt, U. de Faire and K. Berg (eds.): *Genetic Factors in Coronary Heart Disease.* 1994
ISBN 0-7923-2752-7
157. G. Leonetti and C. Cuspidi (eds.): *Hypertension in the Elderly.* 1994
ISBN 0-7923-2852-3
158. D. Ardissino, S. Savonitto and L.H. Opie (eds.): *Drug Evaluation in Angina Pectoris.* 1994
ISBN 0-7923-2897-3
159. G. Bkaily (ed.): *Membrane Physiopathology.* 1994
ISBN 0-7923-3062-5
160. R.C. Becker (ed.): *The Modern Era of Coronary Thrombolysis.* 1994
ISBN 0-7923-3063-3
161. P.J. Walter (ed.): *Coronary Bypass Surgery in the Elderly.* Ethical, Economical and Quality of Life Aspects. With a foreword by N.K. Wenger. 1995
ISBN 0-7923-3188-5
162. J.W. de Jong and R. Ferrari (eds.), *The Carnitine System.* A New Therapeutical Approach to Cardiovascular Diseases. 1995
ISBN 0-7923-3318-7
163. C.A. Neill and E.B. Clark: *The Developing Heart: A "History" of Pediatric Cardiology.* 1995
ISBN 0-7923-3375-6
164. N. Sperelakis: *Electrogenesis of Biopotentials in the Cardiovascular System.* 1995 ISBN 0-7923-3398-5
165. M. Schwaiger (ed.): *Cardiac Positron Emission Tomography.* 1995
ISBN 0-7923-3417-5
166. E.E. van der Wall, P.K. Blanksma, M.G. Niemeyer and A.M.J. Paans (eds.): *Cardiac Positron Emission Tomography.* Viability, Perfusion, Receptors and Cardiomyopathy. 1995 ISBN 0-7923-3472-8
167. P.K. Singal, I.M.C. Dixon, R.E. Beamish and N.S. Dhalla (eds.): *Mechanism of Heart Failure.* 1995
ISBN 0-7923-3490-6
168. N.S. Dhalla, P.K. Singal, N. Takeda and R.E. Beamish (eds.): *Pathophysiology of Heart Failure.* 1995
ISBN 0-7923-3571-6
169. N.S. Dhalla, G.N. Pierce, V. Panagia and R.E. Beamish (eds.): *Heart Hypertrophy and Failure.* 1995
ISBN 0-7923-3572-4

Developments in Cardiovascular Medicine

201. P.E. Vardas (ed.): *Cardiac Arrhythmias Pacing and Electrophysiology. The Expert View.* 1998
ISBN 0-7923-4908-3
202. E.E. van der Wall, P.K. Blanksma, M.G. Niemeyer, W. Vaalburg and H.J.G.M. Crijns (eds.): *Advanced Imaging in Coronary Artery Disease.* PET, SPECT, MRI, IVUS, EBCT. 1998   ISBN 0-7923-5083-9
203. R.L. Wilenski (ed.): *Unstable Coronary Artery Syndromes, Pathophysiology, Diagnosis and Treatment.* 1998
ISBN 0-7923-8201-3
204. J.H.C. Reiber and E.E. van der Wall (eds.): *What's New in Cardiovascular Imaging?* 1998
ISBN 0-7923-5121-5
205. J.C. Kaski and D.W. Holt (eds.): *Myocardial Damage.* Early Detection by Novel Biochemical Markers. 1998
ISBN 0-7923-5140-1
206. M. Malik (ed.): *Clinical Guide to Cardiac Autonomic Tests.* 1998   ISBN 0-7923-5178-9
207. G.F. Baxter and D.M. Yellon (eds.): *Delayed Preconditioning and Adaptive Cardioprotection.* 1998
ISBN 0-7923-5259-9
208. B. Swynghedauw, *Molecular Cardiology for the Cardiologist, Second Edition.* 1998
ISBN 0-7923-8323-0
209. G. Burnstock, J.G. Dobson, Jr., B.T. Liang, J. Linden (eds.): *Cardiovascular Biology of Purines.* 1998
ISBN 0-7923-8334-6
210. B.D. Hoit, R.A. Walsh (eds.): *Cardiovascular Physiology in the Genetically Engineered Mouse.* 1998
ISBN 0-7923-8356-7
211. P. Whittaker, G.S. Abela (eds.): *Direct Myocardial Revascularization: History, Methodology, Technology.* 1998
ISBN 0-7923-8398-2
212. C.A. Nienaber and R. Fattori (eds.): *Diagnosis and Treatment of Aortic Diseases.* 1999
ISBN 0-7923-5517-2
213. J.C. Kaski (ed.): *Chest Pain with Normal Coronary Angiograms: Pathogenesis, Diagnosis and Management.* 1999   ISBN 0-7923-8421-0
214. P.A. Doevendans, R.S. Reneman and M. van Bilsen (eds.): *Cardiovascular Specific Gene Expression.* 1999
ISBN 0-7923-5633-0
215. G. Pons-Lladó, F. Carreras, X. Borrás, M. Subirana and L.J. Jiménez-Borreguero (eds.): *Atlas of Practical Cardiac Applications of MRI.* 1999   ISBN 0-7923-5636-5
216. L.W. Klein and J.E. Calvin, *Resource Utilization in Cardiac Disease.* 1999   ISBN 0-7923-8509-8
217. R. Gorlin, G. Dangas, P.K. Toutouzas and M.M. Konstadoulakis: *Contemporary Concepts in Cardiology, Pathophysiology and Clinical Management.* 1999   ISBN 0-7923-8514-4
218. S. Gupta and A.J. Camm: *Chronic Infection, Chlamydia and Coronary Heart Disease.* 1999
ISBN 0-7923-5797-3
219. M. Rajskina: *Ventricular Fibrillation in Sudden Cardiac Death.* 1999   ISBN 0-7923-8570-5
220. Z. Abedin and R. Conner: *Interpretation of Cardiac Arrhythmias: Self Assessment Approach.* 1999
ISBN 0-7923-8576-4
221. J.E. Lock, J.F. Keane and S.B. Perry (eds.): *Diagnostic and Interventional Catheterization in Congenital Heart Disease, second edition.* 1999   ISBN 0-7923-8597-7
222. J.S. Steinberg (ed.): *Atrial Fibrillation after Cardiac Surgery.* 1999   ISBN 0-7923-8655-8
223. E.E. van der Wall, A. van der Laarse, B.M. Pluim, A.V.G. Bruschke:*Left Ventricular Hypertrophy. Physiology versus Pathology.* 1999   ISBN 0-7923-6038-9
224. J.F. Keaney, Jr. (ed.): *Oxidative Stress and Vascular Disease.* 1999   ISBN 0-7923-8678-7
225. R.G. Masters (ed.): *Surgical Options for the Treatment of Heart Failure.* 2000   ISBN 0-7923-6130-X

Previous volumes are still available

KLUWER ACADEMIC PUBLISHERS – DORDRECHT / BOSTON / LONDON

Developments in Cardiovascular Medicine

170. S.N. Willich and J.E. Muller (eds.): *Triggering of Acute Coronary Syndromes.* Implications for Prevention. 1995 ISBN 0-7923-3605-4
171. E.E. van der Wall, T.H. Marwick and J.H.C. Reiber (eds.): *Advances in Imaging Techniques in Ischemic Heart Disease.* 1995 ISBN 0-7923-3620-8
172. B. Swynghedauw: *Molecular Cardiology for the Cardiologist.* 1995 ISBN 0-7923-3622-4
173. C.A. Nienaber and U. Sechtem (eds.): *Imaging and Intervention in Cardiology.* 1996
   ISBN 0-7923-3649-6
174. G. Assmann (ed.): *HDL Deficiency and Atherosclerosis.* 1995 ISBN 0-7923-8888-7
175. N.M. van Hemel, F.H.M. Wittkampf and H. Ector (eds.): *The Pacemaker Clinic of the 90's.* Essentials in Brady-Pacing. 1995 ISBN 0-7923-3688-7
176. N. Wilke (ed.): *Advanced Cardiovascular MRI of the Heart and Great Vessels.* Forthcoming.
   ISBN 0-7923-3720-4
177. M. LeWinter, H. Suga and M.W. Watkins (eds.): *Cardiac Energetics: From Emax to Pressure-volume Area.* 1995 ISBN 0-7923-3721-2
178. R.J. Siegel (ed.): *Ultrasound Angioplasty.* 1995 ISBN 0-7923-3722-0
179. D.M. Yellon and G.J. Gross (eds.): *Myocardial Protection and the K_{ATP} Channel.* 1995
   ISBN 0-7923-3791-3
180. A.V.G. Bruschke, J.H.C. Reiber, K.I. Lie and H.J.J. Wellens (eds.): *Lipid Lowering Therapy and Progression of Coronary Atherosclerosis.* 1996 ISBN 0-7923-3807-3
181. A.-S.A. Abd-Eyattah and A.S. Wechsler (eds.): *Purines and Myocardial Protection.* 1995
   ISBN 0-7923-3831-6
182. M. Morad, S. Ebashi, W. Trautwein and Y. Kurachi (eds.): *Molecular Physiology and Pharmacology of Cardiac Ion Channels and Transporters.* 1996 ISBN 0-7923-3913-4
183. M.A. Oto (ed.): *Practice and Progress in Cardiac Pacing and Electrophysiology.* 1996
   ISBN 0-7923-3950-9
184. W.H. Birkenhäger (ed.): *Practical Management of Hypertension.* Second Edition. 1996
   ISBN 0-7923-3952-5
185. J.C. Chatham, J.R. Forder and J.H. McNeill (eds.): *The Heart in Diabetes.* 1996 ISBN 0-7923-4052-3
186. J.H.C. Reiber and E.E. van der Wall (eds.): *Cardiovascular Imaging.* 1996 ISBN 0-7923-4109-0
187. A-M. Salmasi and A. Strano (eds.): *Angiology in Practice.* 1996 ISBN 0-7923-4143-0
188. M.W. Kroll and M.H. Lehmann (eds.): *Implantable Cardioverter Defibrillator Therapy: The Engineering – Clinical Interface.* 1996 ISBN 0-7923-4300-X
189. K.L. March (ed.): *Gene Transfer in the Cardiovascular System.* Experimental Approaches and Therapeutic Implications. 1996 ISBN 0-7923-9859-9
190. L. Klein (ed.): *Coronary Stenosis Morphology: Analysis and Implication.* 1997 ISBN 0-7923-9867-X
191. J.E. Pérez and R.M. Lang (eds.): *Echocardiography and Cardiovascular Function: Tools for the Next Decade.* 1997 ISBN 0-7923-9884-X
192. A.A. Knowlton (ed.): *Heat Shock Proteins and the Cardiovascular System.* 1997 ISBN 0-7923-9910-2
193. R.C. Becker (ed.): *The Textbook of Coronary Thrombosis and Thrombolysis.* 1997 ISBN 0-7923-9923-4
194. R.M. Mentzer, Jr., M. Kitakaze, J.M. Downey and M. Hori (eds.): *Adenosine, Cardioprotection and Its Clinical Application.* 1997 ISBN 0-7923-9954-4
195. N.H.J. Pijls and B. De Bruyne: *Coronary Pressure.* 1997 ISBN 0-7923-4672-6
196. I. Graham, H. Refsum, I.H. Rosenberg and P.M. Ueland (eds.): *Homocysteine Metabolism: from Basic Science to Clinical Medicine.* 1997 ISBN 0-7923-9983-8
197. E.E. van der Wall, V. Manger Cats and J. Baan (eds.): *Vascular Medicine – From Endothelium to Myocardium.* 1997 ISBN 0-7923-4740-4
198. A. Lafont and E. Topol (eds.): *Arterial Remodeling.* A Critical Factor in Restenosis. 1997
   ISBN 0-7923-8008-8
199. M. Mercury, D.D. McPherson, H. Bassiouny and S. Glagov (eds.): *Non-Invasive Imaging of Atherosclerosis* 1998 ISBN 0-7923-8036-3
200. W.C. De Mello and M.J. Janse (eds.): *Heart Cell Communication in Health and Disease.* 1997
   ISBN 0-7923-8052-5